Introduction to Neuroimaging Analysis

Oxford Neuroimaging Primers

OXFORD NEUROIMAGING PRIMERS

Introduction to
Neuroimaging Analysis

MARK JENKINSON
MICHAEL CHAPPELL

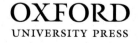

OXFORD
UNIVERSITY PRESS

OXFORD
UNIVERSITY PRESS

Great Clarendon Street, Oxford, OX2 6DP,
United Kingdom

Oxford University Press is a department of the University of Oxford.
It furthers the University's objective of excellence in research, scholarship,
and education by publishing worldwide. Oxford is a registered trade mark of
Oxford University Press in the UK and in certain other countries

© Oxford University Press 2018

The moral rights of the authors have been asserted

First Edition published in 2018

Published in the United States of America by Oxford University Press
198 Madison Avenue, New York, NY 10016, United States of America

British Library Cataloguing in Publication Data
Data available

Library of Congress Control Number: 2017953558

ISBN 978-0-19-881630-0

Printed and bound by CPI Group (UK) Ltd, Croydon, CR0 4YY

Oxford University Press makes no representation, express or implied, that the
drug dosages in this book are correct. Readers must therefore always check
the product information and clinical procedures with the most up-to-date
published product information and data sheets provided by the manufacturers
and the most recent codes of conduct and safety regulations. The authors and
the publishers do not accept responsibility or legal liability for any errors in the
text or for the misuse or misapplication of material in this work. Except where
otherwise stated, drug dosages and recommendations are for the non-pregnant
adult who is not breast-feeding

Links to third party websites are provided by Oxford in good faith and
for information only. Oxford disclaims any responsibility for the materials
contained in any third party website referenced in this work.

This book is dedicated to our parents.

Preface to the Series

The Oxford Neuroimaging Primers are aimed to be readily accessible texts for new researchers or advanced undergraduates in neuroimaging who want to get a broad understanding of the ways in which neuroimaging data can be analyzed and interpreted. All primers in this series have been written so that they can be read as stand-alone books, although they have also been edited so that they "work together" and readers can read multiple primers in the series to build up a bigger picture of neuroimaging and be equipped to use multiple neuroimaging methods.

Understanding the principles of the analysis of neuroimaging data is crucial for all researchers in this field, not only because data analysis is a necessary part of any neuroimaging study, but also because it is required in order to understand how to plan, execute, and interpret experiments. Although MR operators, radiologists, and technicians are often available to help with data collection, running the scanner, and choosing good sequences and settings, when it comes to analysis, researchers are often on their own. Therefore, the Oxford Neuroimaging Primers seek to provide the necessary understanding of how to do analysis while at the same time trying to show how this knowledge relates to being able to perform good acquisitions, design good experiments, and correctly interpret the results.

The series has been produced by individuals (both authors and editors) who have developed neuroimaging analysis techniques, used these methods on real data, packaged them as software tools for others to use, taught courses on these methods, and supported people around the world who use the software they have produced. We hope that this means everyone involved has not only the experience to instruct, but also the empathy to support the reader. It has been our aim for these primers to not only lay out the core principles that apply in any given area of neuroimaging, but also to help the reader avoid common pitfalls and mistakes (many of which the authors themselves probably made first). We also hope that the series is also a good introduction to those with a more technical background, even if they have to forgo some of the mathematical details found in other more technical works. We make no pretense that these primers are the final word in any given area, and we are aware that the field of neuroimaging continues to develop and improve, but the fundamentals are likely to remain the same for many years to come. Certainly some of the advice you will find in these primers will never fail you—such as *always look at your data*.

Our intention with the series has always been to support it with practical examples, so that the reader can learn from working with data directly and will be equipped to use the knowledge they have gained in their own studies and on their own data. These examples, including datasets and instructions, can be found on the associated website (www.neuroimagingprimers.org), and directions to specific examples are placed throughout each primer. As the authors are also the developers of various software tools within the FMRIB Software Library (FSL), the examples in the primers mainly use tools from FSL. However, we intend these primers to be as general as possible and present material that is relevant for all readers, regardless of the software they use in practice. Such readers can still use the example data available through the primer website with any of the major neuroimaging analysis toolboxes. We encourage all readers to interact with these examples, since we strongly believe that a lot of the key learning is done when you actually use these tools in practice.

Mark Jenkinson
Michael Chappell
Oxford, January 2017

Preface

Welcome to this, the introductory primer in the Oxford Neuroimaging Primers series. This primer is aimed at people who are new to the field of MRI neuroimaging research. Over the past few decades magnetic resonance imaging (MRI) has emerged as an increasingly popular and powerful way of studying in vivo brain structure and function, in both healthy and pathological individuals. MRI is a highly flexible imaging method and there are a lot of different types of images that can be acquired (e.g., structural, diffusion, functional, perfusion, etc.). Although this is a great strength, it can also make for a steep learning curve for those entering the field. Our intention for this primer is to provide a general and accessible introduction to the wide array of MRI-based neuroimaging methods that are used in research—an introduction suitable for people from a broad range of different backgrounds and with no previous experience with MRI or neuroimaging. The main emphasis is on ways of analyzing images, but as this interacts greatly with both image acquisition and interpretation, each of these aspects is also covered in this primer. To make this primer as helpful as possible, we also illustrate the text throughout with examples from real datasets; you will find these datasets, along with instructions on how to visualize and analyze them, on the primer website (www.neuroimagingprimers.org).

The text contains several different types of boxes that aim to help you navigate the material or find out more information for yourself. To get the most out of this primer, you might find the description of each type of box below helpful.

Example box These boxes either contain additional written illustrations of key points or direct you to the Oxford NeuroImaging primers website (www.neuroimagingprimers.org), where you will find examples that allow you to directly interact with real data and perform practical exercises to apply the theory described in this primer. These examples are intended to be a useful way to prepare you for applying these methods to your own data; but you do not need to carry out such exercises immediately as you are reading through the primer. The examples are placed at the relevant places in the text, so that you know when you can get a more hands-on approach to the information being presented.

> **Example Box: Look at your**
>
> Enthusiasm to gather lots of dat
> simply failing to appropriately pil
> is that of an experimenter who

Box 1.1: B₀ field inhomoge

Imperfections in the scanner in
lead to a range of artifacts. The
coil should ideally be perfectly ...

Box These boxes contain more technical or advanced descriptions of some topics covered in the primer or information on related topics or methods. None of the material in the rest of the primer assumes that you have read these boxes, and they are not essential for understanding and applying any of the methods. If you are new to the field and are reading this primer for the first time, you may therefore prefer to skip the material in these boxes and come back to them later.

Group Analysis Box

In neuroimaging research studies,
to the larger population rather tha
clinical practice, where the interes

Group analysis box This primer includes one longer box on the topic of Group Analysis. This box describes some general statistics material needed to prepare you for running your own analyses; hence this box should not be skipped. It contains material that is relevant to many topics covered in different chapters of the primer and it is therefore written in relatively general terms.

SUMMARY

■ MRI is very flexible and there a
■ Signals are detected from hydr
■ MRI scanners consist of many
  to or from the water molecule

Summary Each chapter or major section contains, toward the end, a box of summary points that provide a very brief overview, emphasizing the most important topics discussed. You may like to use these boxes to check that you have understood the key points in each chapter or section.

FURTHER READING

■ Huettel, S. A., Song, A. W., & M
  (3rd ed.). Sinauer Associates.
  ■ *This is an accessible, introdu*
    acquisition as well as on fun

Further Reading Each chapter or major section ends with a list of suggestions for further reading, which contain both articles and books. A brief summary of the contents of each suggestion is included, so that you may chose which references are most relevant to you. The primer does not assume that you have read any of the further reading material. Rather these lists represent a starting point for diving deeper into the existing literature. These boxes are not intended to provide a full review of the relevant literature; should you go further in the field, you will find a wealth of other sources that are helpful or important for the specific research you are doing.

Neuroimaging is a dynamic field and will continue to see developments in the coming years, as new acquisition and analysis options become available. Thus this primer will not cover all aspects of neuroimaging or neuroimaging analysis; it is intended as a preparatory text that builds up a framework for understanding the important analysis and acquisition principles for the common neuroimaging modalities, in order to enable new researchers to enter the world of neuroimaging more easily. We hope that it will provide a good preparation for anyone who delves deeper into specific modalities and their analyses, through other primers in this series, or more generally into the vast literature on neuroimaging.

Mark Jenkinson
Michael Chappell

Acknowledgments

There are a great many people who have helped make this primer what it is today, and we are grateful for all their support and assistance. To start with, we would like to thank our editor at OUP, Martin Baum, for enthusiastically getting behind this project and making the whole series a reality. For this primer, special thanks are due to Matteo Bastiani, Janine Bijsterbosch, Jon Campbell, Liv Faull, and Sam Harrison for their huge amount of help, proofreading, and advice with the overall content, the datasets, and innumerable details. We would also like to express our thanks to Iman Aganj, Jesper Andersson, Zobair Arya, Holly Bridge, Mark Chiew, Stuart Clare, Alexandra Constantinescu, Gwenaëlle Douaud, Uzay Emir, Matthew Glasser, Sezgi Goksan, Doug Greve, George Harston, Caroline Hartley, Saad Jbabdi, Sarah Jenkinson, Renée Koolschijn, Saloni Krishnan, Jacob Levenstein, Bradley MacIntosh, Paul McCarthy, Clare O'Donoghue, Thomas Okell, Martin Reuter, Ged Ridgway, Emma Robinson, Adriana Roca-Fernandez, Michael Sanders, Zeena-Britt Sanders, Stamatios Sotiropoulos, Charlotte Stagg, Sana Suri, Eelke Visser, Joseph Woods, Mark Woolrich, and Eniko Zsoldos for invaluable proofreading, advice, and support that helped shape and improve this primer. Much of the material for it developed through the FSL Course and the FMRIB Graduate Programme. We are also thankful to all the participants, lecturers, and tutors on these courses, especially for their feedback over the years, as this has been crucial in developing and honing this material.

Mark Jenkinson
Michael Chappell

Contents

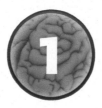

Introduction

Acquiring an image of the brain is difficult, particularly in a living subject, since the brain itself is made up of soft tissues but is surrounded by a hard casing—the skull. Magnetic resonance imaging (MRI) is a very powerful and versatile method, with the ability to safely and noninvasively measure a wide range of properties within the living brain. MRI is able to capture images that provide information about gross anatomy, neuronal activity, connectivity, pathologies, and more. As a single imaging device, it is far more flexible than any of the alternatives—such as positron emission tomography (PET), computed tomography (X-ray/CT), ultrasound, electroencephalography (EEG), and magnetoencephalography (MEG)—although each method still has its own specific strengths and weaknesses. In fact, combining methods can be even better (see section 2.7).

The great flexibility of MRI is due to the fact that there are many ways in which it can be used to manipulate and measure signals from the tissues of the brain (or of other body parts or objects placed in the scanner). As a consequence, there are many choices to be made in the setup of the MRI scanner—and also many different types of image that can be acquired. This means that a large number of different methods are available to analyze MRI data and, as a researcher in neuroimaging, you will need to know how to make the appropriate choices. When acquiring data, there are often other experts on hand (radiographers, physicists, etc.) to help you with acquisition decisions; however, it is less common to have experts on hand to help specifically with your analysis, and so you need to be more self-sufficient. The aim of this primer series is to explain how you can make the right choices when analyzing MRI data.

In this primer we will mainly describe human in vivo neuroimaging using MRI, although a lot of the material also applies to postmortem imaging or to the imaging of other species. In addition, we will discuss clinical research methods along with basic neuroscience, but will only occasionally touch on things related to clinical practice. Diagnostic radiology, which largely involves structural MRI, is beyond the scope of these primers and we refer the interested reader to the many excellent textbooks on diagnostic radiology and clinical brain imaging.

To begin with, the rest of this chapter will provide a very broad introduction to MRI-based neuroimaging research. This starts with a general overview of some common types of images and analysis methods, mainly for those who are new to the field or have dealt only with a narrow specialty. The overview is followed by a walk-through of a typical study, which illustrates the many different stages and considerations to be taken into account when conducting neuroimaging research. In particular, we highlight how interwoven the analysis, acquisition, and experimental design options are. It is important to appreciate that, although these may be presented elsewhere in a compartmentalized way, it is necessary to consider their constraints and trade-offs jointly in order to do good quality research. The last section of this chapter covers, at a very broad level, some aspects of MRI physics and scanner hardware that are helpful when discussing acquisition and analysis.

In the rest of this primer we will go through the more common image acquisitions in a little more detail, giving some explanation of their basic principles as well as of the broad concepts related to how the data are analyzed. We will concentrate mainly on what the basis of the measured signals is and what limitations exist for each type of imaging, since this is crucial for understanding the type of analysis that can be done and for being able to interpret results. The remaining chapters focus on analysis methods that are commonly required by almost any neuroimaging study, regardless of the actual modalities involved, including registration, standard spaces, and surface-based analyses. By the end of this primer you should have a good understanding of the important analysis and acquisition principles for the common neuroimaging modalities. This will provide you with a solid basis for doing neuroimaging research, equipping you to go into more depth in the specific modalities you want to use and into their analyses using other primers in the series, other textbooks, and papers.

1.1 Main MRI modalities and analysis techniques

There is a wide variety in the types of images that can be acquired on an MRI scanner, where different types of images capture different information about the brain and are also called *modalities*. However, there are three modalities that are by far the most commonly used in neuroimaging research: *structural*, *diffusion*, and *functional* imaging—see Figure 1.1. The first, structural imaging, provides information about gross anatomical structures in the brain—e.g., by showing the boundaries of the cerebral cortex and the borders of other structures like the hippocampus (do not worry if you are not familiar with these anatomical terms, as the basics are covered in Appendix A and we encourage you to read this appendix if you are new to brain anatomy). The second modality, diffusion imaging, diffusion-weighted imaging, or diffusion MRI (dMRI), provides information about microstructure and anatomical connectivity within the brain and spinal cord. The third, functional imaging or functional MRI (fMRI), provides information about the activity of the neurons in the brain, either in response to specific stimuli or tasks that the experimenter applies to the participant (task fMRI) or in relation to the spontaneous activity of the participant's neurons (resting state fMRI).

There are also other MRI modalities used in neuroimaging, including those that more deliberately seek to measure physiology. A good example is perfusion MRI, which is often considered a form of fMRI, as it can be used to provide information about brain activity, but is also useful in more clinically oriented studies, such as those measuring the physiological

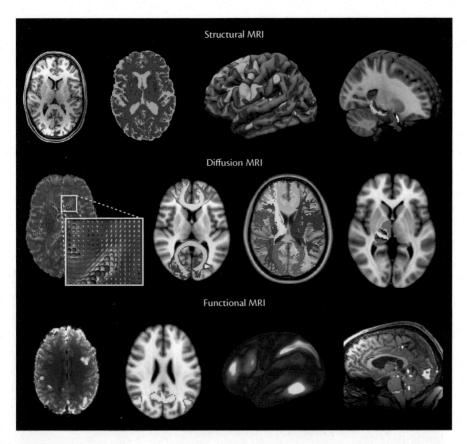

Figure 1.1: Illustrations of the three main MRI modalities to be covered in this primer and examples of various analysis outputs. These include tissue and structure delineation (structural), estimation of white matter tracts and connectivity-based parcellation (diffusion), and functional activations and connectivity networks (functional). Further details about these types of images and analyses will be discussed later in this primer.

response to drugs. Often a number of modalities will be used within a single study, for various reasons. For example, one modality may be used to correct for a limitation in another (e.g., for calibration or artifact correction). Alternatively, information from several modalities can be combined to calculate a different quantity (e.g., the anatomical connectivity associated with a particular functional area) or to provide a clearer, more precise, interpretation—the result of such combinations usually being greater than the sum of its parts.

In research it is also typical for data to be acquired in a group of participants,[1] since looking at an individual alone will not be sufficient for drawing any general conclusions, due to the

---

[1] Participants are often referred to as "subjects," especially in terms such as "between-subject differences," though it is often preferable to use the term "participant" when you address a participant directly, for example when you are talking to someone in your study.

considerable structural and functional variability between individuals. This is a major way in which neuroimaging research differs from clinical practice. The analysis of groups of individuals is thus often a final stage in the analysis—the "group analysis." This kind of analysis can look for a common effect across a single group or can compare different groups (e.g., patients and controls), or even look for a relationship with some other factor (e.g., reaction time). Performing a group analysis requires the alignment—or *registration*—of all of the individuals within the group to a common anatomical *template*. Most research studies use the *MNI152 template* (see Figure 1.2), which comprises an average of 152 healthy adults and has become the standard in neuroimaging research (more details on standard templates will be presented in Chapter 5).

A common theme in neuroimaging analyses is the use of statistics, due to both the noise in the MRI signal and the considerable biological variation between individuals. Statistics make it possible to have a measure of whether the result was just due to random (or chance) selection

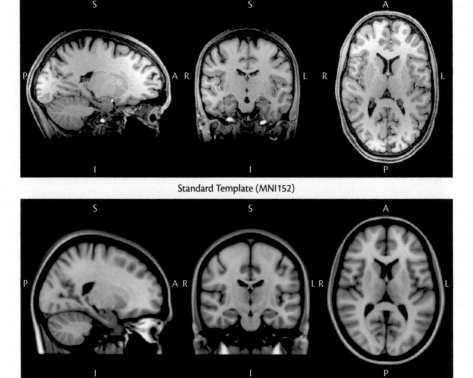

Figure 1.2: Example of a structural MRI of a single individual (top row) and of the MNI152 template (bottom row). In each row the sagittal, coronal, and axial planes (these terms are explained in Appendix A) are shown from left to right. The MNI152 template is built from an average of 152 healthy subjects, though due to individual anatomical variability some areas of the brain are blurry (show less definition), since regions where the folding patterns are very different do not align well between subjects.

or not. This is true for the analysis of all modalities—structural, diffusion, functional, and others. In neuroimaging the statistics are usually based on a single model, called the general linear model (GLM).[2] This is a linear model that can express a very wide range of statistical tests and hypotheses (unpaired and paired t-tests, F-tests, ANOVA, etc.) and is used in both individual and group analyses. The GLM is of fundamental importance in neuroimaging and many of the subsequent examples use the GLM, although at this point you do not need to know more details in order to continue reading. (The GLM is also covered in the online appendix *Short Introduction to the General Linear Model for Neuroimaging.*)

MRI is a very flexible technique and new analyses and modes of investigation are being developed all the time. The most common analysis methods that are applied differ according to the modality used. In this section we will very briefly outline them with the help of some examples. The purpose of these examples is just to give a flavor of the possibilities of MRI in neuroimaging for readers who are new to the field, and maybe to broaden the horizons of those who are familiar with only a subset of the options. If you are new to MRI, then do not worry about the fine details in the rest of this section; just consider the broader picture of what MRI is able to do.

Structural MRI

In structural MRI the main research interest is in determining the shape and size of anatomical structures by finding their boundaries in the image; examples of structures include the cerebral cortex and deep gray matter structures such as the hippocampus or the thalamus (anatomical terms such as these are described in Appendix A). The basic analysis tool used for this operation is *segmentation*, which delineates where different tissues or structures are in the image. Different types of segmentation methods are used for general tissue type (e.g., white matter), for the cerebral cortex, or for individual deep gray matter structures (this is covered in more detail in section 3.2). Once segmentation has been done, various quantities can be calculated and analyzed, such as cortical thickness, local gray matter density, or structural volume and shape.

A commonly used analysis technique for examining differences in local gray matter density is *voxel-based morphometry* (VBM). VBM can be used to find regions in the brain where the amount of local gray matter is different either between groups or in a way that relates to some other parameter, such as amount of time spent learning a task. For example, in a famous paper by Maguire and colleagues, it was shown that there was an increase in the gray matter in the hippocampal region as London taxi drivers learnt how to navigate around the city (see Figure 1.3). VBM allows experimenters to investigate, with statistical tests, the effects of diseases that alter the gray matter or the effects of healthy plasticity related to learning, exercise, and other factors. Additional tools are also available to investigate the effects of disease or plasticity on particular anatomical structures through more specific, biologically related quantities, such as by measuring cortical thickness or structural shape (see Chapter 3 for more details).

---

[2] This model is different from the *generalized* linear model.

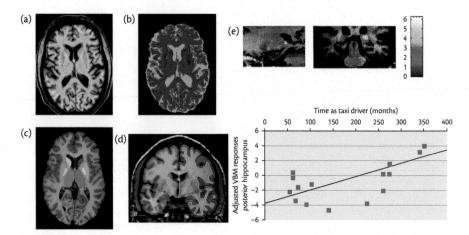

Figure 1.3: Examples of structural imaging and analysis: (a) structural image; (b) tissue-type segmentation (color-coded green for cerebrospinal fluid, red for gray matter, blue for white matter); (c) segmentation of deep gray matter structures; (d) cortical modelling (red for outer gray matter surface and yellow for gray–white matter border); (e) results from Maguire et al., 2000, showing a VBM analysis that demonstrated how changes in the hippocampal area (top) correlated with length of time the participants had been a taxi driver (bottom).

(e) Reproduced with permission from Maguire EA et al., "Navigation-related structural change in the hippocampi of taxi drivers," *Proceedings of the National Academy of Sciences*, Volume 97, Issue 8, pp. 4398–403, doi: 10.1073/pnas.070039597, Copyright © 2000 National Academy of Sciences.

Diffusion MRI

In dMRI, or diffusion MRI, there are two main research interests: microstructural properties and anatomical connectivity. In the first case, measurements can be made with dMRI that are sensitive to aspects of the tissue microstructure, such as axon size, axon density, degree of myelination, and so on (anatomical terms such as these are described in Appendix A). Statistical tests can then be performed to look for changes in these measurements between different groups (e.g., patients and controls) or for correlations with other variables (e.g., neuropsychological test results). The results of these tests can then support existing hypotheses about microstructural change or can help in understanding mechanisms for disease and plasticity.

The other common type of investigation that uses dMRI is the examination of ana-tomical connectivity (i.e., the "wiring" of the brain). This involves a type of analysis called *tractography*, which traces how a particular location in the brain is connected to the rest of the brain through the main axonal fiber bundles in the white matter. Although tractography does not provide quantitative measures of the "strength" of connections (e.g., number of axons), it does delineate the paths of the connections and can give valuable information for surgical planning, and also for detailed in vivo *parcellation* of regions of the brain (i.e., for the breaking up of a large region into individual units or *parcels*; see Figure 1.4). Tractography is currently the only way to probe the structural connectivity of the human brain in vivo. It also provides information that is crucial for interpreting the more global implications of local changes in brain tissue; and the direct analysis of the anatomical

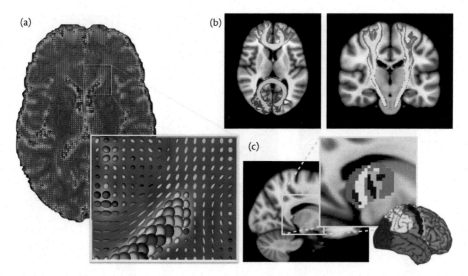

Figure 1.4: Examples of dMRI analysis: (a) illustration of local directional diffusion estimates made from dMRI, where each voxel shows a color-coded spheroid indicating dominant directionality (red = left–right, green = front–back, blue = head–foot); (b) examples of tractography, showing different anatomical pathways through the white matter; (c) parcellation of the thalamus into distinct regions on the basis of connectivity information, with color representing the area of cortex that the thalamic region is most connected to (colors of target regions shown on the brain in the bottom right).

connectivity of brain regions is of ever growing interest, as is its relation to functional connectivity.

Functional MRI (fMRI)

In fMRI there are two main research interests: investigating task-related activity using task fMRI; and functional connectivity using resting state fMRI.

Task fMRI

For task fMRI, the participant is asked to perform a task within the scanner and the objective is to locate and analyze the brain activity in response to it. There can be a very wide range of tasks, from passive stimulation (e.g., visual, auditory) to cognitive tasks (e.g., reading, memory, decision making) to simple motor tasks (e.g., finger tapping). The statistical analysis of changes in the MRI signal in time, using the GLM, creates a map of the locations of brain activity. This analysis is very flexible and can be set up to compare activity during the task with a baseline state, or to investigate relationships with other variables, such as neuropsychological test results. The resulting statistical maps show which locations in the brain have significant changes in relation to the questions of interest (see Figure 1.5), and a wide variety of studies have mapped out the location and nature of brain activity in relation to specific stimuli and tasks. Such studies are not only useful in the context of understanding the way the healthy brain works but are also valuable for probing changes due to diseases and as biomarkers for evaluating therapies and drug discovery.

INTRODUCTION

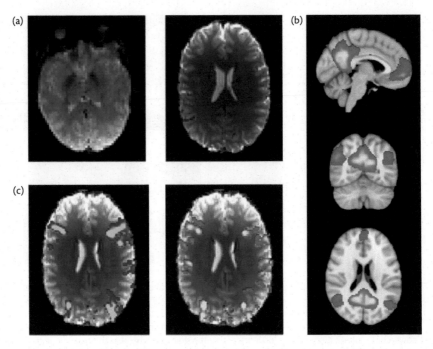

Figure 1.5: Examples of functional imaging and analysis: (a) two functional images of different participants, taken with different scanners and sequences; (b) results from a resting state analysis showing a "default mode network" (on top of the standard template—MNI152); (c) results from a task-fMRI study, showing localized activation to two slightly different stimuli (on top of functional images).

Resting state fMRI

Resting state fMRI uses the same type of MRI acquisition as task fMRI, the only difference being that the participant is not asked to perform any specific task. In fact participants are usually asked to "not think about anything in particular" and just "rest," although they are often asked to keep their eyes open and to look at a fixed point (which helps stop them from falling asleep). The signal in these resting state scans reflects spontaneous brain activity; and it is the correlation of this spontaneous activity between different locations in the brain that provides a measure of functional connectivity, in other words it tells us which regions of the brain are communicating with each other. To determine the network—that is, the set of locations that are correlated—requires specific analysis methods, for example seed-based correlation or independent component analysis (ICA). These techniques can find networks that involve particular regions or can discover the set of functional networks present in the brain (see Figure 1.5). Alternatively, connectivity matrices, which summarize connectivity between a set of regions, can also be extracted from resting state fMRI data and are analyzed with methods such as *network modeling* or *graph theory*. The analysis and interpretation of resting state-based functional connectivity is a relatively new field and much remains to be understood about the meaning of patterns and changes in connectivity (a more detailed account can be found in a separate primer titled *Introduction to Resting State fMRI Functional Connectivity*). Nonetheless, there are many uses of this connectivity information already, including uses for the connectivity-based parcellation of the cortex and for biomarkers of disease.

Perfusion MRI

There is also another variant of functional imaging—perfusion MRI—which can be seen more broadly as an example of physiological MRI. Perfusion MRI provides direct information on the delivery of blood (and, by imputation, of oxygen and nutrients) to the brain tissue. It can, in many cases, offer quantitative measurements; that is, at every voxel it gives a measure of perfusion in physical units (e.g., ml of blood delivered per 100 g of tissue per minute). This is unlike other fMRI modalities, which detect a change in signal with arbitrary units that is then converted into a statistical measure of whether the change could have happened by chance. Arterial spin labeling (ASL), which magnetically labels the blood that flows into the brain, is becoming a popular noninvasive method of obtaining quantitative perfusion images in a relatively short amount of time. The analysis of these data involves the use of a specific physiological model that describes the flow of magnetically labeled blood-water into tissues and the MRI signal that is obtained. From this, quantitative information on *cerebral blood flow* (CBF) and even other hemodynamic parameters can be obtained. This information is particularly useful for medical purposes, especially in investigating pathology and in drug studies. (A more detailed account can be found in a separate primer titled *Introduction to Perfusion Quantification using Arterial Spin Labeling*.)

1.2 Walk-through of a typical study

In order to get a broad understanding of the whole neuroimaging process, we will now describe a typical study (or experiment), which is helpful for understanding how issues in analysis, acquisition, and experimental design relate to one another. However, there is a wide range of experimental protocols and situations, and the subsequent descriptions should serve as illustrative examples only; they are not to be considered rules for the "right way" to do experiments.

Planning

A long time before any scanning happens, you should sit down, think about your experiment, and formulate some questions, hypotheses, or investigations (as not all experiments are hypothesis-driven). This stage requires a considerable amount of time and effort, including reading relevant literature and having discussions with colleagues, especially experienced ones. It is useful to have discussions at this stage, before the details are planned, because misguided and unfocused experiments, which are mainly the result of an easy way to set up an experiment (e.g., by copying a previous experiment with a small change), often produce poor and underwhelming results. Planning is the key to a good experiment and this stage is one of the most important, and often interesting, scientific phases.

Once an appropriate plan has been made, the details of acquisition, experimental design, and analysis need to be decided. And yes, you really did read *analysis* here, even at this early stage, since the analysis can constrain some possibilities, and other things (type of acquisitions, length of experiment, etc.) can be manipulated at this point to improve the analysis results.

This is a general principle that we will come across many times in this and others primers: all of the different parts of an experiment interact, and each has constraints and trade-offs for some choices versus others. Conflict between the different stages of an experiment occurs often, and so good compromises must be reached during this planning phase. Without considering all of the different stages in this early planning phase, it is easy to end up with data that cannot be analyzed or contain too much noise or artifacts. Equally, it is all too easy to end up with an experiment that is so complicated for the participants that not many of them can perform it properly, or is so boring that the participants fall asleep; this is especially important for patients. Only by taking into account all the factors that affect the analysis, the psychology and physiology of the participants, and the acquisition can good compromises be found and an appropriate design be made.

There are many factors that need to be considered, and many of them will be discussed further in this and other primers. To give you a flavor for what is involved, here is a partial list of considerations: How long should the experiment be? What stimuli (if any) need to be provided, in what order, and with what timing? What type of participants should be recruited and what are the exclusion criteria? What sort of scans are needed (e.g., do I need any calibration scans)? How many participants are needed? What analysis software or tools will be required? Do the numbers of participants in the different groups need to be balanced?

Thinking carefully, talking to your colleagues, reading the literature, giving presentations at formal or informal meetings in your lab or group are all things that are helpful when planning. Also remember that good plans are normally the result of an initial attempt that is improved by taking on board feedback and suggestions from others, as well as revisions based on further considerations over a period of time. The more you understand the whole process, the better and quicker you will be at designing valuable studies.

Ethics

Around the same time as this planning phase, the ethics application should be written and submitted, which can often be done in parallel once you have an idea of the basic setup of the experiment. Most experimenters need to complete an ethics approval for their experiments, although occasionally experiments might already be covered by existing ethics applications. The details of this process vary enormously by country, but be aware that the process itself can take a substantial amount of time (e.g., many months); hence it should be done as early as possible. It might require knowing what the participants will be doing in the experiment, so some of the planning (but not all the details) described in the preceding paragraphs usually needs to be decided upon first.

Piloting

It is always advisable, where possible, to run a pilot study on one or two participants before the main study starts. This will involve getting volunteers to be scanned (experienced and cooperative friends and colleagues can often be a good choice here), as long as it complies with the ethics. A pilot stage is very useful, since it offers an opportunity to optimize and improve experiments, increasing the chances of obtaining a strong result; however, it is often neglected. What is involved in a pilot is running through one or more scanning sessions, as if that were the real experiment; checking the time taken to set up and scan the participant; checking the quality of the data, visually and quantitatively; talking to the participants, to make sure that the experiment is understandable and easily tolerable; and running as much of the analysis as possible (often up to, but not including, the group analysis). This is all done in order to spot problems with any aspect of the design—though do not expect great analysis results from a single participant; it is rather the act of going through the whole process that highlights problems. This is a good time to tweak anything in the design that could be improved, and often some things become clear at this stage that were not foreseen or considered carefully enough previously. It is also worth emphasizing that one of the most important tasks in this phase (and in future phases too) is to *look at your data* (see the Example Box "Look at your data!") in order to check that they do not contain any unusual artifacts and that the crucial features of the image are present (this varies depending on whether it is a structural, functional, diffusion, or another type of image).

Example Box: **Look at your data!**

Enthusiasm to gather lots of data in a hurry can easily lead to huge waste, often from simply failing to appropriately pilot and check the acquisition and analysis. One example is that of an experimenter who had planned his study, scanned a whole group of participants, and then did not get any significant results; so he came to ask someone to check his analysis. A senior colleague started off by opening an image in a viewer to see what the data were like, only to discover that there was no brain at all: the whole image was just noise—it was like looking at a picture of a snowstorm! And all the images were just like that. Not only is this embarrassing but it is a big waste of time and money, whereas if the experimenter had looked at the first dataset on the day it was acquired he would have realized that something went horribly wrong. In this case, one of the acquisition parameters had been mistyped in the initial setup, but then saved and used for each session thereafter. Although the data from that first scan would still have been useless, he could easily have fixed it for the next participant (or even rescanned the first participant during the session, if he had checked on the scanner console), and hence got good data for the rest of his study.

Recruiting

After the plans for the experimental design, acquisition, and analysis have been made and the ethics has been approved, it is time to recruit your participants. Your inclusion and exclusion criteria for participants play a major role here in terms of the methods you use to recruit, as well as what is specified in your ethics; the methods may involve posting flyers, sending emails, making phone calls, sending requests to a central database or service, or approaching patients in clinics or outpatient services. When talking to participants at this stage, it is a good idea to perform a pre-screening check to ensure that they are safe to be scanned. Although participants will still need to be screened on the day, pre-screening can prevent wasted visits from those with unsafe implants or bad claustrophobia. (More information about MR safety and screening can be found in the online appendix *Short Introduction to MRI Safety for Neuroimaging*.) It is worth clarifying at this point that being told by a participant that she has previously been scanned does not necessarily mean that she is still safe to be scanned, as the field strength may be different, her previous scan may have been of a different body part, she may have had surgery or other changes in the meantime, and she may not even realize that MRI is different from computed tomography (CT) or other types of scanning. In addition, you can also start the process of obtaining consent, especially if it requires a guardian or other party to be involved. Obtaining consent is absolutely necessary and involves explaining the experiment, answering any questions that arise, and giving the participants time to think further about their participation—they should never feel pressured. It is often necessary at this stage to think about balancing recruitment for different groups, too, in order to achieve the desired numbers per group and to ensure that they are "matched" in appropriate ways when possible (e.g., for particular pathologies or genetic populations you may not have much control over age, sex, IQ, handedness, etc., but you can target recruitment of controls to match this other group).

Scanning

After you have satisfactorily looked at and analyzed the pilot data, made any desired adjustments to the experimental protocol, and recruited at least your first participant, it is time for the experiment to properly start and get into full swing. You might start by getting the participants to attend pretraining sessions, which can involve familiarization with the tasks, taking baseline performance measures, starting some form of training, or getting used to the scanner environment—possibly by using a mock scanner if available (this can be very useful for participants who are very young, confused, or nervous; and, in the absence of a mock scanner, even playing back recorded scanner noise can be helpful). Once the pretraining sessions are completed, you would schedule a time for the scanning session and meet the participants when they arrive, comfortably before the allocated start time. At this point you would explain how the experimental session will run and would make sure that they are fully screened for MRI safety, in case anything changed since the pre-screening.

You will have to organize appropriate radiographer or operator cover for the scanner sessions (with radiographers or operators who are able to deal with your specific participants and acquisition needs) and to ensure that all experimental equipment is set up and tested (e.g., stimuli presentation, button boxes, physiological monitoring recordings) in time for the start of the session. It is important to allow enough time to be able to sort out problems with missing or misconfigured equipment, and not just the minimum amount of time needed when all things are going well. As there are many things to do during an experiment, it is a good idea to have a checklist to run through each time, covering things that need to be done before, during, and after the actual scanning. Taking notes during the experiment (e.g., whether the participant seemed sleepy, confused, or fidgety, and whether any different equipment was used, any setup changed, or anything else was unusual) can be very valuable at a later date if something odd is noticed in the data.

It is important to *look at the data* for each scan of each participant, both during the session (on the scanner console) and after the scan has finished and has been downloaded. This visual inspection, together with running the data through the initial stages of analysis, when appropriate, is vital for checking that the quality is acceptable (see the Example Box "Keep looking at your data!"). If any problems are spotted, then it is crucial to point them out to an appropriate person (e.g., the radiographer, the physicist, the center manager) as soon as possible. Corrective actions can then be taken immediately (hopefully during the scanning session itself), which can help with your particular dataset or with the general scanner setup and hardware for everyone. In some cases simple corrections will be available either through rescanning, reconstructing, and preprocessing the data or within the subsequent analysis, but in other cases it may be that nothing can be done to correct an artifact and, if the problem is severe, then the data might be unusable.

Occasionally, when you or the operator or radiographer looks at a scan of the participant, a potential pathology or anatomical abnormality may be spotted; these are known as *incidental findings*. Each country or center should have a defined procedure to follow when this happens, so be aware of what this is and seek immediate advice if you are not sure what to do. However, the good news is that, beyond some common everyday artifacts that will be explained in subsequent chapters, incidental findings and artifacts are quite rare. In the vast majority of cases there will be nothing to worry about and you can proceed directly with your analysis.

Example Box: Keep looking at your data!

It is important to look at the data after the first participant has been scanned, in order to check that it all worked correctly; but do not stop looking at the data during the main phase of acquisition. An example of what can go wrong was a case when, partway through a study (around the tenth participant), a problem occurred with the wiring in a part of the scanner's head coil, and this resulted in corrupted images where the signal was extremely low in one part of the brain. This persisted for a couple of days before another experimenter noticed it when checking her own data from a separate experiment. As a consequence, a number of datasets that contained this artifact had to be discarded, whereas, if the first experimenter had noticed the problem quickly, it could have been fixed straightaway (the head coil required repair, but a spare was available and only took minutes to swap in). Immediate repair would also have saved other people from losing data acquired through the same faulty coil (people who were clearly not checking their data either). So, even if the first session's data look fine when you check them, you still need to check them every time; so get into the habit of looking at your data. And, for a third time, because it is so important, please make sure that you *look at your data!*

Analysis

Finally, when all this has been done and the data are collected, a full analysis can be run. Its aim is typically to extract quantities of interest (volumes of structures, perfusion values, path of a white matter tract, etc.) or to test a statistical hypothesis (e.g., that patients have reduced functional activity compared to controls), with the outcome often presented as a map of where statistically significant results were obtained (where there was a difference in functional activity, or microstructural measures, or structural boundaries, etc.). Setting up this analysis should be straightforward at this point, as you have already been through the exercise of thinking it through and setting it up as part of the planning and piloting stages. Some people make the mistake of leaving it until this point to think about the group analysis, but that can be a recipe for disaster, as there is only limited scope for fixing problems in a study design during the analysis stage, after all the data have been collected. This is particularly true when crucial scans have not been taken (structural scans, fieldmap scans, an expanded field of view functional scan for partial brain studies, etc.: see later chapters for more details). So make sure that you do think about all the aspects of your study early on in the design phase (see the Example Box "Think through your analysis early").

Example Box: **Think through your analysis early**

We have emphasized how important it is to think about the final analysis at the outset. There are numerous stories of people approaching analysis only to discover that a simple oversight in the acquisition has limited what they can get out of the data (or means that they cannot get useful results at all). This occurs for instance when using ASL perfusion imaging, where it is far too easy to get a perfusion-weighted image, but the experimenter has overlooked that he needs another "calibration" image (typically, of only a few seconds duration) to convert that image into an absolute measure of cerebral blood flow. In this case an experiment can often be "rescued" by looking at relative measures of perfusion, but global changes between individuals (which are common) are lost. Thankfully, this error is becoming rarer, as ASL becomes more standardized.

Interpretation

Once the data are analyzed, all that remains to be done is to interpret the results, which requires careful thought. In fact, some knowledge of acquisition and analysis methods is crucial for a correct interpretation of the results. This does not mean that results cannot be interpreted unless you are an expert in both acquisition and analysis (as almost no one is); but certain limitations in the acquisition and analysis need to be understood and brought to bear on the interpretation. For example, interpreting differences in widely used quantitative diffusion metrics, such as mean diffusivity (MD), requires an understanding of how they relate to biological structures such as axon density and to image quality, for instance signal-to-noise ratio (SNR) or presence of artifacts. Another example is when further investigation of a result is required in order to try to tease apart the underlying driving force, or to check that it was not driven by errors such as misalignment or mis-segmentation (potential problems in VBM studies). This is yet another instance of a point in the process where having a broad understanding of various aspects of neuroimaging is crucial.

The main focus of this primer, and of the whole series, is on the analysis of neuroimaging data. However, given the interconnectedness of all the aspects of neuroimaging, we will also be covering elements of acquisition, experimental design, and interpretation in various places in these primers. Furthermore, despite the fact that the analysis of different MRI modalities will be covered in separate sections, there are ways in which these also interact. This is especially true in interpretation, where there can be substantial benefits to additionally using different modalities (including non-MRI ones: see section 2.7), as such studies can combine advantages from these modalities, which leads to stronger and more clearly interpretable findings.

1.3 MR physics and scanner hardware

It is not necessary to understand everything there is to know about MR physics and how an MRI scanner works in order to run neuroimaging experiments successfully. However, some basics are necessary if you want to be able to design good experiments and to interpret their results carefully. In addition, a working knowledge of MRI safety is essential if you are running experiments. In this section we will outline the basics of MR physics and how MRI scanners work. (More details about MR physics and MRI safety can be found in the online appendices *Short Introduction to MRI Physics for Neuroimaging* and *Short Introduction to MRI Safety for Neuroimaging*.)

The fundamental principle of MRI is that certain atomic nuclei (also called "spins") act like tiny bar magnets and interact with magnetic fields in a way that allows us to both measure and manipulate their magnetic state. Although this interaction is with the nuclei, we do not call it "nuclear" (as in nuclear medicine), as that term would suggest the use of radioactive substances and MRI has nothing to do with radioactivity. It is only the magnetic state of the nuclei that is measured and manipulated, and this does no damage to the nuclei and has no effect on any of the biological processes involving the molecules in which they are contained. For brain imaging, it is the hydrogen nuclei (i.e., protons) within water molecules that are principally targeted, as they are so abundant, though hydrogen nuclei in fatty molecules also contribute signals and show up in some types of scans. Although imaging water may sound uninteresting, it is actually far from it, as there are many different properties of the water molecules that MRI can detect and this is what gives MRI the ability to examine the brain in so many different ways.

In order to create and measure magnetic fields, the MRI scanner uses a collection of different coils, made from electrically conducting wire (see Figure 1.6). Coils are used because passing electric currents through a coil creates a magnetic field and changing magnetic fields inside a coil induces an electrical current in the coil; and both of these properties are used in MRI. That is, since the hydrogen nuclei in water molecules behave like tiny bar magnets, they can be manipulated by the magnetic fields created when currents are passed through these coils. In addition, the nuclei produce small magnetic fields of their own, which are sufficient to generate small electrical currents in some of these coils, particularly the closest one—the head coil.

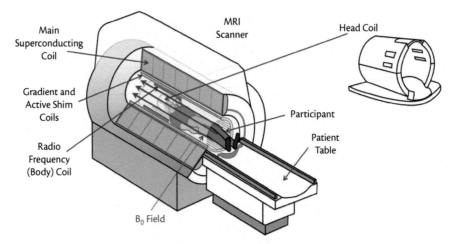

Figure 1.6: Schematic of an MRI scanner, showing the main coils and the B_0 field in relation to the participant inside the scanner. The head coil (top right) is placed around the participant's head prior to them being moved into the center of the scanner (the bore).

M is for Magnetic (B_0 Field)

To interact with the hydrogen nuclei, a very strong static magnetic field is required. It is only in a very strong magnetic field that the tiny bar magnets of the nuclei will tend to point in the same direction (along this main field). If they do not point in the same direction (on average), then the sum of the magnetic fields from them is nearly zero and cannot be detected. This strong magnetic field, known as the B_0 field, is established by a large superconducting coil that is always on and is cooled with liquid helium. It is this field that defines the strength of the scanner, as reported in units of tesla (T); for example, a 3T scanner is one where the B_0 field is 3T. To give you a sense of how "strong" this is, we can compare it to the large electromagnets used in scrapyards to pick up cars, which are approximately 1T, or the magnetic field you are in all the time, generated by the Earth's magnetic core, which is between 25 and 65 micro teslas (μT). Ideally the B_0 field is very uniform within the middle of the scanner (the "bore" of the scanner), which is where the object being scanned (e.g., the head) is located. Outside the bore of the scanner the field falls away rapidly, by design, to avoid stray fields stronger than 5 gauss (or 500 μT) being present in any areas outside the room that houses the scanner. This is important for safety reasons, as magnetic fields stronger than 5 gauss can interfere with pacemakers and other medical equipment.

In order to make the B_0 field more uniform within the head (or whatever object is being scanned) the MRI scanner also contains *shim coils* that create fields that try to cancel the bulk of any nonuniformities in the main B_0 field (see Box 1.1 for optional technical details of magnetic field inhomogeneities). It is important to minimize any nonuniformities in the B_0 field in order to avoid image artifacts, and so a procedure called "shimming" is applied at the start of every scanning session. Shimming is designed to adjust these shim coils so that the field within the brain is much more uniform.

Box 1.1: **B$_0$ field inhomogeneities**

Imperfections in the scanner inevitably affect the images that are created and can lead to a range of artifacts. The main B$_0$ field that is created by the superconducting coil should ideally be perfectly uniform and homogeneous, but in practice it has very small inhomogeneities, some of which are created by the presence of the object being scanned, due to the geometry and magnetic properties (susceptibility) of the materials; these are sometimes called susceptibility-induced inhomogeneities. For the head, it is the air-filled sinuses that always cause minor inhomogeneities, while metallic materials, such as major dental work, can cause greater inhomogeneities. Metals used in most dental work and for surgical implants are not ferromagnetic and are typically safe to introduce into the scanner (though this must be decided by the radiographer or operator on a case-by-case basis; for more information, see the online appendix *Short Introduction to MRI Safety for Neuroimaging*). However, even if they are safe, the metals can often cause such large changes in the B$_0$ field that they render the scans essentially useless due to the sizeable artifacts created. These artifacts are mainly geometric distortions and signal loss, as these are associated with inhomogeneities in the B$_0$ field.

R is for Resonance (B$_1$ field)

A crucial property of the hydrogen nuclei in a strong field is that the little bar magnets (magnetic fields) *precess* or rotate around the axis of the B$_0$ field, but in such a way that the frequency of rotation is proportional to the strength of the external magnetic field. This rotation is important because it creates oscillating fields (B$_1$ *fields*) that we can detect and manipulate externally, at a known frequency. This frequency, called the *resonance frequency* (see Box 1.2), is what the nuclei are tuned to, allowing us to manipulate them by transmitting at this frequency (to "excite" them) and also to receive signals coming back from them at (or near) this frequency. The resonance property is thus the key feature of MRI that allows us to obtain signals. This interaction occurs through *radio frequency (RF) coils* (so named because the frequencies are in the range used for broadcasting radio and TV signals)—the two most common examples being the *body coil* and the *head coil*.

Box 1.2: **Resonance frequency**

The relationship between the resonance frequency (also called *Larmor frequency*) and the field strength is governed by the Larmor equation: that is, the frequency of precession for a hydrogen nuclei is 42.58 MHz times the B$_0$ field strength in tesla. This is 63.9 MHz for a 1.5T scanner, 127.7 MHz for a 3T scanner and 298.1 MHz for a 7T scanner. These frequencies are all in the RF range, as used to broadcast radio and TV signals.

The head coil is placed around the participant's head immediately before they go into the scanner and is the only coil not built into the machine. The main reasons why this coil is not built in is that it is helpful to place it as closely as possible to the object being scanned (in our case, the head) and that there are several types of coil that are useful in different situations, so they are designed to be easily interchangeable (i.e., "plug and play"). The purpose of the coil is to transmit or receive signals (or both) around the resonant frequency of the nuclei—the B_1 (or RF) fields.

The body coil is built into the scanner and performs the same function as the head coil: to transmit or receive RF signals (or both). The body coil is typically a lot further away from the participant's head, and so is less sensitive for receiving the weak signals that are emitted by the hydrogen nuclei within the brain. As a consequence, it is not normally used for receiving signals in neuroimaging; we use the head coil instead. However, the body coil can provide a strong and uniform field for manipulating the magnetization state of the hydrogen nuclei (the "tiny bar magnets"), and because of this uniformity it is usually the preferred coil for transmitting. One exception is in 7T scanners, as these do not have a full body coil, although they still have a separate transmission coil (localized to the head) with better homogeneity than the receiver coil array (also localized to the head). See Box 1.3 for more information on the effects of inhomogeneity in RF (B_1) fields.

Box 1.3: RF inhomogeneity and bias fields

For transmitting RF fields (or B_1 fields), it is the greater uniformity of the signal from the body coil that makes it more appealing for the task, since the head coil can also transmit a strong signal but it is less homogeneous or uniform. This is also true for receiving signals: the body coil is more homogeneous than the head coil. Any departure from a uniform RF field (when transmitted or received) results in the intensities being scaled differently and shows up as lighter and darker areas in the image (this is often called a bias field, or RF inhomogeneity). The extra sensitivity of the head coil in receiving the weak signals typically makes for a worthwhile trade-off versus inhomogeneities when receiving or measuring signals. Since the strength of the transmitted signal is easy to increase by putting larger currents through the coils, the body coil is normally used for transmitting the necessary RF signals in an MRI sequence, in order to get better homogeneity during transmission. Various techniques exist to estimate and correct for the effects of bias fields; we consider them in more detail in section 3.2.3.

There are different varieties of head coils that are used in practice; see Box 1.4 for more details on common variants. One final note about head coils is that they are tuned to a narrow frequency range around the desired resonant frequency. This means that they can only be used at a particular field strength (e.g., 3T) and for a particular type of nuclei (e.g., hydrogen). However, it is possible to get head coils tuned to the frequency of different nuclei (e.g., phosphorus or sodium, which are the most common medically) in order to do imaging or spectroscopy that targets other molecules. One drawback of imaging other nuclei is that they are much less abundant than the hydrogen nuclei in water, and so the total signal is much weaker. Consequently it is harder to get good images, and hence this kind of imaging is not as common.

Box 1.4: Head coils and accelerated imaging

One of the most important aspects of a head coil is the number of individual coil elements that are included, as most modern head coils are *coil arrays* rather than single coils (though single coils, using a "birdcage" design, were originally more common and can still be found in use). Coil arrays are now typically used, as they are more flexible in their geometry and provide overall better sensitivity, and also because they are fundamental for accelerated imaging, or parallel imaging, methods. Using multiple coils, in a coil array, can reduce the noise in an image by increasing the SNR or can reduce the amount of time needed to acquire an image by using parallel or accelerated imaging—or both. Whether the method is used to speed up the acquisition or to reduce the noise is up to the user, as speed versus noise is a standard trade-off in MRI and can be applied to any sequence. The big advantage of accelerated imaging is that it provides a way of getting more images in the same amount of time by comparison to non-accelerated imaging methods. Most methods of acceleration— including in-plane methods, such as SENSE and GRAPPA, as well as simultaneous multi-slice ones, such as multi-band—rely on having multiple coils in the head coil array and being able to measure from these in parallel. The outputs from these coils are often called *channels*; thus it is common for head coils to be referred to as 32-channel head coils, or as 32 elements or 32 coils. It is common to find head coils with 8, 12, 16, 32 or 64 channels, and using ones with more channels is becoming increasingly common, due to the capacity for better SNR and higher accelerations.

I is for Imaging (Gradient Fields)

The resonance property is true for every individual hydrogen nucleus (e.g., those within the water molecules). This means that the observed MR signal is made up of contributions from all the nuclei inside the bore of the scanner, all summed together. In order to determine where the signals are coming from in space (i.e., the location within the head), we need a way of separating out the individual contributions to this summed signal. The way this is done in MRI is to use the fact that the resonant frequency, and thus the frequency of the signal, depends on the field strength. Since it is possible to separate out the contributions of different frequencies to a combined signal (a bit like in listening for different instruments in an orchestra), the location of the signal can be determined if the frequency can be linked to the location.

To relate frequency to location, we deliberately add extra, carefully controlled, magnetic fields that vary with location. We add these fields while acquiring the signal measurements, so that the signals from different locations have different, and known, frequencies. This then allows us to measure how strong the signal is at each frequency and, from that, work out how much signal came from a given spatial location (in practice this involves some advanced mathematics, but this is the basic principle that is used). These extra fields are called *gradient fields* and are created by three different *gradient coils* in the scanner (see Figure 1.7 and, for extra

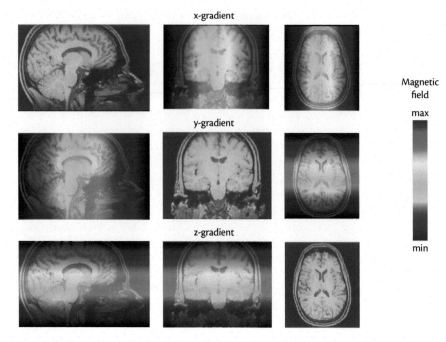

Figure 1.7: Illustration of the three gradient fields: x, y, and z. The colors represent the strength of the magnetic field at each location, which is present throughout the head and makes the signal frequency depend on the spatial location. In these examples the gradients are applied independently, although in practice they are applied in combinations (this results in the colors/gradients changing at an angle: see the online appendix *Short Introduction to MRI Physics for Neuroimaging* for more details).

details, Box 1.5). The most important thing to take from this is that, by applying the gradients, the field is made to vary with location (e.g., one gradient coil can create a field that is small at the bottom of the brain and large at the top of the brain, varying linearly in between). Having a field that changes with location leads to the signals from the hydrogen nuclei having a frequency that depends on their location; thus measuring the frequency content of the received signals lets us work out their location and form an image.

Box 1.5: **Gradient fields**

The spatial location of the signal from specific nuclei is determined on the basis of their resonant frequency, and this is the fundamental principle behind how images are formed. In order to make this work, it is necessary to have a way of making the magnetic field strength change with position in a simple and known way. The gradient coils in the scanner are used to create precisely this kind of field. They create fields that change linearly with position using three coils: one for creating fields that vary with the x position (typically, left to right), one for fields that vary with the y position (typically, anterior to posterior or front to back), and one for the z position (typically, superior to inferior or head to foot). This is enough to determine the spatial locations of all signals by making a series of different measurements with different combinations of gradients. The way that this works relies on advanced mathematics (using Fourier analysis), but the important principle here is that only three different gradient coils (and a lot of measurements) are needed to make this work.

It is important for the gradient fields to be almost exactly linear. That is, if you measured the field strength at different locations and plotted the strength against the position, then the plot should look like a perfectly straight line. Any departures from this result in signals being mislocated in the image, which is a form of geometric distortion, since it is the changes in magnetic field strength with location that are used to work out where the signals come from. Similarly, when the main B_0 field is not perfectly homogeneous, this leads to mislocations as well. In practice the fields are actually very accurate; however, even imperfections and inhomogeneities on the order of one part per million (or less) can cause noticeable distortions, and that is why shimming is so important, as is the careful design and construction of these various coils.

Any inhomogeneities in the B_0 field, or imperfections in the gradient fields, lead to distortions in the final image. These distortions are usually mislocations of the signal, as the spatial locations are calculated (from the frequencies) assuming that the B_0 field is perfectly homogeneous and the gradient fields are perfectly linear (see Box 1.5). Hence, when the field is not at the right value, neither is the frequency of the signal, and so the location is miscalculated. In addition, large inhomogeneities in the B_0 field can cause loss of signal, whereas inhomogeneities in either the transmitted or received RF (B_1) fields result in changes in the image intensity, manifesting themselves as brighter or darker areas in the images. The effects of all of these inhomogeneities are routinely dealt with by the analysis methods (more details in Chapter 3).

In summary, the MRI scanner consists of a set of coils that create and measure magnetic fields in order to interact with and measure the magnetic fields associated with the hydrogen nuclei in water molecules. It uses the property that frequency depends on field strength to determine location of the signal, by creating magnetic fields where the strength varies with location. Radiofrequency fields are transmitted throughout the brain using a coil, usually the body coil, to manipulate the magnetic properties of the hydrogen nuclei (which are like tiny bar magnets), and a coil, usually the head coil, is used to receive signals created by the precessing magnetic fields of these nuclei. From analyzing the frequency content of the measured signals and doing some mathematical analysis, an image can then be formed.

1.4 Overview

This chapter introduced some common types of experiments and analyses, provided an overview of the whole process of conducting a neuroimaging experiment, and gave a brief outline of the fundamentals of MR physics and scanners. The aim of these sections was to provide a framework that is designed to help you learn about the other aspects of neuroimaging in more detail throughout the rest of this primer, in other primers, and beyond that. If this is your first introduction to neuroimaging, then you should not expect to understand everything at this point, and be assured that everything presented so far will be elaborated upon in greater detail elsewhere. The main thing is for you to have a broad understanding of how things interrelate, since in the rest of this primer we will consider specific topics one at a time, although there are many situations where these topics relate to each other. For example, acquisition choices impact on possible analysis options (e.g., not acquiring a fieldmap or a calibration scan leads to not being able to correct for some artifacts) and vice versa (e.g., needing to have enough statistical power requires having a sufficient number or quality of scans). In practice you will need to make a number of choices when designing and analyzing studies, and you need to consider how these choices interact in order to find the best compromise for your particular needs.

SUMMARY

- MRI is very flexible and there are many available types of acquisitions, or modalities.
- Signals are detected from hydrogen nuclei in water molecules throughout the brain.
- MRI scanners consist of many coils that create magnetic fields and send or receive signals to or from the water molecules.
- Neuroimaging research studies use groups of individuals, aligning the images of the brains with registration methods and applying the GLM for statistical analysis.
- There are many choices in analysis and, in order to make appropriate choices, you need to understand the fundamentals of the analysis methods as well as the acquisition principles and the experimental design, since they are all interrelated.
- Noise is always present in MRI scans, along with certain artifacts, which need to be accounted for in the analysis or minimized in the acquisition—or both.
- *LOOK AT YOUR DATA!*

FURTHER READING

- Huettel, S. A., Song, A. W., & McCarthy, G. (2014). *Functional Magnetic Resonance Imaging* (3rd ed.). Sinauer Associates.
  - *This is an accessible, introductory-level textbook, with more of a focus on the physics of acquisition as well as on functional physiology and task fMRI studies.*
- Maguire, E. A., Gadian, D. G., Johnsrude, I. S., Good, C. D., Ashburner, J., Frackowiak, R. S., & Frith, C. D. (2000). Navigation-related structural change in the hippocampi of taxi drivers. *Proceedings of the National Academy of Sciences, 97*(8), 4398–4403.
  - *This is one of the earliest VBM studies to demonstrate healthy plasticity in the human brain—as mentioned in Figure 1.3.*

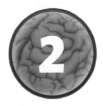

MRI Modalities for Neuroimaging

As you have seen in Chapter 1, there are many different types of images, or *modalities*, within the realm of MRI. At the broadest level this diversity covers structural, diffusion, functional, and perfusion images, but within each of these categories there are more specific modalities or types of acquisitions (a specific type can also be referred to as a *pulse sequence* or just *sequence*). For example, within structural imaging we will discuss modalities such as T_1-weighted and T_2-weighted images, which are both used to examine the gross anatomy but have different characteristics. In this chapter we will discuss a wide range of modalities, mainly those related to structural, diffusion, functional, and perfusion MRI, but also MR spectroscopy and some non-MR modalities that are complementary and can be highly beneficial when combined with MRI.

Modalities differ in what properties of the tissue they are sensitive to when forming an image, and there is a wide range of different physical properties that can be exploited in MRI. For example, there are magnetic interactions with neighboring molecules, motion of molecules, local concentration of materials with magnetic properties like iron deposition or deoxygenated hemoglobin, and more. This diversity allows us to make images that highlight tissues, structures, and processes within the brain—including gross anatomy, functional activity, microstructure, and chemical composition. In the remainder of this chapter we provide an introduction to a range of modalities, and for each one we will cover measurement principles, fundamental aspects of acquisition, limitations, and artifacts associated with that modality. Such information is essential if you want to be able to plan good experiments, to know how to analyze data correctly, and to interpret the results well.

2.1 Image fundamentals

Before we go any further, there are a few fundamentals of MR imaging that you need to know. First, a 3D image (i.e., a volume) is what we consider to be a single image and it is made up of *voxels*—the 3D equivalent of the 2D pixels that make up digital photos. Typical voxel sizes are between 0.5 mm and 4 mm, but voxels do not have to be the same size in each direction. The term *anisotropic* is commonly used to describe voxels with different sizes in different directions; for example, a voxel may be 1.0 × 1.0 × 3.0 mm, which means that it measures 1 mm along two directions but 3 mm in the third direction (see Figure 2.1). Voxels with equal side lengths in all three directions are referred to as *isotropic*; and these are usually better suited to quantitative analysis. Sometimes there are trade-offs that make anisotropic voxels more desirable, such as for speed in clinical practice, where they are very common (thick slices with smaller in-plane voxel sizes are often used: see Figure 2.1). However, for research purposes, isotropic or nearly isotropic voxels are preferred in order to reduce directional biases.

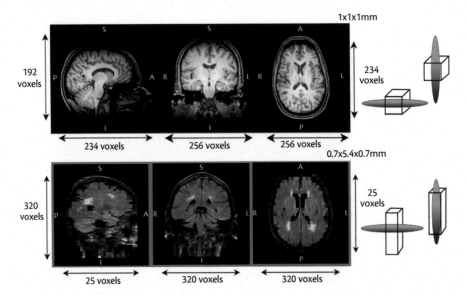

Figure 2.1: Illustration of two different structural images, one with isotropic voxels (first row) and one with anisotropic voxels (second row). In the first case the dimensions of the image are 256 × 234 × 192 voxels (in L–R, A–P, S–I directions) and each voxel is 1 × 1 × 1 mm, which makes the total FOV 256 × 234 × 192 mm³. In the second case the dimensions are 320 × 25 × 320 voxels and each voxel is 0.7 × 5.4 × 0.7 mm, which makes the FOV 224 × 135 × 224 mm³. This second case is an example of a clinical scan designed to have high in-plane resolution and fewer slices (this reduces both the scan time and the number of slices that a radiologist needs to examine). On the right is an illustration of the orientation bias caused by anisotropic voxels—since the MR signal from a voxel is proportional to the volume occupied. The illustration shows a thin elongated object (e.g., a vessel or lesion) in two orientations, passing through either an isotropic voxel (top) or an anisotropic voxel of the same overall volume (bottom). It can be seen that the amount of the voxel volume occupied by the object is moderate and equal for the isotropic voxels, regardless of the object's orientation, whereas it varies from a very small volume overlap (bottom left) to a very large overlap (bottom right) for the anisotropic voxel. Consequently, objects are much easier to detect in certain orientations for anisotropic voxels (bottom right). Such a bias is undesirable in research imaging and analysis.

The term *resolution* also relates to the voxel size, with high-resolution images being made of small voxels and low-resolution images being made of larger voxels. In MRI this resolution can be varied a lot; and it is common to vary it, as there are many trade-offs in acquiring MR images, for example acquisition time and resolution. Therefore it is not unusual to find a structural image with high resolution (e.g., isotropic voxels of 0.9 mm) but functional images with lower resolution (e.g., voxels of 2.5 mm), as the functional images need to use a faster imaging sequence.

Another important property of an image is the *field of view* (FOV) or *coverage*, which is just the voxel size multiplied by the number of voxels in an image. For example, an image with a voxel size of 0.8 × 0.8 × 1.2 mm and consisting of 320 × 288 × 256 voxels would have a coverage or FOV of 256.0 × 230.4 × 307.2 mm³. It is common to specify these values just for a 2D slice of the image, where the number of voxels is called *matrix size* (e.g., the matrix size would be 320 × 288 in the previous example) and to specify separately the *slice thickness* (e.g., 1.2 mm) and the number of slices. The FOV may refer either to a 2D slice or to the 3D volume.

Unlike the voxel sizes and the FOV, the intensities stored in an MR image do not have any physical units; the intensity is the number associated with a voxel that determines the shade of gray when displaying an image. This is different from other types of images, such as computed tomography (CT), where there are real physical units (Hounsfield units, which quantify X-ray absorption). In MRI the signals are arbitrarily scaled and there are no units, so that an isolated numerical value from one voxel (e.g., 105) has no useful meaning. It is only the relative relationship of the intensities between voxels that contains useful information. This makes some aspects of MRI analysis harder, as you cannot rely on images from different scanners—or even from the same scanner at different times—to have a consistent range of intensity values. One of the roles of analysis can be the conversion of voxel intensities into a measure with physical units that uses other information, like a calibration image. For example, arterial spin labeling (ASL) produces a perfusion-weighted image where each voxel's intensity is a relative measure of perfusion, but with a separate calibration scan it is possible to calculate values that have meaningful physiological units (e.g., ml of blood per 100 g of tissue per minute).

It is also common to acquire a series of images in one scan, such as in functional or diffusion imaging, where we acquire an image every few seconds, one after the other (see Box 2.1 for some extra details about the format, either now or on a second reading). Each single image is a volume, while the set of images can be considered to form a 4D image, where the fourth dimension is time. In functional imaging this corresponds straightforwardly to the time dimension that we are interested in; that is, it corresponds to capturing the changes in brain activation over time. We often refer, then, to the set of values over time that come from a single 3D voxel location as a *timeseries* or *timecourse* (see Figure 2.2). For other imaging modalities, such as diffusion imaging, multiple volumes are still acquired sequentially in time, during the scanning session, but the interesting and useful association is not with time but with some other quantity, such as diffusion direction. So, although each image is acquired at a different time, each image is also acquired with a different setting (e.g., different diffusion directions). In this case the set of values from a voxel is not used to examine changes over time but is used instead to investigate differences related to the other settings. However, it is still common to loosely refer to such a set of values as a "timeseries."

Box 2.1: Image formats

For standard 2D images, such as digital photos, there is a large range of file formats for storing them, for example jpeg, tiff, png. For 3D and 4D medical images there are also a range of file formats. In neuroimaging the two most common volumetric formats (for storing 3D and 4D images) are DICOM and NIfTI. In clinical practice the DICOM format is the most commonly used, while in research it is the NIfTI format. Both are capable of storing either 3D or 4D MRI scans, but DICOM stores a lot of other information too (*metadata*), including identifiable information regarding the participant and details about the scanner settings, whereas the the NIfTI format only stores a minimal amount of extra information, mainly relating to resolution and spatial orientation. Very few neuroimaging research tools work directly with DICOM, but a number of tools exist for DICOM to NIfTI conversion. Although other neuroimaging formats exist (e.g., MINC), the NIfTI format is currently the most universal and useful for exchanging images between labs and between software tools. One downside of the NIfTI format is that some of the acquisition information contained in the DICOM files is lost, and so certain values related to the acquisition (such as TE, TR, echo spacing, etc.) need to be separately noted down and kept track of by you, the experimenter.

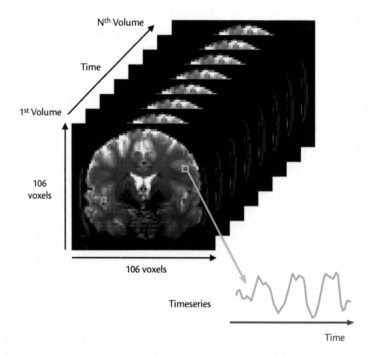

Figure 2.2: Example of a 4D functional MRI dataset. For illustration purposes only, a single slice of each volume is shown, but the 4D image contains a full 3D image (106 × 128 × 106 voxels) for each volume. Extracting the intensities from a single voxel location gives a timeseries (a set of intensities over time, with N time points), as illustrated on the bottom right.

A final point to mention before moving on to consider individual modalities is a general principle of MR acquisition: there is always a trade-off in MRI between having a short scan time, a good resolution, and a low amount of noise (more details about noise will be covered later in the chapter). Each of these characteristics—scan time, resolution, and noise—can be varied, but they interact with one another. That is, you can shorten the scan time by reducing the resolution or by accepting that there will be more noise. Similarly, you could get less noise by either increasing the scan time or reducing the resolution (i.e., having bigger voxels). Or you could increase the resolution (i.e., have smaller voxels) and end up with more noise. The one thing you typically cannot do is have your cake and eat it too; something has to give. Since we always want to reduce the noise in MRI, it is common to sacrifice other things to keep the noise down and improve the *signal-to-noise ratio* (SNR). This will be discussed in more detail in section 2.2.3 (in the part on limitations and artifacts).

One way in which the SNR can usually be improved without sacrificing resolution or time is by increasing the numbers of coils used in the head coil array (e.g., by using a 32-channel rather than a 16-channel head coil). As each coil in the array acquires signal independently, the combination results in a greater SNR for the same acquisition time. However, this is only possible through the use of specific hardware (the head coil) and the amount of benefit depends on the number of coils and the nature of the hardware. Once this hardware is in place, the standard trade-offs between SNR, resolution, and time still apply, hence finding the best compromise is still something you need to do. Using parallel (or accelerated) imaging methods with a head coil array can reduce the acquisition time, but with a penalty in SNR by comparison to the unaccelerated case of using the same head coil. The SNR is of great importance, as care has to be taken to make sure that there is sufficient signal versus noise in any acquisition, so that we have enough statistical power to detect effects, or just to see differences visually. MR physicists spend a lot of time making sure that they get as much SNR from their sequences as possible, and parameters are often tuned on particular scanners to improve the SNR—which is an important reason why it is good to talk to the local physicist, radiographer, or scanner operator to make sure that you use the sequences that give the best results on your particular scanner. We will have more to say about this, as well as about noise and artifacts in acquisitions, in various sections throughout this and later chapters.

2.2 Structural MRI

In neuroimaging, structural MR images are typically used to show the gross anatomy of the brain: that is, mainly gray matter, white matter, and cerebrospinal fluid (CSF). In a clinical setting these are the most commonly used images and a radiologist typically inspects them visually, looking for pathological lesions, anatomical deformations, and so on. It is not uncommon for these clinical images to have very small in-plane voxel sizes but be large through plane (i.e., have thick slices, such as 0.5 × 0.5 × 4 mm). For visual inspection this can be helpful, although it biases the observer to see structures in certain orientations better than others (see Figure 2.1). In research it is much better to remove such biases and to get images with isotropic voxels (equal voxel sizes in the three directions). The typical resolution of a structural image in research is therefore around 1 mm isotropic, but it is becoming more common for this value to be pushed down to 0.8 mm or even lower, with advances in scanning sequences and hardware. Scanning times for structural MR images vary between a few minutes to around 15 minutes, or occasionally more, although the most common timings are around 3–5 minutes. The timing depends on the scanner, the desired resolution, and the quality of the image.

A structural image is a vital component of any research study. It is used for identifying details of individual anatomy and is essential for getting an accurate alignment of brains from different subjects, which is necessary for any group study, including studies that use other modalities such as diffusion, functional, or spectroscopic data. Without a good structural image it is very difficult to do a group study, as poor alignment of subjects will typically ruin the ability to locate changes of interest and will decimate the statistical power. Therefore every study should include a structural image of reasonable quality, which is possible to obtain with 3–5 minutes of scanning.

If you are interested in analyzing the anatomy directly then it is more important to get a structural image of higher quality in terms of resolution and tissue contrast, although with good hardware this does not need to take much longer. The kind of studies we are talking about here are ones that are looking for changes in brain anatomy associated with processes such as neurodegeneration or plasticity and will involve quantifying cortical thickness, local gray matter content, or the shape and size of deep gray matter structures. Accurately calculating cortical thickness or finding structural boundaries requires good-quality images, with good resolution and contrast (i.e., with sizeable differences in intensity between tissues or structures).

2.2.1 Varieties of acquisition

T_1-weighted images are the most common variety of structural image, but there are many other varieties that are available too, such as T_2-weighted, proton density (PD), or FLAIR (which is like a T_2-weighted image but with fluid signal suppressed), as illustrated in Figure 2.3. All of these can be acquired on any MRI scanner and all show the gross anatomy but are not sensitive to other things such as neuronal activity, blood flow, or direction of axonal bundles. Thus these kinds of images are all referred to as structural images, even though their appearance might be quite different.

The reason for having multiple types of structural images in common usage is that each type highlights different aspects of the tissues present, thus providing a very valuable way of investigating the anatomy in vivo. This is particularly important when looking at pathology, as some changes show up much more clearly on certain images; for example, lesions in multiple sclerosis are often very faint on a T_1-weighted image but are much more obvious on a PD or FLAIR image (see Figure 2.3). It is also possible to highlight certain pathologies even more by injecting contrast agents (e.g., certain gadolinium compounds), which are commonly used diagnostically for certain clinical conditions but rarely used in research. For research studies with healthy participants, it is most common to acquire only a T_1-weighted image, as this normally is the best quality, especially for differentiating healthy tissues (gray matter, white matter and CSF), for a given amount of scan time.

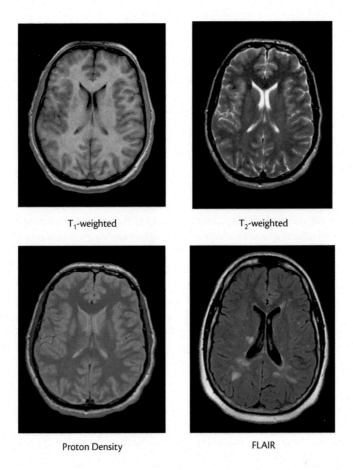

T_1-weighted T_2-weighted

Proton Density   FLAIR

Figure 2.3: Examples of four of the most common structural MRI modalities or varieties. The T_1-weighted, T_2-weighted, and PD (proton density) images are from one subject and the FLAIR image comes from a different subject, where you can see that there are lesions that appear as bright areas within the white matter.

2.2.2 Measurement principles

It is the magnetic properties of the hydrogen nuclei in the water molecules that determine the MRI signal, and for structural imaging there are only three crucial properties that are important: proton density and two relaxation processes, described by T_1 and T_2 relaxation constants. These properties are determined by the local microscopic environment of the water molecules and are different within the different tissue types (i.e., gray matter, white matter, and CSF). The relaxation constants describe how the magnetization of the hydrogen nuclei changes over time, but you do not need to understand (especially on a first reading) precisely what these relaxation times mean or in what way the magnetization is affected (more details can be found in the online appendix *Short Introduction to MRI Physics for Neuroimaging*). The important thing to know is that these three properties are quite different in the different tissues and, due to this, we are able to get MR images that have marked contrast between these tissues.

Proton density is a simple property—it is just the density of the protons that contribute to the MRI signal. This is essentially the concentration of water, given that almost all of the signal in the brain comes from the hydrogen nuclei (protons) of water molecules. The relaxation constants, T_1 and T_2, are determined by many other aspects of the water molecules and their environment, such as the geometry and arrangement of nearby cells, the surrounding chemicals, and more. As a consequence, we can design MRI sequences that are sensitive to these changes, giving us large intensity differences between different tissues, especially by comparison to many non-MRI modalities. However, knowing the value of these three physical parameters (proton density and the two relaxation times), or the numerical value of the signal intensity determined by them, is not enough information to allow us to figure out all the biological characteristics of the tissue. Therefore the signal that we measure in a structural image (i.e., the intensity of the image) highlights the structural boundaries of interest (between the tissues), but only acts as a surrogate of the tissue type rather than providing quantitative information about specific biological properties.

Although many of the microscopic biological characteristics are not uniform within tissue (e.g., across all areas of "gray matter" there are differences in cell type and density that affect the proton density and relaxation constants), the variations of the relaxation constants within a given tissue are much smaller than the differences between tissues (e.g., between gray matter and white matter). This means that the image intensities are relatively constant within a type of tissue but show much larger differences at the boundaries between tissues, which is what allows us to see these tissues in the structural images.

Image contrast and relaxation times

The visibility of the boundaries between tissues is what matters most for structural images, if they are to show the gross anatomy; and having substantial intensity differences between tissues is crucial for this. *Contrast* in an image is defined as the intensity difference across a boundary between two tissues or structures of interest. We need the contrast to be strong in order to detect and measure the geometry of structures in the image (e.g., cortical thickness or hippocampal boundaries). More precisely, it is the magnitude of the contrast with respect to the magnitude of the noise that matters most, and this is measured by the *contrast-to-noise ratio* (CNR). For structural imaging the CNR is one of the most important properties of the image, along with the spatial resolution.

It is possible to obtain different types of structural image by manipulating the sequence to change how much influence each of the three parameters (proton density and T_1 and T_2 relaxation constants) has on the signal intensity. Unsurprisingly, a T_1-weighted image, as the name suggests, is dominated by the influence of the T_1 relaxation constant. However, proton density also has an influence, even in a T_1-weighted image. Actually proton density is the most fundamental property of the three, since zero proton density means that there are no water molecules to contribute signal, and so the signal is always proportional to proton density, regardless of the type of image. A *PD image* is one that is largely independent of the T_1 and T_2 relaxation constants and happens to have the least contrast, as there is only a relatively small difference in water density between the different tissue types (see Figure 2.3). To get a better contrast, the relaxation properties need to be used; and this is what happens in T_1-weighted and T_2-weighted images, as well as in other structural imaging varieties and modalities.

The way that the intensity is made sensitive to the relaxation properties (i.e., in a T_1-weighted or a T_2-weighted image) is by changing the timing of the various magnetic fields applied by the scanner, as specified in the pulse sequence (each type of image acquisition is defined by a pulse sequence). It is these timings, along with the tissue properties, that determine the image intensities, and hence the contrast. The main timing parameters that are adjusted in structural pulse sequences are the *repetition time* (TR) and the *echo time* (TE). These are very important MRI parameters; they are specified in all sequences and are usually quoted in papers. It is not important at this point to know more about them (though interested readers can find details in the online appendix *Short Introduction to MRI Physics for Neuroimaging*). What is important is to know that changing these sequence parameters is enough to vary the amount of T_1 and T_2 weighting, and also the CNR, which results in very different images (see Figure 2.4).

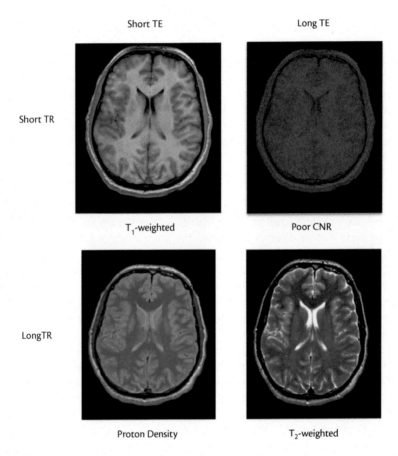

Figure 2.4: Example of how structural MRI modalities relate to the two main sequence parameters, TR and TE. Note that, in the image in the top right, both the SNR and the CNR are very low, and hence this setting is not used in practice. The terms "short" and "long" are relative to the values of the relaxation parameters of the tissue. For instance, a short TR is one that is shorter than the relevant T_1 constant, and a short TE is one that is shorter than the relevant T_2 constant.

Even small changes of TR and TE in a sequence can be useful for improving tissue contrast, and it is possible to tune sequences to give better contrast in certain areas. For example, some deep gray matter structures, such as the globus pallidus, can have quite weak contrast in some T_1-weighted images but can be improved through relatively small changes in TR and TE. However, there is normally a trade-off, and so improving deep gray matter contrast often comes at the expense of worse contrast in other areas, such as at the cortical boundaries. For some subjects, such as infants, the relaxation times can be quite different from those of typical healthy adult subjects, and in these cases specifically tuning the structural sequences to give better contrast can be extremely useful. In addition, different field strengths (e.g., 1.5T vs. 3T vs. 7T) influence the relaxation constants, and so sequences always need to be tuned separately for each field strength.

2.2.3 Limitations

In this section we will discuss a number of limitations of MRI, many of which are common across all MRI modalities. This primer presents (in the following section) quite a range of limitations and artifacts, as having some knowledge of them is important for getting the best acquisitions, for optimizing your analysis, and for correctly interpreting your results. The good news is that in practice you can avoid and correct for many limitations and artifacts. While it might not be possible to eliminate their effects altogether, there is rarely a reason why they should prevent you from using MRI, which is a highly flexible and sensitive method for investigating the brain. We will discuss methods for compensating for and correcting various limitations and artifacts in the following chapters.

SNR, CNR, and resolution

A common limitation across all MRI modalities is noise. We are always fighting against noise, as the signal that we detect is quite weak. This is not much of a problem in other types of imaging (such as optical photography—at least with good lighting), but in MRI the noise is often a limiting factor and a lot of effort in developing acquisition sequences goes into reducing the relative amount of noise. The keyword here is "relative," since it is the magnitude of noise compared to the magnitude of the signal of interest that really counts. This value is sometimes measured by SNR (signal-to-noise ratio), but in structural imaging it is the CNR (contrast-to-noise ratio) that is more important.

Both SNR and CNR are important factors; and they are intrinsically linked to spatial resolution, which is also a crucial factor in structural imaging. How accurately we can find the boundaries of different structures is obviously limited by spatial resolution, but improving this resolution is not easy. That is because the number of hydrogen nuclei in a voxel is proportional to its volume and therefore reducing the size of a voxel reduces the available signal. This brings us back to the general trade-off between SNR (or CNR), spatial resolution, and acquisition time. That is, the longer the acquisition the better the SNR will be, while the better the spatial resolution the lower the SNR. In fact any of these can be traded off against any of the others, as illustrated by the following principles (see also the Example Box "SNR, resolution, and acquisition time trade-offs"):

- SNR is proportional to the voxel volume, and hence strongly impacted by changes in resolution;

■ SNR is proportional to the square root of the acquisition time, and hence only weakly impacted by increases in acquisition time.

Example Box: **SNR, resolution, and acquisition time trade-offs**

We will illustrate the trade-offs between SNR, resolution, and acquisition time with two examples.

First, consider increasing the resolution of an image by a factor of 2 in each dimension—for example, changing from a 1 × 1 × 1 mm voxel size to a 0.5 × 0.5 × 0.5 mm voxel size. The volume of an individual voxel in this case decreases by a factor of 8 (from 1 mm³ to 0.125 mm³), hence the SNR also decreases by a factor of 8. This would typically result in a very noisy image, often with unusably low SNR and CNR. To restore the SNR to the original level (the same as in the 1 × 1 × 1 mm image) would require the acquisition time to increase by a factor of 64 (as the SNR only increases by the square root of this factor and √64 = 8). This would normally be way too long to be practical—for example, a 2-minute scan would end up lasting over 2 hours!

Second, consider increasing the resolution of an image by 10 percent—for example, from a 1 × 1 × 1mm voxel size to a 0.9 × 0.9 × 0.9 mm voxel size. The volume of the voxel in this case only changes from 1 mm³ to 0.729 mm³, and hence the SNR is only reduced to 73 percent of the original value. This may be good enough for practical purposes, but the SNR could be maintained by increasing the acquisition time by a factor of 1.88 (as √1.88 = 1.37 = 1/0.729). Or, more simply, doubling the acquisition time would result in an SNR increase of √2 = 1.41 (a 41 percent increase), which would more than compensate for the reduction due to the change in resolution. That is, a 10-minute scan with an isotropic resolution of 0.9 mm would have an SNR that is approximately equal to that of a 5-minute scan with an isotropic resolution of 1 mm.

Also note that we could just change the acquisition time on its own, without changing the resolution, if we wanted to increase the SNR, but the gain in SNR is not very large when compared to the valuable scanner time. Typically, larger SNR benefits can be achieved by changing other aspects, if available (e.g., by using a head coil array with more coils, or a different type of MRI sequence). However, decreasing the SNR in order to shorten the acquisition time is commonly done; and it is done either by changing the parameters for a given sequence (such as sampling speed or bandwidth) or, more often, by using parallel or accelerated imaging methods (which require a coil array) or fast imaging sequences. These methods are covered in more detail later on in this primer and in the online appendix *Short Introduction to MRI Physics for Neuroimaging*.

Consequently, spatial resolution is normally only changed in relatively small amounts (e.g., by 10 percent) in order to reduce the SNR or acquisition time penalties (or both). Conversely, spatial resolution can be sacrificed in order to speed up acquisitions or improve SNR, and this is one of the trade-offs that are often made. These trade-offs are general principles that are true for all MRI modalities, not just for structural imaging, and so the same considerations apply in many instances (in fact functional and diffusion images have lower resolution largely because of the need to improve SNR in this way).

Partial volume

No matter what the spatial resolution ends up being, it will still be relatively large with respect to the structures of interest. For example, the cerebral cortex is only a few millimeters thick but is highly folded, and this means that in many voxels there is not a single tissue but a mixture of tissues (e.g., some gray matter from the cortex and some neighboring white matter or CSF). The resulting signal from such a voxel ends up being a weighted average of the signal from each tissue, with the weighting being proportional to the fraction of the volume associated with each tissue (see Figure 2.5). This is known as the *partial volume* effect and is another limitation common to all MRI modalities. In structural imaging the partial volume influences how precisely boundaries can be located or volumes calculated.

Other limitations

Another limitation of structural imaging is that it does not provide quantitative information. That is, a given intensity value has no useful meaning on its own (as the intensities are arbitrarily scaled

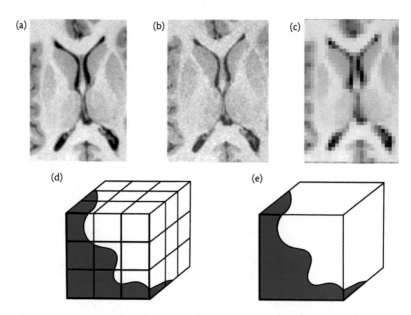

Figure 2.5: Illustration of noise, resolution, and partial volume. Top row shows the same region around the lateral ventricles, with (a) good SNR, CNR, and spatial resolution; (b) reduced SNR and CNR; (c) reduced resolution but good SNR and CNR. Bottom row shows an illustration of partial volume of gray and white matter for (d) higher resolution (27 voxels, each 1 × 1 × 1 mm) and (e) lower resolution (1 voxel, 3 × 3 × 3 mm). In both cases there is a mixture of tissues within the voxels, but in (d) there are also voxels that only contain a single tissue. Intensity in a voxel is a weighted average of the pure tissue intensities by the proportion of volume occupied; for example, if gray matter was 30% of the volume in (e), then the intensity would be $I = 0.3 \times I_{GM} + 0.7 \times I_{WM}$.

by the scanner), and it is only its relationship with other intensity values, typically at boundaries, that conveys useful information. Furthermore, the intensities are only surrogates of the things that we are interested in, such as tissue type, and these intensities reflect a wide range of different processes that affect the relaxation times, such as cell density, chemical environment, microscopic geometry, and so on. As previously mentioned, these vary even within one type of tissue (e.g., not all the parts of the gray matter have the same type of cells or cell density), and such variations make it more difficult to use the intensity for labeling the tissue type. However, in some cases this can be a strength rather than a limitation, as it provides some indication of biological variations within tissues.

A very specific limitation of most structural MRI is that the bone is not visible in the image, as there is not enough water content to provide an appreciable signal. Hence the skull ends up being as dark as air, which also has no appreciable signal, although the muscles and fatty tissues outside the skull, and sometimes the marrow within the bone, are visible. This means that it is not possible to distinguish clearly between air in the sinuses and the bone nearby, or to see fractures or trauma in the skull. If such information is needed, then a CT scan is really required; and, for clinical cases, this is routinely done.

Similarly, for certain other pathologies, such as multiple sclerosis (MS), a single T_1-weighted image does not highlight all of the useful information very well. In particular, lesions are far more prominent on PD or T_2-weighted images, whereas the T_1-weighted images often provide the best overall anatomical description. Therefore using the T_1-weighted image in conjunction with the PD or T_2-weighted images allows for the pathologies to be more clearly interpreted. This is just one example of a situation where having a single modality or structural sequence is limiting, whereas having multiple ones provides richer information.

2.2.4 Artifacts

Unfortunately there are also a number of artifacts in MRI, most of which occur rarely, although some are always present but well compensated for in the analysis phase. It is not particularly important that you understand the details of the physics behind these artifacts, or even that you know what the complete range is. What is important is to recognize the most common types, to know what to do about them, and to be vigilant in checking your data and in seeking advice about other artifacts as soon as you notice them.

There is considerable variety among the root causes of these artifacts, which can be due to scanner hardware imperfections, equipment malfunctions, operator error, subject movement and other physiological confounds. Each of these factors affects the physics of acquisition in different ways, but the details of these processes are beyond the scope of this primer and are not necessary to understand in order to recognize the artifact or correct for it when possible. We say "when possible" because not all artifacts can be corrected, and there is a wide range of possibilities when it comes to correction. There are cases where the artifacts can be simply and easily fixed on the scanner console or in image reconstruction (a stage that normally happens automatically on the scanner before you get your images), or cases that can be dealt with very well in standard or specialized analyses. However, there are also cases that can be only approximately corrected for in the analysis, and cases where nothing can be done and either the artifacts have to be tolerated or the acquisition thrown away.

In structural imaging the most common artifacts are motion-induced artifacts, bias field or radio frequency (RF) inhomogeneities, ghosting, gradient nonlinearity distortions, and wrap-around. Figure 2.6 shows examples of all of these artifacts. Most of them are normally very minor or nonexistent in typical scans. Table 2.1 gives some information about the basic cause, the prevalence, and the recommended action for each of these.

There is also a range of additional artifacts, such as RF interference, RF spiking, susceptibility artifacts, parallel imaging artifacts, inflow artifacts, reconstruction errors, and so on; Figure 2.7

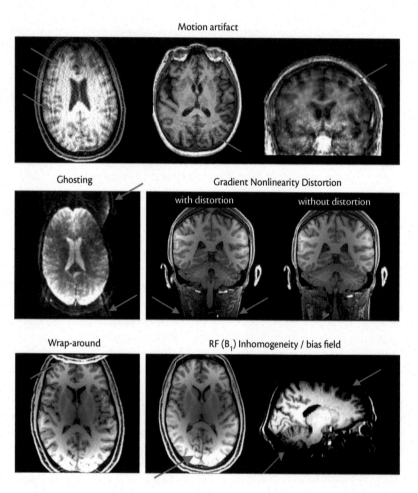

Figure 2.6: Illustration of common structural artifacts. Top row: motion-induced artifacts, where additional edges, or ripples, can be seen. Middle row: ghosting (shifted and wrapped version of the image superimposed on the original) and gradient nonlinearity distortion (neck is compressed horizontally towards the bottom of the image by comparison to a non-distorted image). Bottom row: wrap-around (back of the head wraps around to the front, and the signal from the scalp clearly ends up overlapping with brain tissue) and bias field (or RF inhomogeneity), where there is either brightening or darkening, such as at the back of the brain or at the top and bottom of the brain. See Table 2.1 for more information about these artifacts.

Table 2.1 Common artifacts in structural MRI: causes, prevalence, and recommended actions.

Artifact Name	Cause	Prevalence	Recommended Action
Motion	Subject moving in the scanner	Extremely common: often weak but can be strong—can be seen on a detailed inspection even if weak	Ask subjects to remain still; make them comfortable; pad the head with cushions or similar; rescan for bad artifact (ones creating obvious edges/ripples) or exclude data if cannot rescan
Bias Field (RF Inhomogeneity)	Standard imperfections in RF coils	Always present to some extent: normally noticeable by eye	Corrected well by standard analysis methods
Ghosting	Complex MR physics reasons	Extremely common but usually very weak; strong cases are unusual and may signify a problem with the scanner or sequence	Potential for improvement with alternative reconstruction (see physicist/radiographer); for bad cases need to rescan or exclude data
Gradient Nonlinearity Distortion	Standard imperfections in gradient coils	Always present but sometimes corrected in reconstruction on the scanner; not that strong within the brain but more noticeable in the neck and spine	Check if brain is centered at magnet isocenter; or redo reconstruction with the gradient nonlinearity correction turned on (see physicist/radiographer); can also fix with specialized postprocessing
Wrap-around (Aliasing Artifact)	FOV (field of view) set too small by the radiographer/operator	Very uncommon but very obvious	Rescan (with larger FOV) or exclude data; OK to ignore if wrap-around does not reach the brain

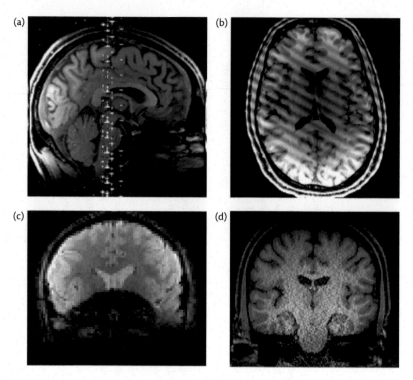

Figure 2.7: Less common structural artifacts: (a) RF interference; (b) RF spiking; (c) susceptibility artifact (in this case it is due to an MRI-safe, nonferrous dental implant); (d) parallel imaging reconstruction noise, typically due to the use of very high acceleration factors (note the high levels of noise in the central regions by comparison to the periphery).

shows examples of some of these. They vary in cause and appearance, but all share a common characteristic: they lead to brain images that do not look normal. The best way to detect these artifacts is described in Figure 2.8, which we strongly, strongly encourage everyone to follow—*both* during the scanning session (when you can spot some of these artifacts immediately on the console and can then do a rescan if there is time) *and* as soon as possible afterwards, when you get your reconstructed data. If you do spot a potential artifact, then the best thing to do is seek advice straightaway from scanner operators, radiographers, MR physicists, or other experienced colleagues who will be able to help determine what the artifact is and how to correct it. Timing is important since, as pointed out in Chapter 1, some artifacts are caused by equipment problems that will continue to affect the scanner until they are fixed, and so, if everyone is vigilant with their scans, then these problems, when they do happen, will have a minimal impact.

Remember that you do not need to be an expert in these artifacts, their causes, or the required actions to take—especially to begin with. As you gain more experience you will become familiar with common artifacts and will know how to deal with them and whether they are problematic or not; but you will not become an expert on all types of artifacts—leave that

LOOK AT YOUR DATA!

Figure 2.8: How to detect artifacts.

for others. Instead, just get into the habit of looking at your data, learn how to recognize when a brain does not look normal, and seek advice on artifacts when needed (see the Example Box "MRI artifacts" for real examples to view).

The artifacts covered here for structural imaging are actually quite general artifacts that are common to all MRI scans. Hence all of these artifacts can also occur in other MRI modalities (e.g., diffusion or functional imaging), although in those modalities there are also some additional artifacts. We will see examples of these later on in this chapter. It is not all bad news though, as problematic artifacts are relatively rare, so most of the time you will only need to do a quick check and then will be able to get on with the rest of your analysis.

Example Box: **MRI artifacts**

On the primer website you will find a set of structural images to view, with instructions on how to do that. These images are a mixture of the structural modalities discussed in this chapter, with and without artifacts, so that you can learn what images should look like and practice finding artifacts by looking at your data.

2.2.5 More acquisition varieties

There is a wide variety of other structural images, or sequences, that are available on an MRI scanner. These include fluid attenuated inversion recovery (FLAIR), white-matter nulled images, double-inversion recovery (DIR), susceptibility-weighted imaging (SWI), quantitative susceptibility mapping/imaging (QSM/QSI), magnetization transfer (MT), angiography, venography—and more. Some of these images are illustrated in Figure 2.9 and a few details are provided in Table 2.2. These images can all be considered "structural," since they are designed to depict aspects of the gross anatomy, although they are targeted at different properties, such as blood vessels in angiography and venography or iron deposition in SWI. Many are common in clinical practice (especially FLAIR and SWI), as they highlight specific pathologies well (e.g., lesions in the case of FLAIR and microbleeds in the case of SWI), although bear in mind that clinical acquisitions are not always suitable for research studies (e.g., due to very anisotropic voxel sizes) and vice versa. We will not go into the details of these types of imaging here; we just want to make you aware that they exist and are options to be considered when you plan your studies, especially if you have subjects with pathologies.

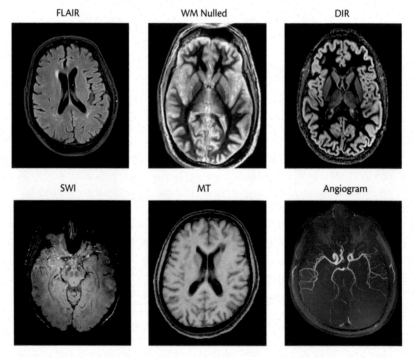

Figure 2.9: Examples of other structural modalities: FLAIR (fluid attenuated inversion recovery); white-matter nulled image; double-inversion recovery (DIR); susceptibility-weighted imaging (SWI); magnetization transfer (MT); angiogram.

Table 2.2 Structural image varieties.

Sequence	Sensitive to	General Use
FLAIR	Gray matter and white matter (suppresses fluids, especially CSF; otherwise it has a T_2-weighted contrast)	Clinical and research: especially for highlighting lesions
WM nulled	Gray matter and CSF (suppresses white matter)	Research: especially for studying subcortical anatomy such as external/internal globus pallidus
DIR	Gray matter (suppresses white matter and CSF)	Research and clinical: especially for cortical lesions and details of the cerebral cortex
SWI or QSM/QSI	Iron content in tissue	Clinical and research: especially for microbleeds or iron accumulation in tissue
Magnetization Transfer	Bound versus free water and thus the chemical environment of the water	Clinical and research: highlights lesions and generally abnormal tissue
Angiography / Venography	Blood vessels	Clinical and research: mapping out normal and abnormal cerebral vasculature (larger vessels only, i.e., not capillaries)

One technique used by several of these sequences is that of nulling specific tissues, as this technique can substantially improve the contrast in both healthy and pathological tissues. It is used by FLAIR (to null CSF), by DIR (to null both CSF and white matter) and in white-matter nulled imaging. One common method used for nulling or suppression involves adjusting the time when RF fields are transmitted and received in the sequence: the scan parameters are modified so that there is one point in time when there is no signal from one particular tissue but there is signal from the other tissues. Fat suppression is also applied (using this technique or an alternative one) in some T_1-weighted images and in almost all functional and diffusion images. However, you do not need to know the details of how the techniques work—just that it is possible to perform tissue suppression (for more detail, see the online appendix *Short Introduction to MRI Physics for Neuroimaging*). Effective suppression of the signal often relies on the tissue(s) to be suppressed having relaxation times that match those targeted by the sequence; as a result, departures from these relaxation times (e.g., due to variation in the composition of the tissue) can result in only partial suppression. However, even partial suppression is often very helpful (e.g., for improving tissue contrast) and sufficient for a lot of purposes.

The reason why fat suppression is used in functional and diffusion images is that, if no suppression were done, the fat signal would be shifted spatially and would overlap substantially with the brain tissue in the image. This is due to an artifact known as the chemical shift artifact, and results in large shifts, of many voxels, of the fat signals from where they should appear. For structural images, there are methods for making the chemical shift artifact small (smaller than a voxel); but in functional and diffusion images, because of other compromises made for speed, these methods are not viable. As a consequence, fat suppression is essential in order to prevent this overlapping signal from corrupting the brain images.

Finally, there are types of images that can measure some physical properties of the scanner that prove useful (such images are not really "structural" images, but we will mention them here). This includes images that measure, quantitatively, the magnetic fields in the scanner, for example the B_0 and B_1 (RF) fields. Since these fields always contain some degree of nonuniformities and those cause artifacts, being able to quantify and map them spatially can be very important for correcting certain artifacts. For instance, a B_0 *fieldmap* is important for correcting geometric distortion and this, or some equivalent, is recommended whenever acquiring functional or diffusion images (see sections 2.3 and 2.4). Such images are rarely acquired in clinical practice but are extremely useful in both neuroscience and clinical research.

SUMMARY

- Many varieties of structural images exist, each of which can highlight different aspects of the anatomy, including pathological tissue.

- T_1-weighted images are the most common structural images, used for getting good CNR (contrast-to-noise ratio) and tissue discrimination, especially in healthy subjects.

- Isotropic or nearly isotropic acquisitions are better for neuroimaging research.

- Image intensity depends mainly on the proton density and on the T_1 and T_2 relaxation times, which in turn depend on many aspects of the local microstructure and chemical environment.

- Structural images are not quantitative but provide intensities that are a surrogate for the main tissue types in the brain.

- Other types of structural images exist that highlight other characteristics of the tissue, such as the presence of lesions, iron deposition, and vessels.

- Many artifacts can occur in MRI acquisitions and these need to be detected as soon as possible; you should do this by *looking at your data*.

- Some artifacts can be corrected for easily, others cannot be corrected for at all, so if you find an artifact (or an incidental finding) in your data you should seek advice on what to do from an expert.

- Structural images are needed in all types of experiments, including functional and diffusion experiments.

FURTHER READING

- Huettel, S. A., Song, A. W., & McCarthy, G. (2014). *Functional Magnetic Resonance Imaging* (3rd ed.). Sinauer Associates.
  - *This is an accessible, introductory-level textbook, with more of a focus on the physics of acquisition, as well as on functional physiology and task fMRI studies.*
- Toga, A. W. (2015). *Brain Mapping: An Encyclopedic Reference.* Academic Press.
  - *Extremely comprehensive reference covering all aspects of MRI acquisition and analysis, with separate in-depth chapters written by individual experts in each area; chapters available separately.*
- Buxton, R. (2009). *Introduction to Functional Magnetic Resonance Imaging: Principles and Techniques* (2nd ed.). Cambridge University Press.
  - *A more detailed introduction to both MR physics and neural physiology, which also offers an overview of the principles of ASL and BOLD fMRI.*
- Symms, M., Jäger, H. R., Schmierer, K., & Yousry, T. A. (2004). A review of structural magnetic resonance neuroimaging. *Journal of Neurology, Neurosurgery & Psychiatry, 75*(9), 1235–1244.
  - *A general review of a range of structural MRI modalities and of their use in both research and clinical practice.*

2.3 Diffusion MRI

Images that are acquired with diffusion MRI (dMRI) sequences are typically used to examine the "wiring" of the brain (i.e., anatomical connectivity) as well as to investigate tissue microstructure (to detect differences related to disease or healthy plasticity). For example, dMRI has proven to be extremely useful at quantifying changes due to stroke and is a sensitive early marker of tissue damage. Investigations using dMRI are normally restricted to the white matter, where the axons are concentrated, but certain acquisition and analysis techniques allow dMRI to be used to probe gray matter as well.

2.3.1 Measurement principles

The principle that dMRI is based on is that water molecules, which are the ones that provide most of the signal, are always in random motion and bumping into structures and into each other, as described by physical diffusion processes (i.e., Brownian motion). What makes this feature useful is that this diffusion is significantly altered by the presence of bundles of elongated axons, as the water molecules cannot pass easily through the cell membranes. Consequently the water molecules preferentially move (diffuse) along the direction in which the axons are oriented, in both the extracellular and intracellular spaces. An illustration of this is shown in Figure 2.10. The more the axons are packed together, the greater the difference between diffusion (movement) along the (axial) direction of the axons and the other (perpendicular or radial) directions.

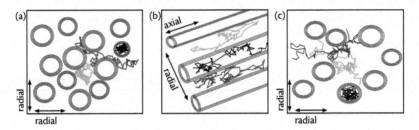

Figure 2.10: Three separate examples of water molecules diffusing in axonal fibre bundles (differently colored paths represent individual water molecules; black inside an axon and blue and green in the extracellular space). There are more restrictions to diffusion (a) in the cross-section (radial directions) than (b) along the axons (axial direction). This is true for both intracellular and extracellular water molecules. When the axons are less tightly packed (e.g., due to neurodegeneration), as shown in (c), the extracellular water is more free to diffuse in radial directions, which leads to observable changes in the MRI signal.

Instead of biological quantities of interest, dMRI analysis quantifies the physical properties of the diffusing water molecules. For instance, dMRI can measure how far water molecules have moved (diffused) in different directions, on average, within a given period of time. Typical dMRI sequences only measure the diffusion of water molecules over a short time interval, where the molecules typically move over distances in the range of tens of micrometers. This is what makes dMRI useful as a probe of microstructure. For example, the average of the diffusion in all directions can be measured and, when there are more boundaries (e.g., cell membranes) in the local environment, the average diffusivity will be smaller. When there are fewer boundaries (e.g., in the fluid-filled ventricles, or in an area with a low axon/cell density), the average diffusivity will be larger. Interpreting what exactly a change in average diffusivity might mean biologically is left to the researcher.

Many physical quantities are derived from the dMRI signal by using a particular type of analysis model: the diffusion tensor, as in *diffusion tensor imaging* (DTI). This model is a mathematical description of the diffusion process and we will briefly discuss it here, as its relationship to the physical diffusion can be understood without knowing the details of the image acquisition process. The DTI model falls short of other, more realistic biophysical models of tissue microstructure, as it cannot represent more than one axonal fiber bundle running through a voxel, which is a relatively common occurrence anatomically. However, it is a useful model, very widely used, and a large proportion of the diffusion MRI literature is based on quantities that are derived from this model.

The two most commonly used quantities that are derived from the diffusion tensor model are *mean diffusivity* (MD) and *fractional anisotropy* (FA)—see Chapter 3. We have already discussed average diffusivity and this is essentially the same as MD, while FA (which is completely separate from whether the voxel dimensions are anisotropic or not) is a measure of how different the diffusion is in different directions. That is, low FA represents nearly equal diffusion in all directions (isotropic), whereas high FA represents preferential diffusion in some directions but not in others (see Figure 2.11). In addition, the diffusion can be divided into diffusion along the strongest direction—*axial diffusivity* (AD)—and diffusion perpendicular to the strongest direction—*radial diffusivity* (RD).

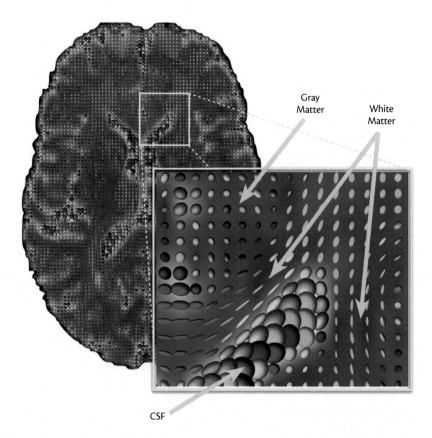

Gray
Matter

White
Matter

CSF

Figure 2.11: Visualization of diffusion in each voxel using results from fitting the diffusion tensor model. Spherical shapes represent isotropic diffusion (low FA), whereas shapes that are thin represent highly anisotropic diffusion (high FA), with the size representing the mean diffusion (MD). The color indicates the principal diffusion direction (red for left–right, green for posterior–anterior, and blue for inferior–superior). Voxels in the ventricles, which contain CSF, appear as large spheres with low FA, high MD, and highly variable principal directions (they are nearly spherical, so the principal direction is governed by noise). Voxels in the gray matter are similar to CSF but with lower MD, so smaller spheres, while voxels in the white matter appear as elongated shapes with high FA and more consistent directions.

Anatomical connectivity is primarily based on using the direction of the axonal fiber bundle(s) at each location. Various models are used to estimate this information from the dMRI signal and include the diffusion tensor model as well as more biologically inspired models or models based on signal deconvolution principles. The algorithms for determining connectivity use the estimated direction of the axon bundle(s) at each voxel and trace this direction from voxel to voxel, stepping along a white matter tract, which can then show how gray matter in one region connects to gray matter in other regions. This process of tracing the tract is called *tractography* and is the fundamental tool in investigating anatomical connectivity using dMRI.

2.3.2 Acquisition

At this point you should have some idea about how measuring the diffusion can give information about microstructure and anatomical connectivity. What has not been mentioned yet is how this information is acquired in the MRI scanner. There are two main differences between the types of acquisitions used for dMRI and those previously described for structural MRI. One difference is that special gradient fields are applied during dMRI in order to sensitize the image to diffusion in a particular direction. Without these gradient fields there would be negligible diffusion information in the image intensities. The second difference is that many separate 3D images of the brain need to be acquired. This is because each single image is sensitive only to diffusion in one direction, and therefore a set of images is needed to capture diffusion over a range of directions. In order for this acquisition not to take a huge amount of time, each image needs to be acquired very quickly, in a matter of seconds, and this requires special *fast imaging sequences*.

By far the most common fast imaging sequence is the *echo planar imaging* (EPI) sequence, which is also used for functional imaging. The physics behind how the sequence works is not important at this point (if you want more details, then see the online appendix titled *Short Introduction to MRI Physics for Neuroimaging*), but it is important to know that the extra speed comes with certain penalties. These penalties include decreased spatial resolution (e.g., typical diffusion images have voxel sizes of 2 mm or more) and increased sensitivity to artifacts, particularly geometric distortion. As a consequence, a single 3D volume from a diffusion MRI acquisition will appear to have limited spatial fidelity and will be distorted (see Figure 2.13 for examples of some images). However, as we typically need to acquire between 30 and 200 images for useful dMRI data (depending on the type of experiment being run), it is necessary to bring the acquisition time for each volume down to around 3 to 4 seconds, which leads to total scanning times between 5 and 15 minutes.

Recent developments in fast imaging, such as parallel imaging and simultaneous multi-slice imaging, can further reduce the scanning time (by using the signals from multiple coils in a head coil array) with relatively minor penalties in SNR or resolution, though artifacts still persist and tend to increase with larger acceleration factors. The speed, from either a standard EPI sequence or one with accelerations, is crucial for dMRI and therefore it is worth the trade-off in terms of resolution and artifacts. For this reason, a lot of work goes into developing preprocessing techniques designed to minimize the artifacts, which we will discuss further in Chapters 3 and 6.

The other major difference in comparison to structural imaging (and also, in this case, comparison to functional imaging) is the use of special gradient fields, called *diffusion-encoding gradients*. These magnetic fields are created by the gradient coils in the scanner (the same ones used to figure out the spatial locations of the signal) but are made especially strong and applied right at the beginning of each slice acquisition (if you would like more information, see the online appendix titled *Short Introduction to MRI Physics for Neuroimaging*). What these gradients do is make the magnetic field change strongly along one direction in space.

The water molecules that do not move in this direction cannot tell that there is any magnetic field change, and so are unaffected by it. However, the water molecules that do move along this direction experience different magnetic fields as they move, and this affects their resonant frequency. The changes in frequency lead to changes in *phase* (i.e., in how far the magnetic orientation has rotated), and this is crucial for the dMRI signal. Molecules that do not move stay in phase with each other and emit precisely the same signal as if no encoding gradients were present, whereas molecules that have moved by different amounts due to diffusion will be out of phase with each other to some degree, and their signals will partially or totally cancel. Hence the more movement or diffusion there is in the direction of the gradient, the smaller the measured signal will be.

Due to these effects, there are areas in the image that are darker than they would normally be if no diffusion-encoding gradients were applied, and these dark areas correspond to places where the water molecules moved (i.e., diffused forwards or backwards) along the diffusion-encoding direction (see the Example Box "Diffusion signal in different tissues"). There must be a substantial proportion of water molecules in a voxel that diffuse in that direction if they are to be detected, which is why only fiber bundles can be detected, rather than just a small number of axons. It is also necessary for the axons to be reasonably well aligned with one another, in order for the effect to be consistent and to come out in the average. However, this does not prevent dMRI from being able to detect voxels containing two or more different fiber bundles, which may be crossing each other.

Since each single 3D image only gives information about diffusion in one direction, we need to acquire many images with different diffusion-encoding directions, in order to build up a picture of how the diffusion varies with direction. For applications where measuring simple microstructural properties is the main interest, a relatively small number of 3D volumes is needed, where each has a different diffusion-encoding direction: typically 30 or more, though the more you have the better the SNR will be. For applications involving connectivity it is crucial to distinguish the fine details of the axon directions, and hence more 3D volumes (and directions) are needed: typically, 60 to 200—though, again, the more you have the better. Note that clinical applications, where speed is of the essence, might only use 3 or 4 directions to get an even simpler diffusion measure for examining pathological tissue.

It is not only the number of directions that needs to be specified, but also their orientation in space. Directions should be spread evenly and can be visualized as points on a sphere (where the direction is along the line from the center of the sphere to the point on the surface). Since water diffusing either way along a line causes a reduction in the signal, it does not matter whether a diffusion direction is pointing one way or the exact opposite way. As a consequence, it is not uncommon to just distribute directions around half the sphere, as the opposite points give the same information and could be considered redundant. This is only true when there are no artifacts, whereas some of the artifacts in diffusion imaging, such as geometric distortions, do behave differently in the two cases (for a direction and its 180° counterpart). For this reason, it is generally better to distribute directions over a full sphere (see Figure 2.12), in order to give the artifact correction methods richer information.

Full Sphere   Half Sphere

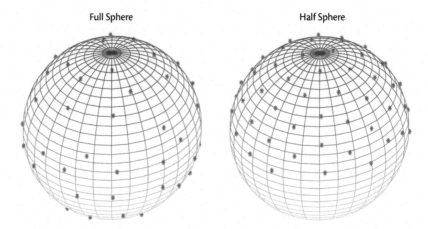

Figure 2.12: Example showing a set of 64 diffusion encoding directions (red stars) that are evenly distributed on a full sphere (left), and the same directions on a half-sphere (right) where all those in the lower half of the full sphere are reversed. Both formats are common, but the full sphere version has advantages when it comes to artifact correction.

Example Box: **Diffusion signal in different tissues**

Let us consider a concrete example of three separate voxels: one voxel in the CSF, which is full of fluid with no fixed cells; a second voxel in white matter, in the middle of a large axonal fiber bundle where it is full of axons and associated myelin sheaths that are all aligned in one direction (we will go even further and say that it is part of the corticospinal tract and the fibers are running in an inferior–superior direction); and a third voxel in gray matter, where there is an array of neuronal cell bodies and some axons, but with no particular orientation on average across the voxel. You may find Figures 2.11 and 2.13 useful to refer to. Start by considering the acquisition of one image where the diffusion-encoding direction is in the superior–inferior direction. In the CSF voxel there will be quite a lot of diffusion in this direction, as in CSF there is quite free diffusion in all directions, since the water is not restricted by any fixed cells. As a consequence, the intensity in this voxel will be low for this direction, since the greater the diffusion is the smaller the signal is. In fact, for a CSF voxel, this will be true of all diffusion-encoding directions, as the water diffuses equally in all directions. Hence in Figure 2.13 the ventricles are dark in all the diffusion images; and they are associated with large spheres in Figure 2.11. The same is true of the gray matter, in that the water diffuses in the same amount in any direction, but here it does have a lot of fixed cells around that hinder the diffusion (i.e., the distance that the water manages to move is smaller), and so the intensity in this voxel is higher than in the CSF, and the visualization in Figure 2.11 shows smaller spheres in the gray matter than in the CSF. For the white matter voxel, this particular diffusion-encoding direction aligns well with the axonal fiber bundle; thus the water is able to diffuse well in this direction, being only minimally hindered, and hence the intensity is low, like the intensity in the CSF voxel. However, for a different diffusion-encoding direction, such as anterior–posterior, water in the white matter voxel experiences a lot of obstructions or restrictions when moving in that direction (i.e., perpendicular to the axons). Therefore it will not diffuse as far and the intensity will be much higher. This variation with the diffusion-encoding direction is highlighted in Figure 2.13 and results in elongated shapes in the visualization of white matter in Figure 2.11.

You can see from this example that the direction of the diffusion-encoding gradient has the largest effect on the intensity in the white matter voxel, and this is how the crucial information about fiber direction is encoded in diffusion images. It is also worth noting that the amount of time that matters for diffusion, from the point of view of a dMRI acquisition, is typically of the order of 10 ms. Thus the distance that water molecules diffuse during this time is roughly 10–30 μm, which means that the water molecules only have time to interact with their local microscopic neighborhood. This is why diffusion imaging is sensitive to the local microenvironment.

In addition to the directions, the acquisition is affected by the strength and the timing of the diffusion-encoding gradients. The key combination of these is measured by the *b-value*, which expresses how strongly a given amount of diffusion will affect the MR signal (i.e., the image intensity). Typically b-values of 1000–1500 s/mm^2 are used as a trade-off between having high sensitivity to diffusion and good SNR. Higher b-values have greater sensitivity to diffusion but lead to less signal overall in the image (as even small amounts of diffusion lower the signal), whereas they have little effect on the noise and hence the SNR is lower. However, the better sensitivity to diffusion creates better angular contrast, and hence more precise estimates of direction, if there is not too much noise. Lower b-values, on the other hand, have good SNR but poorer sensitivity to diffusion and hence lower angular contrast.

Box 2.2: HARDI

Certain types of sequences try to get the best of both worlds by acquiring images with different b-values as well as with different directions. These acquisition schemes are known in general as HARDI (high angular resolution diffusion imaging) methods and include multi-shell acquisitions as well as more general approaches. In multi-shell acquisitions a small number of distinct b-values are used for all the encodings, for example, one can use only two b-values, but with many directions per b-value, which can be visualized with each set of directions on a sphere (see Figure 2.12) where the radius is proportional to the b-value, resulting in two nested spheres or shells. Other alternatives can use a greater number of distinct b-values, with one variant effectively forming a 3D grid of different b-values and directions rather than having them lie on a set of spheres. It is worth noting that not all scanners can get to higher b-values, as the strength and speed required for the gradients is beyond some scanners, with older or clinical scanners being the most likely to be restricted. Such sequences, when they can be acquired, need different approaches to analysis, but the methods for doing this are readily available.

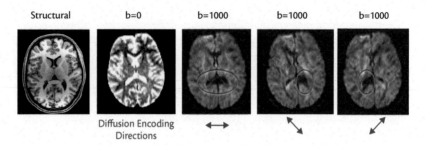

Structural   b=0   b=1000   b=1000   b=1000

Diffusion Encoding ⟷   ↙   ↗
Directions

Figure 2.13: Example of axial images from a dMRI experiment. From the left: T_1-weighted structural image; non-diffusion weighted (b = 0) image; and three diffusion MRI images (all with b = 1000 s/mm² but with different diffusion encoding directions, shown below). Red circles show some examples (in the corpus callosum) of where strong diffusion contrast exists (i.e., reduction in signal): left–right fibers in the first and fibers at ±45°, matching the encoding direction, in the latter two.

Regardless of the type of acquisition scheme used, it is also necessary to collect several images without using the diffusion-encoding gradients—that is, images that contain no diffusion weighting. These are referred to as "b = 0" or just "b0" scans, and should not to be confused with the B_0 field, which is totally different. Such images provide a crucial baseline for being able to fit models and extract quantitative information (such as MD, FA, etc.) from the diffusion MR intensities. This baseline is necessary in order to know how much the diffusion of the water molecules has reduced the signal intensity when the diffusion-encoding gradients are used. Without such a baseline it would not be possible to calculate the relative reduction in intensity and hence the amount of diffusion, since the intensity also varies throughout the brain due to other confounding factors—for example the amount of water present (the proton density) and relaxation-related changes, as can be seen in the intensities of the b = 0 image in Figure 2.13 (also see the Example Boxes "Diffusion signal in different tissues (revisited)" and "Viewing diffusion images"). Therefore it is important to get a good baseline, and so normally several such non-diffusion-weighted (b = 0) images are acquired to get a less noisy average. This allows the changes due to proton density and relaxation times, which are not of interest for diffusion imaging, to be factored out when the models are fit in the analysis stage. It is only the proportion of the signal that is reduced when the diffusion-encoding is applied that counts, as this is determined by the diffusion alone. So, although the raw images will still show tissue contrast and other variations, the diffusion models compensate for this and provide quantitative measurements that are independent of these factors, by using the b = 0 baseline images.

Example Box: Diffusion signal in different tissues (revisited)

Let us again consider our example voxels from before. The non-diffusion-weighted (b = 0) images will all have higher intensities than any of the images where diffusion-encoding gradients were applied, but the relative difference varies. For the CSF voxel, there is a large difference between the intensity in the b = 0 image and that in the diffusion-encoded images, which indicates a large amount of diffusion (and this can be seen by how bright CSF is in the b = 0 image in Figure 2.13 versus how dark it is in the b = 1000 s/mm² images). In the gray matter voxel there is a smaller difference between the intensities in the b = 0 images and the diffusion-encoded images, while in the white matter voxel there is a fairly minimal difference for the encoding directions that are not well aligned with the axons and a very large difference for directions that are aligned well with the axons. Information from both the b = 0 images and the diffusion-encoded images is needed in order to extract the desired quantitative information about diffusion and axon fiber directions.

Example Box: **Viewing diffusion images**

On the primer website you will find instructions for viewing an example diffusion dataset. This will allow you to become familiar with how the intensity varies with both diffusion-encoding direction and tissue type. Furthermore, it will provide examples of typical artifacts that are to be expected in all diffusion images.

2.3.3 Limitations

As with structural imaging, a limitation of diffusion imaging is that it does not provide a direct measure of the properties of the biological tissue that are of most interest, such as the axon size, axon density, degree of myelination, and so on. Instead, the measured signal is an indirect measure of all of these things, and more. The signal is still sensitive to changes in these properties (e.g., decrease in axon cell density associated with neurodegeneration), but it does not allow us to easily pinpoint what biological change is associated with the observed change in intensities. For this we require additional hypotheses and an understanding of the biological mechanisms and of how they affect the diffusion images, in order to come to a valid interpretation. There is also a lot of research activity in trying to develop dMRI techniques that can infer these kind of biologically meaningful values more directly; but at present these are less common, cutting-edge techniques, whereas here we will describe the much more common type of dMRI acquisition.

Due to partial voluming, it is only possible to measure what happens in axonal fiber bundles where there are thousands or millions of axons aligned in the same direction. Small fibers, or groups of axons, do not change the diffusion imaging signal enough to be measurable, unless the voxel size is very small. For in vivo imaging it is difficult to obtain a high enough resolution with sufficient SNR to be able to measure small fibers, but in postmortem studies it is possible to go much further due to the trade-off of resolution with acquisition time. In addition, when large fibers cross each other it is harder to get clear information from the raw diffusion images. In such situations, or even when fibers touch and move apart but do not cross (called "kissing" fibers), it is still possible to extract useful information from the diffusion images, but only when the SNR, resolution, and number of directions are sufficiently high.

It is also difficult to obtain clear information from regions where there is pulsatile motion, such as the brainstem, since diffusion imaging is sensitive to the movement of the water molecules. Normally this movement is due to diffusion and that is the information we want, but it is not possible to disentangle it easily from other movements. A lot of effort is made in acquisition to decouple the bulk motion of the head from the diffusion movement, and this is effective at stopping the diffusion signal from being strongly influenced by the movement of the head. However, local, pulsatile motions have different characteristics and are not compensated for in the same way. Therefore acquiring good diffusion images in areas like the brainstem requires extra effort, such as denoising, recording extra physiological information about cardiac and respiratory processes, or synchronizing the image acquisition to the cardiac cycle (a process called *cardiac gating*). These are all additions to the standard diffusion acquisition and need to be planned for specially.

Diffusion MRI also requires much higher performance of the gradient coils than other imaging modalities. That is because the diffusion-encoding gradients need to be both strong and rapidly switched on and off. On older scanners, or on ones built to lower specifications, these gradients might be quite limited and the quality of the dMRI that is possible on such scanners is likely to be restricted.

Finally, another limitation is that connectivity information obtained from tractography is not quantitative. Measures of the biological or physiological "strength" of a connection (e.g., of the number of axons) cannot be obtained quantitatively from dMRI for the same reason that other biological quantities, such as axon density, cannot be obtained at a local level.

2.3.4 Artifacts

Fast imaging is crucial for both diffusion and functional imaging, and the EPI sequence (or an equivalent) must be used to make these acquisitions feasible. Consequently there are trade-offs to be made for the speed, and these include lower spatial resolution, reduced tissue contrast, and also additional artifacts. The most important artifact induced through the use of EPI in dMRI is the *geometric distortion*. This is caused by inhomogeneities or nonuniformities in the B_0 field that mainly arise from perturbations caused by nearby air pockets in the sinuses (these are called B_0 *distortions* or *susceptibility-induced distortions*, as it is the different magnetic susceptibility of the air in the sinuses, by comparison to other tissues, that causes the majority of B_0 inhomogeneities). Any difference between the local B_0 field and the ideal, uniform B_0 field introduces a change in the frequency of the signal emitted by the hydrogen nuclei in that area (for this reason they are also sometimes referred to as *off-resonance* fields or effects, given that the frequency is no longer the normal resonant frequency). Since frequency is used to calculate the spatial location, these changes in frequency result in mislocation of the signal, that is, geometric distortion. The B_0 inhomogeneities themselves are not influenced by the use of EPI (i.e., they also exist when using structural imaging sequences), but the distortions they create in the image are much larger when using EPI, as EPI is more sensitive to these inhomogeneities.

The distortion is at its worst in the inferior frontal and inferior temporal areas of the brain, as these are nearest to the sinuses and other air cells that cause the B_0 inhomogeneities. One good thing is that we do know what direction the distortion occurs along—it is along the phase-encode axis, which is one of the axes of the image and is chosen by the operator during the

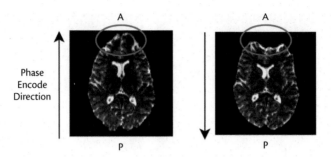

Phase
Encode
Direction

Figure 2.14: Example of axial images from a dMRI experiment. Two b = 0 images with opposite phase encode directions (P-A and A-P), demonstrating the reversed geometric distortions (red circles)—as discussed in the section on artifacts.

setup of the scan. We can also reverse the direction of the distortion by changing the sign of this phase-encode direction in the scanner setup, and a pair of scans taken using these two phase-encode directions are often referred to as a *blip-up–blip-down* pair or a *phase-encode reversed* pair. An illustration of such a pair is shown in the Figure 2.14, and is a good way to visualize the amount of geometric distortion. Acquiring a pair of images like this is very useful for correcting the geometric distortion in the analysis (see section 3.3.2 and Chapter 6).

Another artifact that is common in diffusion imaging is *eddy-current distortion*. This is a consequence of using strong diffusion-encoding gradients that are rapidly turned on and off, which then induce electrical currents in the nearby metallic surfaces of the scanner. These currents are known as eddy currents and they arise for the same reason why moving a magnet in a coil of wire can generate electrical current. The eddy currents then, in turn, create unwanted magnetic fields (using the same principle as an electromagnet), and these fields linger and interfere with the imaging gradient fields that we need in order to determine the spatial locations of the signals. As a consequence, the spatial locations are incorrectly assigned and the images are geometrically distorted, which needs to be corrected for in the analysis (see Figure 2.15).

Along with correction methods that can be applied during the image analysis phase, there are several types of dMRI acquisition sequence that exist for minimizing the eddy currents or their effects. These sequences are widely used, but typically have a penalty in acquisition time or SNR. As analysis methods have improved in their ability to correct for eddy-current distortions, the use of these sequences has begun to decrease and some of the simpler sequences, with worse distortions but faster acquisitions and better SNR, are gaining favour.

2.3.5 Analysis

To get the information of interest from the diffusion images (e.g., mean diffusivity values, or tractography-based connectivities), it is necessary to run a number of preprocessing stages, and then a final model-fitting stage. Many of these preprocessing stages are common to functional imaging as well, due to the same fast imaging sequence (EPI) being used, but a number of the preprocessing stages are specific to dMRI. Different tools will implement slightly different

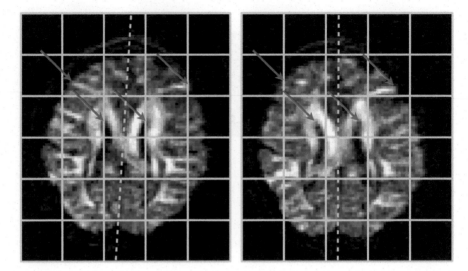

Figure 2.15: An example of eddy current distortions in dMRI. Two diffusion-encoded images (from the same 4D acquisition) with different diffusion encoding directions are shown, demonstrating the geometric distortions caused by the different eddy currents on the image (predominantly in the left–right direction in this case). The red arrows indicate corresponding anatomical locations that are clearly shifted due to the eddy current distortions (easiest to see with respect to the fixed image grid in yellow). The blue dotted line indicates the approximate inter-hemispheric plane, which illustrates the magnitude of the geometric distortion as well as the fact that it is largely a global, linear distortion.

processing steps, and potentially in different orders, but the basic principles are very much the same for all. More details about the analysis are given in Chapter 3; in this section we will give a brief overview.

The main aim of the preprocessing stages is to remove, as much as possible, the artifacts that are present in the images. In dMRI these are principally motion- and distortion-related artifacts, and so motion correction, eddy-current correction, and B_0-distortion correction are the standard preprocessing stages. As these artifacts interact with one another, it is becoming more common for the preprocessing corrections to be combined together into a single step, depending on the software package used for analysis. No matter how it is implemented, the desired results are the same: a set of images where the geometric and motion-induced distortions have been corrected for and the changes in intensity between the different 3D images just reflect the changes induced by diffusion.

After the preprocessing, a model-fitting stage is usually applied, which operates at each voxel separately, since the information at each voxel is independent and only related to that voxel. For microstructural analysis the most common model that is used is the *diffusion tensor model*, which assumes that the diffusion in different directions follows a simple mathematical model. This model can be visualized as an ellipsoid (like a rugby ball or american football) and covers a range of possible shapes, from a sphere to a thin, elongated (prolate) ellipsoid—as illustrated in Figure 3.11. These shapes illustrate the diffusion that would occur inside voxels containing CSF (sphere) or a single axon fiber bundle (thin and elongated), intermediate shapes being able to represent different fractions of axons. However, it is a very simple model and does not represent very well other biological cases, such as crossing fibers. Nonetheless, it has been applied extensively in the literature and is still used routinely.

Other models for microstructure also exist, such as CHARMED (composite hindered and restricted model of diffusion) and NODDI (neurite orientation dispersion and density imaging). These require more sophisticated acquisitions (e.g., a multishell acquisition; multiple nonzero b-values, with many directions for each—if you are interested, see Box 2.2). Such models can provide more detailed descriptions of the water diffusion. For example, NODDI separately quantifies three different water compartments—free water (isotropic component) and those in or near the axons and other cells (intra- and extracellular)—as well as estimating the degree of axonal fiber dispersion within a voxel. Having these separate values makes it possible to improve interpretation of what might be happening to the tissue biologically, although this model is still a simplification that provides surrogate measures for the underlying biological quantities of interest.

In addition to voxelwise information relating to the microstructure, the directional information can also be used to trace the path of the axonal fiber bundles through the white matter, to estimate anatomical connectivity between gray matter regions. The estimation of these pathways, or tracts, is done using tractography algorithms, which start at an initial location and take small steps along the locally estimated direction, to trace out a tract. There are two main varieties of tractography algorithm, depending on how they treat the estimates of the directions: *deterministic tractography* and *probabilistic tractography*. These will be discussed in more detail in Chapter 3.

SUMMARY

- Diffusion of water provides indirect information about local microstructure and axonal fiber directions.

- Quantitative measurements of local physical diffusion processes (e.g., mean diffusivity) can be obtained, but anatomical connectivity (via tractography) is not quantitative.

- Each 3D image provides information about diffusion in one direction, which is specified in the sequence by the diffusion-encoding gradient.

- Many different directions, and hence images, are needed for a dataset (typically 30 or more for microstructural analysis and 60 or more for tractography), and it is better if these are distributed over a full sphere.

- Acquisitions require fast imaging methods: typically the EPI sequence, possibly with acceleration via parallel imaging and/or simultaneous multi-slice acquisitions.

- EPI sequences have limited spatial resolution and SNR and suffer from local geometric distortions, which can be accounted for in the analysis if other supporting acquisitions are made (e.g., phase-encode reversed $b = 0$ scans, or fieldmaps).

- In addition to images with diffusion encoding, it is necessary to acquire images with no diffusion encoding (several $b = 0$ images) in order to establish a baseline for quantifying the diffusion-related intensity changes.

- Eddy currents, induced by the strong diffusion-encoding gradients, create artifacts in the images that can be corrected for in the analysis.

- Preprocessing stages in diffusion analysis include combined or separate steps for motion correction, B_0-distortion correction and eddy-current correction.

- The diffusion tensor model (as in DTI) is a mathematical model that is commonly used to estimate voxelwise quantities from dMRI data.

- Tractography algorithms are used to determine anatomical connectivity by tracing the paths of axonal fiber bundles through the white matter.

FURTHER READING

- Jones, D. K. (ed.). (2010). *Diffusion MRI*. Oxford University Press.
  - *A comprehensive textbook with many individual chapters, written by experts in the field and with variable amounts of technical detail.*

- Johansen-Berg, H., & Behrens, T. E. (eds.). (2013). *Diffusion MRI: From Quantitative Measurement to in vivo Neuroanatomy*. Academic Press.
  - *A comprehensive textbook with many individual chapters, written by experts in the field and with variable amounts of technical detail.*

- Le Bihan, D., & Johansen-Berg, H. (2012). Diffusion MRI at 25: Exploring brain tissue structure and function. *Neuroimage, 61*(2), 324–341.
  - *General overview paper for dMRI.*

- Johansen-Berg, H., & Rushworth, M. F. (2009). Using diffusion imaging to study human connectional anatomy. *Annual review of neuroscience, 32*, 75–94.
  - *A critical review of diffusion tractography and its application to studying connectivity.*

2.4 Functional MRI

Both diffusion and structural MRI focus on the anatomy of the brain, whereas functional MRI (fMRI) highlights dynamic changes in the brain in order to examine neuronal activity. What fMRI is sensitive to is actually the changes in the blood (the hemodynamics), which are known to alter due to changes in neuronal firing. More specifically, it is the hemoglobin that MRI is sensitive to, because of a particularly useful property whereby oxygenated and deoxygenated forms of hemoglobin interact with magnetic fields differently. This induces variation, or inhomogeneities, in the local magnetic field that depend mainly on the concentration of the deoxygenated hemoglobin, and these field changes result in small, but detectable changes in the MRI signal.

This relationship between neuronal activation and MRI signal change is known as the *blood oxygenation level dependent* (BOLD) *effect*, and this style of functional imaging is often referred to as BOLD imaging or BOLD fMRI. This is not the only way to image functional changes in an MRI scanner though, the main alternative being ASL (arterial spin labelling), which is discussed in section 2.5; but BOLD fMRI is currently the most common approach, mainly due to having better SNR. It is always useful to keep in mind that both are still surrogates of neuronal activity and are really measuring a signal that is based on changes in the blood. Other ways of measuring brain activity are also possible with non-MRI methods; see section 2.7 for a discussion of useful complementary techniques.

2.4.1 Physiology

Neurons send signals to one another via electrical impulses called *action potentials*, which travel down the axons. The transmission of this signal to other neurons, however, is not electrical but chemical in nature. Transmission occurs at the *synapse*, which is a junction between an output of an axon—an *axon terminal*—and an input to another neuron—a *dendrite*. Transmission involves the release and uptake of chemical *neurotransmitters*, along with a number of other cellular processes. All of these processes require energy, which is supplied in the form of oxygen and glucose from the blood; thus, when the neurons are more active, they require more oxygen and glucose from the local blood supply.

As a consequence of the need for varying amounts of oxygen and glucose, the blood vessel network in the brain is set up to be able to dynamically change the local blood supply. This is done by manipulating the muscles that surround various *arterioles* (vessels) that feed into the *capillaries*—that is, very small blood vessels that permeate areas of neuronal tissue (gray matter). To make sure that neurons are not starved of oxygen or glucose, increases in neuronal activity lead to relatively large increases in local cerebral blood flow (CBF) and cerebral blood volume (CBV), which overcompensate for the smaller increase in the cerebral metabolic rate of oxygen consumption ($CMRO_2$). The overall result is an oversupply of oxygenated blood, which minimizes the risk of neurons being starved, and also leads to the concentration of deoxygenated hemoglobin going down in areas of greater neuronal activity.

2.4.2 Measurement principles

The deoxygenated form of hemoglobin is the one that disturbs the local magnetic field, making it less uniform, as the magnetic fields interact differently with it by comparison with the surrounding tissues, whereas the oxygenated form of hemoglobin and the surrounding tissues both interact with the magnetic fields in a similar way. Therefore, in the presence of deoxygenated hemoglobin, the local magnetic (B_0) field becomes less uniform, and this leads to a reduction in signal from water molecules inside the capillary and from those in the tissue immediately surrounding the capillary (see Figure 2.16). This is described quantitatively by a version of the T_2 relaxation time called T_2^* (see Box 2.3 for more details), and images that are sensitive to BOLD contrast are also called T_2^*-weighted images.

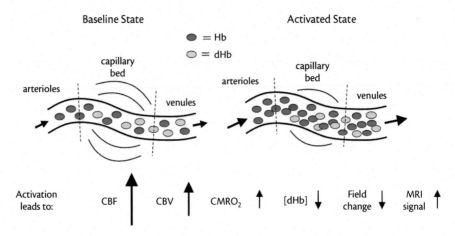

Figure 2.16: Illustration of the BOLD effect: an increase in local neuronal activation (moving from the baseline state, left, to the activated state, right) is accompanied by large increases in cerebral blood flow (CBF) and cerebral blood volume (CBV), more modest increases in oxygen extraction ($CMRO_2$), and thus an overall increase in the amount of oxygenated blood (Hb) present, by comparison with deoxygenated blood (dHb). As a consequence, the concentration of deoxyhemoglobin decreases, as do the magnetic field inhomogeneities that it causes, leading to an increase in MRI signal.

Box 2.3: T_2^* Relaxation and BOLD

Localized B_0 magnetic field inhomogeneities affect how the MR signal decays, as the hydrogen nuclei end up with a range of resonant frequencies. This means that they go out of phase with one another more quickly, which reduces the total magnetization, and hence the signal. This effect is quantified by the T_2^* relaxation time, which incorporates all the T_2 relaxation process, as before (on the basis of many microscopic properties), as well as the extra effect of these localized B_0 field inhomogeneities. The result of increased B_0 inhomogeneities, due to an increased concentration of deoxygenated hemoglobin, is a quicker relaxation process, in which the signal decays away faster. That is, the signal decreases when there is more deoxygenated hemoglobin, and this is the case when there is *less* neuronal activity. Conversely, when neuronal activity increases, the result is an increase in the locally measured MRI signal. These signal changes are detectable, provided that a sequence is used that is sensitive to T_2^* relaxation. This means that *spin-echo* sequences (see online appendix *Short Introduction to MRI Physics for Neuroimaging*) are generally not used (though they are used in dMRI), as the spin echo removes most of the T_2^* component of the change, leaving them primarily sensitive to T_2 relaxation. Thus most functional imaging is based on fast *gradient-echo* sequences that are tuned to be as sensitive to T_2^* relaxation effects as possible, since the changes are actually quite small—typically around a 1 percent change in signal.

The chain of response from a stimulus through to neuronal activity, then finally to a measured signal, is governed strongly by the blood's response and is characterized quantitatively by the

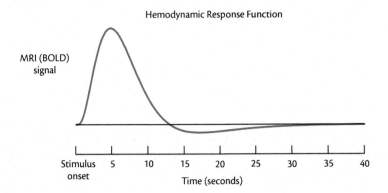

Figure 2.17: Illustration of a typical hemodynamic response function (HRF) for the adult human brain. This shows the change in MRI signal intensity (labeled "BOLD activation" here) as a function of time, as would be expected in response to a very short stimulus. It demonstrates the sluggish nature of the blood response, which takes around 6 seconds to peak and over 20 seconds to return to the original baseline value. By contrast, the electrical activity of the neurons only lasts for tens to hundreds of milliseconds.

hemodynamic response function (HRF). This is the measurement that would be expected in a perfect, noise-free MRI scanner when a subject received a short, sharp stimulus and the brain was only responding to that (i.e., neglecting all other neuronal and physiological changes). One crucial thing about the HRF is that the response is sluggish—it takes about 6 seconds to peak and then around 20 seconds to fall back to baseline (see Figure 2.17). This has two major consequences, one good and one bad. The bad news is that we cannot see the precise timing of the neuronal changes. We are only able to see the delayed and spread-out response due to the hemodynamics (which is on the order of seconds), and not the timing of the neuronal firings (which is on the order of tens to hundreds of milliseconds). However, the good news is that, as a consequence, we do not have to acquire MR images of the brain every hundred milliseconds or so. We can get away with acquiring images every few seconds, without missing the brain responses. This is very helpful, since acquiring brain images every few seconds is relatively straightforward, whereas getting useful images every hundred milliseconds or so is (currently) almost impossible.

2.4.3 Acquisition

Even though we only need images every few seconds, the way we acquire structural images is not suitable, because each image of the brain takes minutes and hence we need to use fast imaging sequences, as we did for dMRI. In fact we normally use the same basic sequence as in dMRI—the EPI sequence—often with accelerations from parallel imaging or simultaneous multi-slice acquisitions (or both). This enables images to be acquired quickly: typically 0.5 to 3 seconds are needed for a whole brain image, and the time taken to acquire one volume in fMRI is the TR of the sequence. For functional images, the sequence is also tuned to make it as sensitive to T_2^* changes as possible—normally by setting the TE (echo time) of the sequence to be similar to the T_2^* of gray matter—so that the subtle BOLD effect can be detected.

The EPI sequence allows us to get images quickly enough to detect the hemodynamically induced changes, but it makes these images prone to most of the artifacts encountered in structural and diffusion images, as well as to additional *signal loss*. This signal loss is essentially an enhanced version of one aspect of the BOLD effect: intensity reduction due to B_0 inhomogeneities, which is much greater near the sinuses and air cells, as they create larger

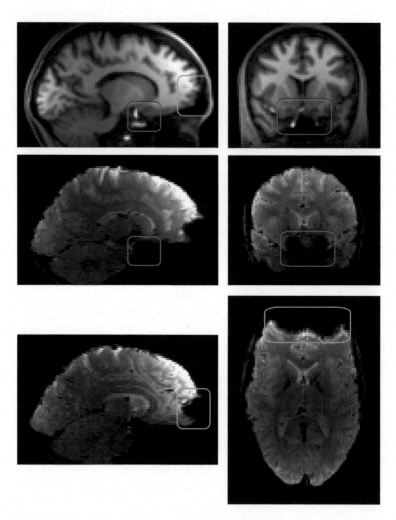

Figure 2.18: Illustration of distortion and dropout in EPI. The first row shows a T_1-weighted structural image that is resampled and reoriented to match the functional EPI acquisitions shown in the second and third rows, in order to provide a comparison with the undistorted anatomy. Dropout (signal loss) is prevalent in the inferior frontal lobes, as highlighted by the red boxes (EPI shown in second row, where a large amount of signal is lost within the boxes by comparison to the T_1-weighted structural in the top row). The geometric distortion is highlighted by the blue boxes and is most prominent in the orbitofrontal cortex (it appears as though a bite has been taken out of the frontal cortex in the EPI: third row). Note that the bright parts in the T_1-weighted structural image in and near the boxes correspond to blood vessels.

inhomogeneities. Technically the $T_2{}^*$ sensitivity for BOLD fMRI is obtained by using a *gradient-echo* version of the EPI sequence rather than the *spin-echo* version used in dMRI. We use a spin-echo version in dMRI because we do not want diffusion images to be sensitive to the BOLD effects and to the associated signal loss artifacts (for those who are interested, more details can be found in the online appendix titled *Short Introduction to MRI Physics for Neuroimaging*). The net result is that typical functional images are low resolution (voxel sizes of around 2–3 mm) and suffer from limited tissue contrast, geometric distortion (like diffusion images), and signal loss (unlike diffusion images), as shown in Figure 2.18, but are exquisitely sensitive to the BOLD effect, so that they can successfully measure changes in neuronal activity.

2.4.4 Limitations and artifacts

One of the main limitations of BOLD fMRI is that it is only an indirect measure of the neuronal activity of interest. That is, we would like to be able to make more direct measurements of the firing of the neurons, but instead we can only measure the induced changes in the blood oxygenation via the BOLD effect. In addition, fMRI is not quantitative and so we cannot simply interpret the intensity values meaningfully by taking them on their own. What we can interpret are changes in intensity over time, either in relation to stimuli or in relation to other measured signals (e.g., timeseries from remote brain regions). Quantitative measurements are available for functional activity but require a different modality—ASL (see section 2.5)—though this modality has its own limitations. Nonetheless, we can still derive a lot of information from BOLD fMRI measurements.

As mentioned before, fast imaging is necessary for fMRI but brings with it several trade-offs, such as limited spatial resolution, low tissue contrast, geometric distortion, and signal loss. These come in addition to the artifacts that can occur for structural MRI, especially motion, which may cause substantial signal changes. In fact this is a major confound in fMRI, and specialized motion correction methods exist both in preprocessing and in the subsequent statistical analysis—methods that aim to compensate for it as much as possible. Thankfully, one artifact that fMRI does not suffer from is eddy-current distortion, since no diffusion-encoding gradients are used in fMRI—and these gradients are the cause of the large, problematic eddy currents. Methods for correcting the remaining geometric distortions and for compensating for the signal loss (both due to B_0 inhomogeneities) are applied in the analysis of fMRI. More detail about these methods is presented later in this section and in Chapters 3 and 6.

Due to the limited resolution and tissue contrast in these functional images, it is often difficult to identify in them detailed anatomical structures directly. It is even harder to precisely align or register functional images that come from different subjects with different anatomies. For this reason it is important to acquire a structural image for each subject, as this allows for greater precision in locating anatomical regions or borders as well as for greatly improved registration accuracy between subjects, which is very important for having good statistical power in a group analysis.

In addition to the structural image, a B_0 *fieldmap* image (often referred to just as a fieldmap) should be acquired in any functional study, as this allows the geometric distortions to be corrected in preprocessing and registration, which substantially improves the precision of localization and statistical power for group analyses. Signal loss can also be predicted from the fieldmap, although the signal cannot be restored; only alternative acquisition methods can restore signal in the areas that are typically affected by signal loss—methods such as reducing slice thickness, angling the slices, or using z-shimming techniques. However, signal loss predictions allow some analysis methods to be able to compensate for the negative effects of the loss of signal, particularly in registration. An alternative to a traditional fieldmap acquisition is to derive the same information from a set of phase-encoding reversed b = 0 scans. More details about fieldmaps and registration will be presented in Chapter 6.

All of this applies equally to functional experiments that involve stimuli and tasks, known generally as task fMRI, and to ones conducted without explicit stimuli, known generally as resting state fMRI. As a rule of thumb, task-based experiments are used to study the nature and location of specific processes in the brain, whereas resting experiments are primarily used to study functional connectivity between different regions of the brain. However, this generalization does not always hold: for example, task-based experiments can also be used to study aspects of connectivity and resting state experiments can be used to investigate localization. The next sections will discuss task-based and resting state fMRI separately, though in limited detail. Readers interested in knowing more about resting state fMRI should consult the primer *Introduction to Resting State fMRI Functional Connectivity*.

2.4.5 Task-based functional MRI

In a task-based fMRI experiment the subject in the scanner is instructed to perform some task, chosen by the experimenter from a wide range of possible tasks, for example sensory (visual, auditory, tactile, smell, taste), cognitive (decision-making, gambling, recognition, memory, reading), physiological (pain, breathing challenges, attention–sleep–arousal, drugs), or motor (button box, finger tapping). It is important to try to avoid any large motions and certainly anything that might move the head. Pressing buttons is fine, but speaking and shoulder movement should be especially avoided; and even leg movement can end up moving the head. The type and timing of the stimuli must be designed in advance and this information is crucial for the analysis. Careful design is needed if you want to make an experiment that is good from a psychological perspective but also has good statistical power.

Experimental design

There are many things to consider when you are designing task fMRI experiments. Two of the most important considerations are: (i) having enough repeats of the stimulus and (ii) using at least two conditions.

Repeating the stimulus is important because we do not have much SNR in fMRI in general, so repetition is used to increase the amount of data and hence statistical power. The principle here is the same as used when averaging multiple measurements in order to get a better mean value estimate, since errors and the effect of noise diminish as more data can be averaged. Having many repeats of a stimulus gives us multiple measurements of the same brain activity and hence a better, less noisy estimate of the true value through averaging (though we let our statistical models do the averaging for us—we do not average raw data).

Using at least two different conditions (e.g., types of stimulus, or anything that evokes a different brain state) is also crucial, since fMRI is not quantitative. This means that we cannot just measure the signal corresponding to one state of the brain and then interpret the number we get from it. The hemodynamic response changes the MR signal, but only by a small fraction (around 1 percent), and we need to calculate this *difference* in signal between two states of the brain to measure what the change in signal was and to infer from it the neuronal activity. There can be more than two different conditions and we can compare all of them, which is common; but there must be at least two conditions. Normally we have one simple, fundamental condition that we describe as the *baseline* condition. This is sometimes "rest" (i.e., something that does not require much neural processing, such as staring straight ahead, often at a fixed point), although the neurons in the brain are always active. However, the baseline condition can actually be as complicated as desired. In fact, it could be a cognitive task, but one not as difficult or rich as the alternative, nonbaseline condition(s); e.g., the baseline condition could be a mental arithmetic task with easier numbers than the nonbaseline condition. As long as there is a difference between the conditions, the experiment can be analyzed and the activity related to this difference can be investigated. Note that this difference between brain states is often assumed to be simple and to relate only to a particular type of task, but when designing the experiments care should always be taken to assess whether this principle is satisfied or valid from a psychological point of view. For example, if subjects use different cognitive strategies for the baseline and for the alternative conditions, it is not easy to interpret the differences in brain activity that result.

There are many other aspects of creating a good design, some of them statistical, others psychological. For example, from a statistical standpoint, long stimuli (boxcars) are more powerful than short, separate ones (single events); see Figure 2.19. Psychological considerations include avoiding habituation and boredom, maintaining the right level of difficulty, and avoiding predictability and unwanted anticipation. In practice there are many considerations and complexities to take into account in an experimental design for task fMRI, but these are beyond the scope of this primer. The interested reader is encouraged to learn more about this from courses and other textbooks (see further reading).

Analysis

In this section we will provide a brief overview of the analysis of task fMRI data, in order to give you a broad picture of what happens in such analyses. This will help you understand the need for different analysis stages and how they relate to one another and to aspects of the acquisition and experimental design. Further details about the analysis are presented in Chapter 3.

Although great pains are taken to ensure that the image acquisitions are as clean as possible, a range of artifacts and undesirable signals are present in functional images. These need to be removed or controlled for in the analysis, so that we can validly use the images to infer something about neuronal processes. There are various forms of artifacts, such as those related to physics or hardware, to physiology, and to a combination of both (e.g., head motion). As a consequence, the analysis of fMRI data includes an extensive set of preprocessing operations that aim to eliminate or reduce most of these artifacts. None of the methods are perfect, but modern preprocessing does a good job at removing the majority of the artifactual signals. There are also alternative methods to deal with some artifacts directly in the statistical modeling (e.g., regressing-out physiological signals), and often a mixture of both methods is employed, though some form of preprocessing is always carried out (see section 3.4).

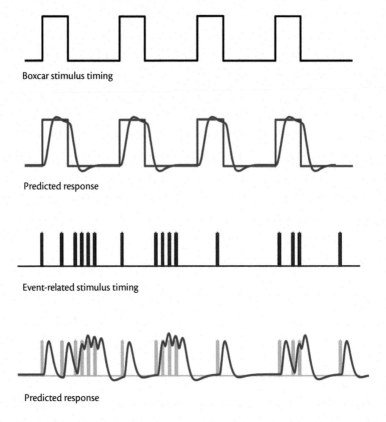

Figure 2.19: Examples of boxcar and single-event designs: stimulus timing and predicted response (a model of the MRI signal in the presence of neuronal activity to the stimulus, which takes into account the HRF—in blue) are shown for each. Boxcar designs, where continuous or dense sets of stimuli are presented for intervals of typically 10 to 40 seconds, alternating with similar periods of the baseline condition, normally have greater statistical power but are limiting with respect to how the stimuli can be delivered.

After the preprocessing is done, the analysis of task-based fMRI is performed using models of the *predicted response* to the known stimuli. This predicted response is calculated using the stimulus timings and what is known about the hemodynamics, that is, the sluggish HRF (see Figure 2.17). However, although the HRF takes around 20 seconds to return to baseline, the stimuli do not need to be separated by 20 seconds in order for us to estimate the effect sizes of interest.

Once a model is built using the predicted responses, the *general linear model* (GLM) is used to look for these responses in the measured MRI signal. The GLM is a crucial part of all neuroimaging analyses, not just for fMRI (a brief introduction to it can be found in the online appendix titled *Short Introduction to the General Linear Model for Neuroimaging*). The GLM helps determine, on the basis of statistics, where there is a significant relationship between the measured signal and the predicted responses. However, the GLM is not tied to any one type of statistics; it can be used equally well with parametric statistics or with nonparametric (e.g., permutation-based) statistics. Furthermore, the GLM is very flexible in the type of tests it can perform, including testing at the group level for single-group averages, unpaired-group differences, paired-group differences, correlations with other covariates, ANOVA-style analyses, and more.

Statistical hypotheses related to the questions of interest for an experiment are formulated in the GLM by using *contrasts*, which define what exactly is being tested statistically, that is, the hypothesis: for example, individual responses, differences between responses, or more complex relationships between responses and other variables. A statistical test is then performed, for each contrast, separately in each voxel. This produces maps that show which voxels contain statistically significant results. In fMRI analysis, as in all forms of neuroimaging, it is extremely important to correct such results for multiple comparisons in order to avoid making a lot of false inferences. For more information, see the online appendix titled *Short Introduction to the General Linear Model for Neuroimaging* and Chapter 3 here, where you will also find more about the rest of fMRI analysis.

2.4.6 Resting state functional MRI

The big difference between task fMRI and resting state fMRI is that subjects in resting state experiments are not asked to do anything specific in the scanner, besides possibly looking at a fixation cross. Hence there is no experiment to design, and resting state data can be acquired across a very wide range of subjects, including infants, severely cognitively impaired subjects, and even sleeping or unconscious subjects. However, the kind of images acquired for resting state fMRI are exactly the same kind as acquired for task fMRI.

Functional connectivity

What makes resting state fMRI particularly interesting is that it can be used to look at the functional relationships between different parts of the brain. This is known as *functional connectivity*, which is different from structural connectivity that looks at the "wiring" of the brain via the axonal connections. The underlying principle behind functional connectivity is that (i) neuronal activity is always going on, even in "rest," and (ii) neuronal activity is linked across different brain areas, as they communicate among themselves and process shared information. The fluctuations due to this activity can be measured using fMRI acquisitions and the signals compared between different regions to see where they are similar. A common way to do this comparison, which is one of many alternatives, is to use correlations of the MRI timeseries from different locations. This is the historical basis of the field, and it is due to Biswal and colleagues' observations of correlated signals in remote but biologically related areas (see Figure 2.20 for a more recent example showing a network derived from correlation with the timeseries from a seed region in the posterior cingulate cortex).

Analysis

One method of analyzing resting state data is to just calculate such correlations, which is known as *seed-based correlation*. This method maps out how one region (the seed) is functionally related to all other locations in the brain. In such an analysis the "connectivity" is inferred by using the correlations of the signal fluctuations, which is an indirect measure of what is happening at the

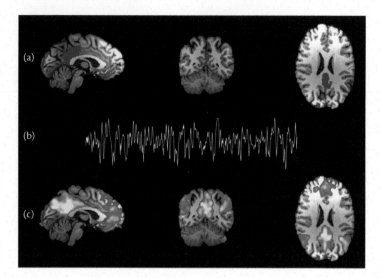

Figure 2.20: Results from a resting state seed-based correlation analysis on a single subject: (a) the seed region of interest in the posterior cingulate cortex (shown in blue); (b) the BOLD timeseries extracted from this region; (c) a thresholded map of the correlation of the timeseries in each voxel with the seed timeseries.

neuronal level, since it is based on the hemodynamics and not on the electrical activity of the neurons. One important problem for functional connectivity methods is that such correlations can also be driven by other causes of signal fluctuation, for example by physiological effects such as the changes during the respiratory and cardiac cycles, or by artifacts induced by head motion. These signals are much more problematic in resting state fMRI than in task fMRI and require much more careful attention in the preprocessing and analysis. The good news is that the current methods do a good job of reducing the impact of these artifacts and physiological confounds when the analysis is done carefully. However, there are several sources of ongoing debate as to the optimal way to deal with these artifacts, and this area of analysis is one of the most changeable and disputed.

Another method of analysis for resting state fMRI data is based on using whole-brain approaches rather than seeds. The most common method in this category is *independent component analysis* (ICA)—a relative of principal component analysis (PCA) and factor analysis—that decomposes the acquired fMRI data into separate components, each of which is described by a spatial map and a timecourse (see Figure 2.21). For each component, the values in the spatial map represent the amount of that component's timecourse that is present in the fMRI data at each location. So voxels with high values (or "weights") in a given map share a relatively large proportion of the same timecourse, and therefore a component can be thought of as showing a network of areas that share a common signal. This is the principle behind how ICA is used to analyze resting data: showing different networks that explain the acquired data. It is also normal for ICA to identify non-neuronal components, and in fact ICA is one of the best tools for separating the interesting (neuronal) from the noninteresting or artifactual (mainly non-neuronal) components. Many methods for "cleaning" or "denoising" resting state fMRI data as

Default Mode Network   Dorsal Attention Network

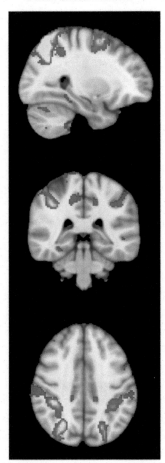

Figure 2.21: Results from a resting state independent component analysis of a group of subjects. Two different networks are shown: the default mode network and the dorsal attention network. Each is shown as a volumetric view using the most representative sagittal, coronal, and axial slices (top to bottom).

a preprocessing step use ICA, although ICA is also used for directly analyzing and interpreting the neuronal networks of interest.

In addition to extracting networks in the form of spatial maps and timecourses, resting state fMRI data are often analyzed at the level of functional regions rather than at the level of voxels. One way of doing this is to create network matrices, which capture the connections between different brain regions. This requires that the regions (or *nodes*) are predefined, though they may be extracted from the same data, using methods such as ICA. Once these regions are defined, the connectivity between them is measured in some way, such as through the temporal correlation of representative timecourses from the regions. These connectivities are then arranged into a *network matrix* where each element represents the connectivity value between a pair of regions. Such matrices can then be analyzed directly or may be used to define a *graph* (usually by thresholding each connectivity to create a binary on/off link or *edge* between regions), and these graphs can be analyzed in different ways.

The analysis of resting state fMRI data is also covered in more detail in Chapter 3, although the interested reader is also referred to a separate primer in this series, titled *Introduction to Resting State fMRI Functional Connectivity*.

SUMMARY

- Functional MRI (fMRI) provides a surrogate measure of neuronal activity by using the BOLD effect, which is sensitive to blood oxygenation.

- Deoxygenated hemoglobin disturbs the local B_0 magnetic field; that changes the T_2^* relaxation times, and fMRI acquisitions must be made very sensitive to T_2^*.

- EPI acquisitions (with possible accelerations via parallel imaging and/or simultaneous multi-slice acquisitions) are required for fast imaging, and the use of gradient-echo sequences makes them sensitive to T_2^*.

- Artifacts include all the artifacts present in structural and diffusion imaging, as well as signal loss, but not eddy-current distortions.

- Correction for geometric distortion and compensation for the negative impact of signal loss (but not restoration of the signal) can be applied in the analysis stages if a fieldmap (or the equivalent phase-encode reversed b=0 pair) is also acquired.

- Task fMRI involves designing experiments with stimuli and/or mental tasks and is analyzed using the GLM, which provides information about the response to the task/stimulus.

- Resting state fMRI does not require stimuli or tasks, and provides information about functional connectivity between regions of the brain. It is commonly analyzed using seed-based correlations, independent component analysis (ICA), or network/graph analyses.

FURTHER READING

- Huettel, S. A., Song, A. W., & McCarthy, G. (2014). *Functional Magnetic Resonance Imaging* (3rd ed.). Sinauer Associates.
  - *This is an accessible, introductory-level textbook with more of a focus on the physics of acquisition as well as on functional physiology and task fMRI studies.*

- Buxton, R. (2009). *Introduction to Functional Magnetic Resonance Imaging: Principles and Techniques* (2nd ed.). Cambridge University Press.
  - *A more detailed introduction to both MR physics and neural physiology, which also offers an overview of the principles of ASL and BOLD fMRI.*

- Amaro, E., Jr., & Barker, G. J. (2006). Study design in fMRI: Basic principles. *Brain and Cognition, 60*(3), 220–232.
  - *General paper describing experimental design for task fMRI.*
- Arthurs, O. J., & Boniface, S. (2002). How well do we understand the neural origins of the fMRI BOLD signal? *Trends in Neurosciences, 25*(1), 27–31.
  - *General paper about the physiological basis of the BOLD signal.*
- Bandettini, P. A. (2012). Twenty years of functional MRI: The science and the stories. *NeuroImage, 62*(2), 575–588
  - *Paper introducing a special issue that covers many aspects of functional MRI acquisition and analysis.*

2.5 Perfusion MRI

Perfusion is the process of delivering blood to the network of capillaries in tissues. This is clearly critical for the delivery of nutrients and for the complementary removal of waste products. In the brain, perfusion is normally quantified in terms of cerebral blood flow (CBF), in units of ml of blood per 100 g of tissue per minute. Confusingly, despite being called CBF, perfusion is not a flow measurement, since it is actually a measurement of the *delivery* of units of volume of blood per volume (mass) of tissue per unit time (rather than the normal units for flow, which would be volume per unit time). Typical CBF values in the brain are 60 ml/100 g/min for gray matter and 20 ml/100 g/min for white matter.

There are two major reasons why we might want to measure perfusion:

- to quantify the "resting" CBF or associated parameters of blood delivery, as a form of physiological MRI—for example, if we are looking for changes in perfusion associated with a disease;
- to investigate changes in perfusion associated with neuronal activity, where the measurement is based on an alternative mechanism to BOLD fMRI, both providing indirect information about activity via changes in hemodynamics.

The fundamental principle of all perfusion MRI techniques is the use of a tracer or contrast agent that is introduced into the bloodstream and made to alter the image intensity in proportion to the blood within, or delivered to, the tissue. These methods normally require some form of baseline image, taken without the tracer agent being present for comparison. It is then possible to interpret the difference between tracer and tracer-free images in terms of perfusion. It is quite common to acquire timeseries data when doing perfusion MRI to track the wash-in (first appearance of tracer) and sometimes also the wash-out (disappearance of the tracer) within the voxels. The timeseries in each voxel can then be interpreted via a model of how the tracer behaves in the tissue—tracer kinetic modeling. This is how other information may be extracted, such as timing information related to transit of the tracer through the vasculature. Perfusion MRI is able to produce perfusion-weighted images, but, when the concentration of the tracer in the blood can be calculated, by using kinetic models and calibration images, quantitative values can also be provided.

2.5.1 Arterial spin labeling

ASL is unique in being the only truly noninvasive way to measure perfusion in the brain. Its uniqueness is due to the way in which the "tracer" is created: RF inversion of the magnetic state of the hydrogen nuclei (see the online appendix titled *Short Introduction to MRI Physics for Neuroimaging*) is used to label blood-water in the arteries in the neck prior to its entering the brain. An image is acquired after a delay, the *postlabel delay*, which allows the labeled blood-water to reach the brain. If this is subtracted from another image, acquired without any label (the control), the result is an image that is related only to the label, and hence to the perfusion. This subtraction is very important because the signal arising from tissue is typically about 100 times stronger than the signal arising from the labeled blood-water. Compared to structural imaging, ASL has a low SNR, due to its reliance on the small difference in signal from the labeled blood-water. Thus it is common to use a low resolution, of the order of 3 mm, and to acquire multiple repeated volumes and combine them through averaging, so as to achieve better overall SNR—trading acquisition time for better SNR.

We will consider here the general principles of ASL, its acquisition, and its analysis. Further details can be found in the primer titled *Introduction to Perfusion Quantification using Arterial Spin Labelling*.

Measurement principles

ASL relies on water as its tracer and water is to a large extent freely diffusable in the brain, which means that it rapidly exchanges between blood, cells, and other extravascular spaces. ASL images are thus a direct measure of delivery: the labeled water accumulates in the tissue. A major limitation of ASL is that the tracer is short-lived, its lifetime being determined by the T_1 relaxation-time constant, which determines the rate at which the label decays. This needs to be taken into account in the quantification, but it also limits the application of ASL in situations where the time for blood to reach the tissue is long by comparison to T_1—that is, longer than a few seconds. This means that ASL can be problematic in patient populations where increased vascular transit times are associated with the disease.

Experiments

ASL can be used just like BOLD fMRI, to look at where greater amounts of blood are diverted to; hence it can act as a surrogate marker for neuronal activity. Its major advantage over BOLD fMRI is that it is a quantitative measurement of a physiological process. It is also potentially better localized in the brain, where greater neuronal activity is happening, by being a measure of perfusion rather than of changes in oxygenation, which are more likely to be seen in the venous circulation, downstream from the site of activity. It is also more suitable for experimental designs that take a long time, since in these experiments the drift in the baseline signal over time reduces the ability to observe activation in BOLD studies but is overcome in ASL by the repeated control images that are acquired. For example, ASL has been used in studies where "rest" and "active" sessions have taken place days or even weeks apart, yet quantitative differences in perfusion could still be identified. The penalty is usually a decrease in SNR, which is the main reason why ASL is less common than BOLD fMRI. It also has a lower temporal sampling rate, since pairs of images are acquired and each image needs around three seconds of preparation (labeling and postlabel delay). ASL can be combined with BOLD, if you want to get the advantages of both, although a penalty is then paid in the acquisition time.

ASL is more widely used to measure "resting" perfusion where an acquisition lasting a few minutes of alternating label and control images will be used. Taking the mean of the subtracted pairs is used to achieve a good overall SNR and to provide a perfusion image in an individual. It is then possible to use these images in group studies in order to create spatial maps of perfusion, not unlike in the group analysis of BOLD fMRI. However, ASL provides quantitative perfusion and thus quantitative inferences can be made about the perfusion differences that are observed. More advanced ASL acquisitions vary the delay between labeling and image acquisition (this is multiple postlabel delay ASL), in order to investigate other aspects of hemodynamics in the brain, such as blood arrival time, or to quantify arterial blood volumes. ASL has also been combined with BOLD in "dual-echo" sequences, in some cases with subjects breathing different gas mixtures, and used to quantify not only perfusion but also cerebral blood volume (CBV), and even $CMRO_2$.

Acquisition

There are different ASL techniques that vary the way in which the blood-water is labeled, as well as the method used for acquiring the brain images. The most important distinctions are pulsed versus continuous labeling and 2D versus 3D image acquisitions. The ASL label is generated using RF (B_1) fields in the neck, and this can be achieved either (i) by applying a pulse of RF over a region of the neck (and upper body)—that is, through pulsed ASL (pASL); or (ii) by labeling blood-water continuously as it passes through a plane located in the neck—that is, through continuous ASL (cASL); see Figure 2.22. For various reasons, cASL typically provides higher SNR than pASL but was not practical in the past on many scanners. However, the pseudo-continuous (pcASL) approach offers cASL-style labeling using pulses that can be achieved on the majority of scanners. It is also increasingly common for ASL data to be acquired using *background suppression*; this adds, prior to the acquisition of the image, extra RF pulses that attempt to suppress the signal arising from the brain tissue that is not the result of labeled blood-water. This suppresses some of the

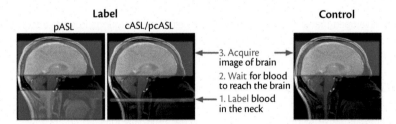

Figure 2.22: ASL acquisition involves labeling the blood-water in the neck either passing through a plane (cASL/pcASL) or in a volume (pASL), followed by a delay to wait for the labeled blood-water to reach the brain, then imaging. A control condition is also required in which no labeling is performed.

common (or static) signal, which has advantages because it reduces artifacts that occur at the point of subtraction due to differences between the images from motion or other physiological effects.

A number of image acquisition sequences can be combined with the ASL labeling and both 2D methods (which sequentially collect slices through the brain) and 3D methods (which build up information to form the whole 3D brain in a different way) have been used. 3D methods are generally able to provide higher SNR, something that is very beneficial to ASL but can suffer from blurring artifacts. This has led to the use of segmented 3D acquisitions, where a subset of the data is collected during one label-control pair, the rest being acquired in subsequent pairs and then recombined. The disadvantage of this approach is the greater sensitivity to motion that occurs during the acquisition of the different segments, which is difficult to correct for in the analysis. Since 2D methods acquire slices sequentially, they do not suffer from the same artifacts, but later slices are acquired with a longer postlabeling delay, and so these slices will have lower SNR.

The ASL community has reached a consensus, primarily for the clinical application of ASL, that pcASL labeling with a 3D imaging method and background suppression should be used. This is likely to become the standard in many studies, particularly where ASL is acquired to complement other modalities. However, some of the other variants have particular strengths for different applications, especially the use of multiple postlabeling delays, and so will continue to be used in neuroimaging studies.

Analysis

The analysis of ASL data follows a fairly standard set of steps, regardless of the variant of ASL used. These are subtraction, kinetic model inversion, and calibration. As we have already noted, subtraction of the label–control pair is sufficient to produce a perfusion-weighted image, although multiple pairs need to be averaged to get a good quality image. Quantification of perfusion requires correction for the processes that change the label, which can be achieved through the use of a kinetic model to describe the ASL signal. A final step to calculate the "concentration" of the label, which can be as simple as using a PD-weighted image for calibration, is required to convert the values in an ASL image into absolute measures of perfusion. Many of the other processes used to analyze ASL data, such as motion correction and registration, are similar to BOLD fMRI data, although the pairwise nature of ASL can produce its own specific challenges and artifacts.

Due to the typically low resolution of ASL data by comparison to the anatomy of the brain, ASL perfusion images suffer quite substantially from partial volume effects. This results in perfusion images appearing to be visually very similar to maps of gray matter distribution and can mean that subtle changes in perfusion are hard to see or detect, even within a group. Methods have been developed that attempt to correct for this effect where independent estimates of partial volumes of gray and white matter can be provided, for example from a structural segmentation.

2.5.2 Dynamic susceptibility contrast

Another alternative to perfusion imaging is to use externally injected contrast agents, which is what *dynamic susceptibility contrast* methods are based on. Popular contrast agents for imaging perfusion using MRI are based on *gadolinium*. This element is chosen because it has specific magnetic properties that means that it has a detectable change on standard

T_1- and T_2-weighted images. Because gadolinium is highly toxic on its own, contrast agents are specifically designed to "shield" the gadolinium from the body yet still allow the magnetic interactions between it and water that are needed to produce an effect. Gadolinium contrast agents are quite widely used in clinical practice for the assessment of perfusion or related changes in vasculature or tissue in disease, but they are less popular in research studies that include healthy individuals. This is increasingly due to fears over the residual toxicity of the available contrast agents; for example, they are now not recommended for use in individuals with poor kidney function due to fears over effective excretion of the agent.

Measurement principles

Gadolinium agents affect both the T_1 and the T_2 relaxation properties of water. It is not important to understand the mechanisms of this process (more details can be found in the online appendix titled *Short Introduction to MRI Physics for Neuroimaging*), but the T_1 change is largely associated with gadolinium when the latter is within the vasculature (e.g., in the capillary bed), whereas T_2 effects dominate when the gadolinium has left the vasculature and has entered the extravascular extracellular space (it generally does not cross cell membranes). These two effects have led to two categories of imaging based on gadolinium contrast agents:

- *dynamic susceptibility weighted* (DSC)—which is based on T_2-weighted images;
- *dynamic contrast enhanced* (DCE)—which is based on T_1-weighted images.

While both can be used in the brain, you will normally find DSC used for perfusion imaging, and you will rarely find it used anywhere else in the body. This has a very simple reason: the brain is (almost) unique in very tightly restricting what is allowed to pass out of the bloodstream and into the tissue, possessing what is called the *blood–brain barrier*. This prevents the gadolinium agents from leaving the blood, because the contrast agent molecules are too large. Thus in the brain a T_2 (or T_2^*) effect is seen, and so T_2-weighted imaging is most appropriate. Elsewhere in the body the contrast agent is normally quite free to leave the blood and to accumulate in the tissue, and commonly DCE is used. This is especially the case for tumours, as they have a more "leaky" vasculature and so show up on DCE images due to a higher accumulation of contrast agent. Therefore, if you find DCE (T_1-weighted imaging with a contrast agent) used in the brain, it will almost certainly be in a study related to cancer.

Acquisition

Typically a DSC MRI would involve repeated T_2-weighted imaging (or T_2^*-weighted imaging) from before the contrast agent is injected until some time later, when it has had time to pass fully through the brain at least once. It will continue to circulate in the bloodstream for some time after injection, but the concentration will become more evenly distributed and provide less useful information about perfusion, although it can still affect any subsequent imaging. Thus a DSC dataset will contain a timeseries of measurements in each voxel. This would look something like Figure 2.23: starting from a baseline before injection, the signal measurement decreases as the agent passes through the voxel before returning (approximately) back to the baseline. A good DSC experiment will seek to sample the dynamics of the contrast agent as regularly as possible, more than once every two seconds, since this is important for quantification. Because DSC relies

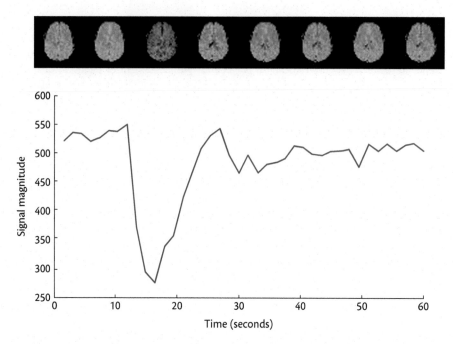

Figure 2.23: Example of DSC-MRI timeseries. Notice that the signal intensity drops during the passage of the contrast agent through the vasculature in a voxel; this results in a darkening of the image in areas of high vascular volume.

on T_2-weighted imaging and on a contrast agent that has quite a marked effect on the signal, the SNR is better than ASL and a higher resolution can be employed; it is not uncommon to find voxels sizes around 1.5 mm. This makes DSC less prone to partial volume effects than ASL.

Analysis

The DSC measurement is related, albeit nonlinearly, to the concentration of the contrast agent; and it is common to do a conversion to (relative) concentration over time. From the concentration timeseries often semi-quantitative metrics, such as time-to-peak, may be calculated as indirect measures of perfusion (or changes in perfusion), and this is especially common in clinical applications. More quantitative measures can be determined via the use of a kinetic model, which commonly entails making a measurement of the contrast agent over time in a major artery, which is selected either automatically or manually from the image data, to get the *arterial input function*. It is then possible, through a simple calculation, to get a measure of cerebral blood volume (CBV) within the voxel. To get a perfusion value, a process commonly called *deconvolution* is required. This only produces a measure of relative perfusion, and further information about the actual contrast agent concentration is needed for conversion to an absolute measure of perfusion. Methods do now exist that attempt to provide absolute perfusion measurements, but they are far less commonly used.

SUMMARY

- Perfusion is defined as the delivery of blood to the tissue, in units of ml of blood per 100 g of tissue per minute.

- ASL magnetically labels water in the neck and the water that is in the arteries (blood-water), then flows up into the brain.

- The images are measured in pairs, one following labeling (the label/tag image) and one with no labeling (the control image).

- Subtraction of label and control images leads to a perfusion-weighted image.

- Quantification of perfusion requires subtraction, kinetic model inversion, and calibration.

- The kinetic model specifies how the magnetic label changes over time, and it does so by modeling the MR physics and physiology.

- Calibration requires the acquisition of an additional image, usually a PD-weighted image.

- Further corrections for partial volume effects can help to considerably improve accuracy.

- DSC relies on the effect of a gadolinium contrast agent on T_2-weighted images.

- The DSC contrast agent stays within the blood and never enters brain tissue; this means that it can measure properties such as cerebral blood volume (CBV).

- Analysis of DSC data ranges from semi-quantitative metrics through to quantification of perfusion, with some methods being reliant on a measurement of signal from a larger artery in the image.

FURTHER READING

- Chappell, M., MacIntosh, B., & Okell, T. (2017). *Introduction to Perfusion Quantification Using Arterial Spin Labelling* (Oxford Neuroimaging Primers). Oxford University Press.
    - *This primer provides an introduction to the acquisition and analysis of ASL perfusion MRI.*

- Buxton, R. (2009). *Introduction to Functional Magnetic Resonance Imaging: Principles and Techniques* (2nd ed.). Cambridge University Press.
    - *A useful and more detailed introduction to both MR physics and neural physiology, which also offers an overview of the principles of both ASL and BOLD fMRI.*

- Alsop, D. C., Detre, J. A., Golay, X., Günther, M., Hendrikse, J., Hernandez-Garcia, L., et al. (2015). Recommended implementation of arterial spin-labeled perfusion MRI for clinical applications: A consensus of the ISMRM perfusion study group and the European consortium for ASL in dementia. *Magnetic Resonance in Medicine*, 73(1), 102–116.
    - *This ASL "white paper" or consensus paper gives a very good summary of common ASL methods and offers recommendations for a simple ASL protocol for routine applications, along with some guidance on more advanced usage for neuroimaging.*

■ Welker, K., Boxerman, J., Kalnin, A., Kaufmann, T., Shiroishi, M., Wintermark, M., American Society of Functional Neuroradiolgy, & MR Perfusion Standards and Practice Subcommittee of the ASFNR Clinical Practice Committee. (2015). ASFNR recommendations for clinical performance of MR dynamic susceptibility contrast perfusion imaging of the brain. *American Journal of Neuroradiology*, 36(6), E42–52.

    ■ *This paper, although aimed primarily at clinical applications, summarizes consensus recommendations on acquisition and analysis of DSC perfusion MRI.*

2.6 Spectroscopy (MRS)

All the MR imaging modalities we have looked at so far have used the signals from the hydrogen nuclei in water molecules to form the image. These modalities have concentrated on different properties (e.g., magnetic relaxation properties, diffusion, local field inhomogeneities) to highlight different aspects of biology in the brain (e.g., cellular environment and tissue type, microstructure and direction of axons, hemodynamic/functional changes). However, it is also possible to get signals back from other nuclei (e.g., from hydrogen nuclei in other molecules, besides water; or, if special coils are used, from completely different nuclei, such as Na, ^{31}P, ^{13}C, F), and this is what *MR spectroscopy* (MRS) is able to do. This can then give information about the amount of other interesting molecules in the brain, for example N-acetylaspartate (NAA), choline, creatine, glutamate, and gamma-aminobutyric acid (GABA). The information provided by MRS is therefore highly complementary to that offered by the other techniques we have discussed and can provide new insights into fundamental processes at work in the brain at the microscopic level (e.g., plasticity or pathology). There are also some challenges, since the concentration of these molecules is far lower than that of water; hence the signals are very weak and some compromises need to be made in the imaging in order to acquire useable data.

2.6.1 Measurement principles

MRS relies on a process called *chemical shift*. This causes the signals from each type of molecule to have a characteristic shift in frequency, which then allows the contribution of each type of molecule to be separated and quantified. Chemical shift occurs because the distribution of electrons around a molecule is characteristic for that type of molecule, and these electrons cause small changes in the magnetic field in different parts of the molecule. Hence the effective magnetic field that each nucleus actually experiences is altered, as the electrons "shield" the nucleus to some degree, and so the frequency of the emitted signal is also altered. As each type of molecule has a different distribution of electrons (the electron "cloud"), its signal has a different, and characteristic, set of frequencies. Therefore, by carefully measuring the frequency components of the signal, the separate contributions of the different molecules can be calculated.

2.6.2 Acquisition

In order to be able to measure the different molecular contributions, it is necessary to have very good SNR and very precise measurement of frequencies. To achieve this, given the very small concentrations of most other molecules in the brain, the signal is usually averaged over a large region, of the order of one to several *centimeters*. Otherwise the signal of interest would be completely drowned out by the noise. Consequently, most MRS acquisitions actually only acquire information in one single "voxel," where this voxel is huge by comparison with other images (e.g., volumes of 1–27 cm³ in MRS as opposed to 0.001–0.03 cm³ in standard MRI) and it is usually very carefully placed to cover a particular region of interest. It is also possible to get whole brain coverage by using similarly large voxels, with MR spectroscopic imaging (MRSI) methods, but these acquisitions are rarely used due to their complexity in both acquisition and analysis. Special expertise is required from the radiographer or scanner operator to perform MRS acquisitions, either for a single voxel or for MRSI, and you should not just assume that this is simply available but check in advance whether it is possible on your system and with the available local expertise.

2.6.3 Limitations and artifacts

One big limitation of MRS is the low SNR, which makes it necessary to use such large voxels and sacrifice spatial resolution. Another limitation is that MRS can only separate out contributions from molecules with frequencies that are sufficiently different (separated) from those of other molecules that are present. Otherwise the signals overlap too much and the different molecule contributions cannot be separated. This limitation, together with the need to have a sufficient concentration of the molecules, is the reason why certain molecules of interest cannot be investigated with typical MRS sequences and scanners (e.g., dopamine, serotonin, and acetylcholine). It is possible to get around this limitation to some degree by using higher field scanners (e.g., 7T), as these have greater SNR and separate frequencies better. In fact MRS is probably the modality that benefits the most from using scanners with higher field strength.

When using an MRS sequence, it is important to pay special attention to two aspects that are normally quite routine. One is the location of the field of view, especially when only a single voxel is being scanned. This is typically looked after by the radiographer or scanner operator, who sits at the console and delimits the field of view on the screen, often carefully rotating the acquisition so as to align it with the individual anatomy. For example, performing MRS in the hippocampal region is normally done by rotating the scan so that the image axis aligns with the main axis of the hippocampus, and then a long but relatively narrow "voxel" (i.e., a rectangular field of view) is drawn around the hippocampus. It is also possible to automate this process, typically by using a structural scan, or possibly the initial localizer scan, to perform automated alignment (registration) with an existing template or previous scan. The latter situation arises commonly in longitudinal imaging, where a subject is scanned once at baseline and then again in a follow-up that could be days, months or years later. In this situation, getting the most consistent voxel placement is important for obtaining accurate quantification of the differences and for reducing biases that could be created from inconsistently imaged areas at the edges of the voxel. Consequently, these automated methods are strongly recommended over manual placements and should be used whenever possible.

The other aspect requiring special attention is the shimming of the region of interest. Although shimming is done in all image acquisitions and is important for obtaining a more uniform magnetic field throughout the brain, it is particularly important for MRS. This is because any local departures from a uniform field result in changes in the frequency of the signal that comes from those locations. In other MR imaging modalities these changes in frequency result in mislocations of the signal (geometric distortions) that either are kept very small through the sequence design (e.g., in structural imaging) or can be corrected for in the analysis (e.g., in functional or diffusion imaging). However, as the frequency information in MRS is crucial for determining which molecules produce the signal, it is even more important to make the field as uniform as possible. Therefore extra effort goes into the shimming for MRS, though this is often done through the same automated methods as those used for other sequences. The difference is that in MRS the shimming is concerned only with the specific region of interest and can sacrifice uniformity in other regions of the brain as a trade-off, which is acceptable here with only one voxel but would not be acceptable in other imaging applications.

2.6.4 Analysis

In addition to the fact that the acquisition is very specialized, some of the analysis tools available to process the data are also very complex and specialized—although simple fits and identification of key peaks can be done visually or with more basic software. The basic principle behind analyzing MRS data is fitting a model to the observed data, where the model is based on the characteristic spectra (set of frequencies) for a set of molecules that are known to occur in the brain. This might be done for a single voxel, where the data consist of a single set of amplitudes at different frequencies, or for an image comprised of such voxels. Either way, the main idea is to fit this model and determine the amount of each type of molecule that is present per voxel. The range of molecules that can be fitted depends on the nature of the scanner, the sequence used, and the sophistication of the software. As discussed previously, limitations related to the frequency precision and SNR of the scanner or sequence, by comparison with the frequency difference between molecules, are the main factors. In practice there are many other complications, details, and nuances that go into both acquisition and analysis, but these are beyond the scope of this primer.

SUMMARY

- MRS can examine the concentration of molecules other than water, such as NAA, choline, creatine, glutamate, GABA, and so on.
- MRS relies on a set of characteristic frequencies from each type of molecule, due to chemical shift, to determine which signals come from which molecules.

- The signal is very weak due to the much lower molecular concentrations, and so voxel sizes are of an order of magnitude bigger in each dimension (typically, a few centimeters) by comparison to those of the other MR modalities.

- Often only a single voxel (or ROI) is acquired.

- Specialized acquisition sequences and analysis methods are needed for MRS (or its imaging equivalent, MRSI) and local expertise is necessary for acquiring and analyzing such data.

FURTHER READING

- Stagg, C., & Rothman, D. L. (Eds.). (2014). *Magnetic Resonance Spectroscopy: Tools for Neuroscience Research and Emerging Clinical Applications.* Academic Press.
  - *This is a comprehensive textbook covering MRS acquisition, analysis, and applications.*

2.7 Complementary techniques

In this chapter we have described most of the common MRI modalities, but there are also other MRI modalities. These include *angiograms* and *venograms*, which highlight the blood vessels within the brain, on the arterial and venous side respectively; *susceptibility-weighted images* (or *quantitative susceptibility images*), which highlight iron deposition in tissue; *magnetization transfer* (MT) images, which highlight certain pathologies; and also modalities that measure the physical properties of the scanner, such as B_1 maps, which measure the B_1 field in each voxel. Depending on your area of interest, you may end up using some of these sequences too.

This section will mainly focus on complementary, non-MRI techniques such as alternative imaging methods, electrophysiology, and stimulation or intervention techniques. The reason why we want to highlight these is that MRI, although it is a very flexible imaging technique that produces high-quality images, cannot do everything; non-MRI modalities can significantly enhance experiments and greatly clarify interpretation. Although this primer and others in the series will concentrate on MRI, we do not advocate neglecting other modalities and actually want to encourage you to think carefully about the possibilities of combining MRI with non-MRI modalities. The rest of this section will briefly outline several of the main additional modalities and techniques, but we leave further investigation of the available and relevant methods to you.

2.7.1 Imaging methods

On the imaging side, the main non-MRI techniques used in neuroimaging are positron emission tomography (PET), X-ray or computed tomography (CT), and ultrasound. These techniques measure information in completely different ways and typically have both advantages and disadvantages by comparison to MRI. These advantages and disadvantages relate to what can be measured, the invasiveness of the imaging procedure, and the achievable spatial and temporal resolutions.

To start with, PET scans are more invasive than MRI scans since they require injections of radioactive tracers and rely on detecting gamma ray photons that result as secondary products from the decay of the radioactive tracer. This leads to lower spatial and temporal resolutions compared to MRI, but can have significant advantages when targeting specific molecular compounds. For example, detecting tau or beta-amyloid (compounds associated with pathology in Alzheimer's disease) is something that PET excels at, while it is not currently feasible with MRI.

CT images are 3D images reconstructed from measurements made using X-rays. They can image the structural anatomy with very high spatial resolution and excellent SNR, but often with very poor contrast between tissues in the brain (low CNR), although this can be altered for some structures by injecting contrast agents. Again, this is a more invasive technique than MRI (due to the tissue damage associated with X-rays); but it is a common clinical imaging technique, and one vastly superior to MRI when it comes to looking at bony structures and intracranial hemorrhage, which is very important when dealing with possible head trauma. However, MRI is much better for investigating the brain anatomy associated with the soft tissues (gray and white matter). On the other hand, CT is quicker and cheaper than MRI, so it is often the first scan obtained in a hospital for neurological patients; and it is invaluable for detecting or ruling out a range of pathologies.

Ultrasound is another common medical imaging modality and has many applications, although it is much more limited in investigations of the brain, due to the difficulty of imaging inside the bony skull and the lack of contrast between the soft tissues in the brain. Hence this is an imaging modality that is rarely applied in adult brain imaging. Currently it has more applications in fetal and neonatal development, including in investigations of the fetal and newborn brain.

2.7.2 Electrophysiology and fNIRS

In addition to imaging modalities, there are other measurement techniques that provide very useful complementary information, as well as some spatial localization. The most common examples are electrophysiology techniques—*electroencephalography* (EEG) and *magnetoencephalography* (MEG)—which measure the electrical activity of the neurons, and functional near-infrared spectroscopy (fNIRS), which measures the hemodynamic response.

MEG is a technique that detects the very tiny changes in magnetic field associated with neuronal firing and its electrical activity. It has much higher temporal resolution (milliseconds or better) compared to fMRI and is able to look more directly at the electrical activity of the neurons, rather than relying on the hemodynamics. However, it cannot localize the signal spatially as well as fMRI does, since it is based on a set of sensors placed near the scalp (see Figure 2.24). It is, however, a noninvasive technique, and actually slightly better than fMRI, as it is virtually silent, unlike the incredibly noisy MRI scanner. It is predominantly used in neuroimaging research

EEG MEG

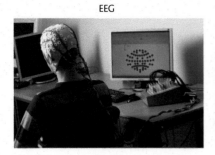 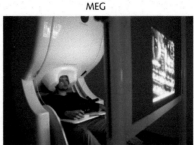

Figure 2.24: Illustrations of EEG and MEG experiments, both of which involve a set of sensors placed on or near the surface of the scalp.

studies and is highly complementary to MRI in the investigation of brain activity, especially with respect to the fast neuronal dynamics.

In EEG a set of electrodes are placed directly on the scalp (see Figure 2.24) and detect tiny changes in voltage that are associated with the neuronal firing (electrical activity) inside the brain. Due to the presence of the skull and interference (such as from activity in muscles in the face, scalp, and eyes), it is difficult to precisely determine where the signal is coming from and to get reliable information from single bursts of activity. However, by averaging across repeated trials, a very detailed picture of activity can be formed, with much higher temporal resolution than fMRI but with less precise spatial localization; the temporal resolution is similar to that of MEG, but spatial localization is somewhat worse than in MEG. The reconstructed signals are usually shown as maps on the surface of the scalp, as EEG is predominantly sensitive to activity in cortical regions near the skull. Some advantages of EEG over MEG are that it is much more readily available, is very cheap, and can even be combined with fMRI in the scanner (though this is quite rare and requires extra equipment and on-site expertise to make it work). It can also be done at a patient's bedside for clinical investigations. In terms of getting precise details about neuronal firing, EEG and MEG provide considerable advantages over fMRI, but combining these with fMRI experiments is even better, as it integrates the high spatial resolution of fMRI and the high temporal resolution of EEG/MEG.

The fNIRS technique measures changes in the hemodynamics on the basis of the difference in absorption of near-infrared light between oxygenated and deoxygenated blood. Specific frequencies are used such that the light penetrates the skin, muscle, and bone well but is largely absorbed by the blood. This provides a way to measure, with high temporal resolution (better than in fMRI), the blood response in areas near the surface of the cortex. Typically sensors are placed around the scalp, like the electrodes in EEG, and so fNIRS is only capable of a limited degree of spatial localization (which is much worse than in fMRI). Again, like EEG, fNIRS can also be combined with fMRI scans in simultaneous acquisitions, though without some of the difficulties associated with simultaneous EEG recordings (where the changing magnetic fields applied by the MRI scanner induce sizeable unwanted currents).

Figure 2.25 gives information about some of these complementary techniques and about others not detailed here, along with their spatial and temporal resolutions and their invasiveness.

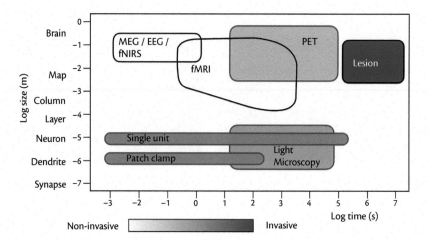

Figure 2.25: Illustration of a range of complementary techniques in neuroscience (imaging and nonimaging) and of how they compare with respect to spatial resolution (vertical axis), temporal resolution (horizontal axis), and invasiveness (shading).

2.7.3 Transcranial brain stimulation methods (TMS and tDCS)

In addition to these extra recording devices there are also additional techniques, which we previously referred to as stimulation or intervention methods. The most prominent of these are *transcranial magnetic stimulation* (TMS) and *transcranial direct current stimulation* (tDCS), which can be used to manipulate the way in which the brain functions. In TMS a large changing current is passed through a coil that is held just above the scalp and induces magnetic fields and corresponding (but small) electrical currents inside the brain. These currents cause action potentials in the neurons and alter the normal function of that part of the brain, allowing experimenters to determine how changes in that region's function affect any overall response or processing of stimuli. This is used widely in neuroscientific studies to gain better understanding of brain regions and networks. TMS can also be used to study cortical excitability or as a technique to induce lasting changes (tens of minutes) in excitability.

The tDCS technique involves placing electrodes on the scalp and passing a small direct current through them that passes through parts of the brain, as determined by the electrode placement. This triggers temporary changes in neural firing in a relatively localized region of the brain that can last for some period of time after the stimulation, which is useful for both neuroscientific study of healthy brain function and clinical application in disorders such as depression. The ways in which both TMS and tDCS affect the brain are topics of ongoing research, but they are increasingly playing a role in basic science and clinical investigations of the brain, offering new insights into brain activity.

Finally, we again encourage you to think carefully about the benefits of combining complementary techniques with your MRI experiments, either the ones mentioned in this chapter or others. The availability of the different techniques varies widely, depending on what equipment is around but also, crucially, on the expertise necessary to acquire good quality data with them. For example, PET and MEG are quite rare, but usually come with highly trained operators, whereas

EEG equipment is much easier to come by, but without some local expertise in setting it up to get good quality recordings and analyze the data it may not be worthwhile. Also, in hospital environments, CT and ultrasound facilities are very common; but they are not seen as commonly in pure research settings. It is advisable to find out what the situation is in your particular institution or in collaborating ones, so that you know what you have access to and how difficult it is to use these techniques. Some of the most interesting and enlightening experiments are those that combine methods in order to benefit from the advantages of different techniques. Therefore it is worth investing some time into thinking about this, not only for your own experiments but also in order to understand the literature better—although you can also do excellent experiments with MRI alone. The main point here is to think broadly about possibilities in the planning stage, and not just to fall back on a method because it is familiar or convenient when another method, or combination of methods, might be even better.

SUMMARY

■ There are a range of non-MRI techniques that can measure aspects of brain structure or function in a complementary way to MRI.

■ Transcranial brain stimulation techniques allow in vivo manipulation of brain processes and can have advantages when combined with imaging.

■ When planning experiments, a wide range of techniques and combinations of them should be considered.

FURTHER READING

■ Zimmer, L., & Luxen, A. (2012). PET radiotracers for molecular imaging in the brain: Past, present and future. *Neuroimage*, 61(2), 363–370.
  ▪ *A general overview of the use of PET in neuroimaging.*

■ Proudfoot, M., Woolrich, M. W., Nobre, A. C., & Turner, M. R. (2014). Magnetoencephalography. *Practical Neurology*, 0, 1–8.
  ▪ *A brief overview of MEG and its clinical applications.*

■ Hansen, P., Kringelbach, M., & Salmelin, R. (eds.). (2010). *MEG: An Introduction to Methods.* Oxford University Press.
  ▪ *A comprehensive textbook on MEG acquisition, analysis, and acquisitions.*

■ Hari, R., & Puce, A. (2017). *MEG-EEG Primer.* Oxford University Press.
  ▪ *A primer, not from this series, covering both EEG and MEG in equal measure.*

■ Sparing, R., & Mottaghy, F. M. (2008). Noninvasive brain stimulation with transcranial magnetic or direct current stimulation (TMS/tDCS): From insights into human memory to therapy of its dysfunction. *Methods*, 44(4), 329–337.
  ▪ *An overview paper discussing theory and applications for both TMS and tDCS techniques.*

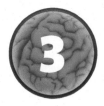

Overview of MRI Analysis

In this chapter we will present an overview of the most common analysis pipelines and of the various individual steps, methods, and stages involved. A *pipeline* is a defined series of analysis steps that are performed one after the other, in an established order. Many standard pipelines exist and software tools often make some conventional pipelines available, as well as offering users the flexibility to specify their own. You will notice that, although the pipelines we outline here are based on the modalities we met in Chapter 2, sometimes a pipeline can require other data as well.

Although many neuroimaging software tools and algorithms are available, most of them use the same broad principles. So, despite the fact that not every tool or pipeline can be covered here, the principles and techniques you will learn about are very widely applicable. The analysis methods also contain various options and adjustable parameters and you, as the user, will need to be able to select the pipelines, methods, options, and parameters that best suit your data and the type of analysis you want to perform. In order to be able to do this well, you need to understand some of the basics of these analysis methods; and the objective of this chapter is to introduce you to the different pipelines and methods that are available as well as to some of the main parameters. More details about specific methods are provided in later sections of this primer, in other primers, or in the Further Reading sections.

Before we move on to discussing the pipelines in more detail, it is worth considering one particularly important aspect of any analysis step or method, namely how robust it is. The *robustness* of a method is a measure of the chances of it "failing" (i.e., producing an unacceptable result) on an individual subject or image rather than a meaure of its accuracy or precision. It is possible to have a method that is highly robust (i.e., almost never *fails*) but has only moderate accuracy or precision. Similarly, it is possible to have a method that has very high accuracy or precision when it works but has poor robustness, failing in a sizeable fraction of cases. The definition of *failure* here depends on the application but represents results which are clearly erroneous and unacceptable. Analysis methods ideally need to be robust as well as accurate and precise. It is difficult to assess robustness, though, since this requires running the method on a wide variety of images, and the types and quality of MRI images keep changing year by year, so you cannot easily assign a number to robustness. Nonetheless, robustness is a crucial aspect of an analysis method and automated, robust methods are especially needed for large cohort studies, where careful manual inspection becomes difficult or impossible to achieve.

Two common aspects of analysis in neuroimaging research that will crop up repeatedly are group analysis and statistics. These are presented in the Group Analysis Box, since the concepts here are common to the analysis of almost every type of neuroimaging dataset. Following this, the rest of this chapter will outline a range of major pipelines and the individual steps or methods that make up those pipelines.

Group Analysis Box

In neuroimaging research studies, group analysis is used so that results can be generalized to the larger population rather than being true only for a single subject. This is different from clinical practice, where the interest is in the particular patient. In research we want to know about findings that are generally applicable, and to do this we need to take into account individual variability, which requires us to use groups of subjects. One consequence of this is that we need to use *registration* methods to geometrically align the brains of different subjects together, so that each voxel refers to a specific anatomical location that is consistent across all subjects. This registration typically uses a *template image* for the alignment, which is an average image of either the group of subjects in the study (a *study-specific template*) or a separate group of subjects (a standard template; most commonly the MNI152, which contains an average of 152 healthy adults).

Once registration has been performed, it is necessary to use appropriate statistics to take into account the noise in the images as well as the biological variability between individuals. Almost all statistical analyses in neuroimaging use the *general linear model* (GLM), as this is extremely flexible and can be used for individual subject and group analyses, as well as with parametric or nonparametric (e.g., permutation-based) statistics. More details about the GLM and imaging statistics can be found in the online appendix titled *Short Introduction to the General Linear Model for Neuroimaging*.

Registration

Aligning the anatomy between images is a crucial component in almost all studies, especially group studies. Registration is the process of aligning images and can be used to align two images from different subjects or an image from a subject and a template image.

In group analyses, registration is typically used to align a structural image of each subject to a template image. This template image is an average image and can either be formed from the group currently under study or be a standard template created previously, from a separate population. Standard templates are usually created from a large group of individuals and represent a common population. The most widely used standard template is the MNI152, which covers an average of 152 healthy adults, but other templates exist for children and other species. If the group under study does not match the demographics of the subjects used to form the template image, then it may be better to use a study-specific template, even though the subjects involved may be

Before Registration

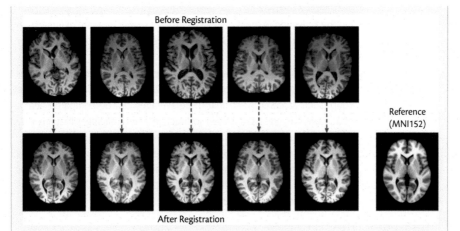

Reference
(MNI152)

After Registration

Figure 3.1: Illustration of registration in a group analysis: five subjects with different brain sizes and folding patterns, each registered to a common reference template (MNI152). The top row shows slices from the original images, while the bottom row shows the corresponding images after registration. Note how similar all the images are in the bottom row and how well matched they are to the reference image.

fewer—however, this can be a tricky trade-off for small groups. Regardless of the template used, the objective of registration for group analysis is to remove individual variation in anatomy and produce a set of images where each voxel corresponds to a consistent anatomical location across the group (see Figure 3.1).

The *spatial transformation* that is created by performing a registration describes how voxel locations in an individual subject relate to voxel locations in the template. Once such a spatial transformation is known, it can be applied to other data from that subject (e.g., diffusion measurements, functional activations) to create a version of the data that is aligned with the template. By doing this for all subjects, you create a dataset that contains the information of interest and has consistent anatomical locations across subjects; this dataset is then ready to be analyzed at the group level (see Chapter 5 for more details).

The GLM

A *group-level analysis* (also called *higher level* or *second-level analysis* in task fMRI) is performed in order to combine data across subjects, and in neuroimaging this analysis is usually done with the GLM. The purpose of a group analysis is to test hypotheses such as whether there is a consistent response in all individuals, or whether the responses relate to other quantities of interest (e.g., individual neuropsychological test results). The standard group-level analysis combines information extracted from individual subjects for the purpose of performing statistical hypothesis tests that take into account the estimates of the quantities of interest, the noise (or variation) within each subject's data, and the variation in quantities between subjects that are due to biological differences. Taking into account both measurement noise and biological variation means that the tests relate to hypotheses about the population that the subjects came from, and not just about the individual subjects in a particular cohort.

For instance, would the activation in the hippocampus (or any other quantity of interest) in an individual *from the population* show a dependency on memory test scores (or any other measure of interest)?

The GLM that is used for group-level analysis contains regressors or explanatory variables (EVs) that model effects across subjects—for example, regressors modeling the average value within a group (such as controls) so that these averages can be compared across groups. One of the reasons why the GLM is used so much in neuroimaging is that it is very flexible, and as a consequence many types of statistical test are possible: single group t-test, unpaired group t-test, paired t-test, ANOVA, and so on. The results from any of these tests take the form of maps that show which voxels are statistically significant, and these maps are usually displayed on the same template image (most often the MNI152) that was used for between-subject registration (see Figure 3.2).

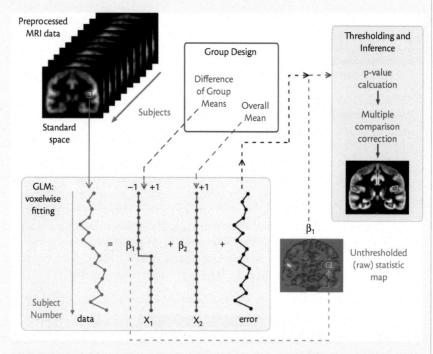

Figure 3.2: Illustration of a group-level analysis using the GLM. Top left shows a set of MRI data, after preprocessing to calculate the quantity of interest (local gray matter content for VBM, fMRI effect size, etc.), all transformed into standard space (aligned with a standard template). A group design has been specified—in this example a simple two-group design is shown (the difference in the means between groups being the quantity of interest). The GLM is fit to the data in each voxel in turn (bottom left box), in order to obtain voxelwise estimates for the parameters β_1 (difference of group means) and β_2 (overall mean), plus an error term. The parameters that are determined from the GLM for each voxel are the main outputs, shown as an unthresholded statistic map (bottom right) and after thresholding and inference (top right). The use of multiple comparison correction in the inference is crucial for obtaining valid statistical results.

One other essential part of any statistical analyses in neuroimaging is the application of *multiple comparison correction* methods whenever a voxelwise analysis is performed (voxelwise analyses are analyses that perform a separate statistical test at each voxel). This is crucial, because the number of voxels in an image is enormous (typically hundreds of thousands, or more) and, if no multiple comparison correction is done, then the number of incorrect inferences (known as *false positives*) will be very large and the results invalid and untrustworthy. Thankfully a number of multiple comparison correction methods are available; and they are built into all neuroimaging software packages—you do not need to understand how they work, just that one of them must be applied to obtain valid results. Knowing further details about statistical testing and using the GLM are not necessary steps for reading this primer, but both will be necessary if you want to continue to learn about neuroimaging. We therefore recommend that, after reading this primer (or now, if you prefer), you also read the online appendix titled *Short Introduction to the General Linear Modelling for Neuroimaging*.

3.1 Early stages

Prior to doing any statistical analysis, the initial stages of most analysis pipelines apply various preprocessing steps designed to reduce or remove artifacts and confounds from the data. In this section we will discuss what comes before all of these steps: some of the very early and common preprocessing steps.

The very first thing that happens to measurements from the scanner is that they are reconstructed into images, which is an operation that is normally performed directly on the scanner without your needing to be aware of it. However, for some kinds of artifacts, it is potentially useful to go back to the reconstruction phase and choose different options there (e.g., gradient nonlinearity correction). This is something that the scanner operator or physicist could do for you, after you have let them know about an artifact and while the raw data are still available. In the vast majority of cases the reconstruction is successful and does not need a second thought. After this the image files are available for the user; the file format used is often DICOM if directly from the scanner, but the files may take other formats. To use the data in neuroimaging analysis tools, you normally need to convert these data to the NIfTI format or possibly to another custom format (see Box 2.1 on image formats). Conversion to NIfTI may be done by your analysis package or may require the use of a separate conversion tool—or, if you are lucky, it may be done automatically for you.

Once you have your images in NIfTI format, or some equivalent, you should check that the quality is good and that they do not contain artifacts, as discussed in section 1.2. Checking the images is usually best done by eye, by just looking at the data. There are also automated quality control (QC) software tools that can help produce reports and highlight certain aspects, but these should be used in addition to visual inspection, not instead of it. One automated tool that is very useful at identifying a range of artifacts, especially in functional data, is independent component analysis (ICA). This tool decomposes the data into different components or sources, but still generally requires manual inspection of these components in order to separate artifacts and components of interest.

After verifying that there are no problematic artifacts in your data, or after getting advice and correcting them, you are ready to start on the analysis. Each modality has its own typical pipeline and set of steps, as outlined in the next sections, but there are two very simple steps that are useful to apply to any images: *reorientation* and *cropping*.

Reorientation is different from registration or alignment, in that it does not aim to align individual anatomical structures in the image. All it aims to do is set the axes to standard directions, so that they approximately match the template being used. In the MNI152 standard template, the first image axis (or, more precisely, voxel axis) is the left–right axis, the second axis is the posterior–anterior axis, and the third axis is the inferior–superior axis. The reorientation simply performs 0°, 90°, 180°, or 270° rotations, to rearrange the axes (see Figure 3.3 and, for extra detail about coordinates and axes, see Box 3.1). There is absolutely no change in resolution or image quality that is associated with such reorientations. However, this step is not essential, although it is generally helpful and some tools have it built into them. By applying this step to each modality, you minimize the work that registration has to do later on and you make it easier to look at all the images in a comparable way. For oblique images (e.g., where an axis might change in both anterior and superior directions), reorientation will not make the axes aligned with a nonoblique template, but it normally does no harm to run it.

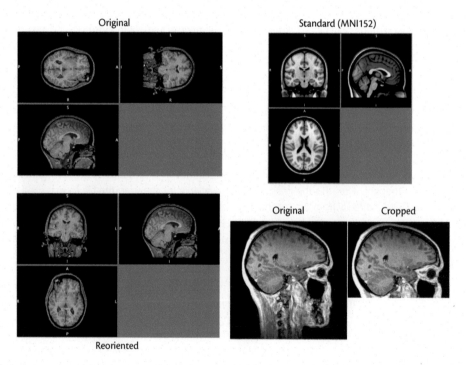

Figure 3.3: Illustration of reorientation designed to match the MNI152 orientation: original image from scanner (top left), reoriented version (bottom left), and standard orientation of the MNI152 (top right). Bottom-right panel shows an image with a large FOV (original) and the cropped version, which helps improve the robustness of brain extraction and registration.

Box 3.1: Voxel and world coordinates

The locations in an image are specified mathematically, with coordinates. However, there are two types of coordinate in common use: *voxel coordinates* and *world coordinates*. These differ in the units used, where their origin is located, and in how their axes relate to the anatomy. For voxel coordinates there are no units; they simply specify voxel locations in terms of their place within the 3D array of numbers that make up the image (which is a bit like specifying a row and column in a spreadsheet). Thus the coordinates take on integer values for each voxel, have the origin at the first (corner) voxel, and can have any relationship with the anatomical axes (determined by how the head was positioned in the scanner and how the scanner operator setup the scanning planes). For world (or mm) coordinates, the coordinates take on real (floating point) values, in units of mm, and it is common that the origin is at a specific anatomical location and that the axes correspond to specific directions—for example, x is left–right, y is posterior–anterior, and z is inferior–superior. This is generally true for world coordinates associated with a standard space (like the MNI152) or for those associated with the scanner space (assuming that subjects are oriented in a standard way in the scanner's bore). More information on coordinate systems will be given in section 5.1.3.

One important property of a world coordinate system is its *handedness*, which relates to the ordering and signs of the axes. In the example in the previous paragraph, + x corresponds to right (R), + y to anterior (A), + z to superior (S), and such a coordinate system is referred to as an RAS system, which is right-handed (since, with your right hand, you can use your thumb to point right, the next finger to point anterior and the next finger to point superior). Swapping the sign of any axis will swap from a right-handed to a left-handed coordinate system, and vice versa. Since keeping track of left and right in a brain image is very important (as it is next to impossible to tell left and right by visual inspection of an image), processing pipelines go to great lengths to avoid flipping image axes and use rotations instead (since all rotations preserve the handedness of the coordinate system). This is why the reorientation step performs 0°, 90°, 180°, or 270° rotations, which is similar to swapping axes around but explicitly avoids any flips (or reflections) that would change the handedness. Both the NIfTI image format and the MNI standard space specify a right-handed coordinate system.

Cropping is a step that aims to cut the image off in such a way that parts of the image that are far from the brain (e.g., in the neck, or the empty space above the head or to the side) are removed. It does not remove nonbrain structures near the brain (this is the job of brain extraction: see Chapter 4), but just defines a box to be placed around the relevant part of the head, so that the rest can be thrown away. This is often helpful in structural imaging, where large areas of neck and even shoulders can be included in the image. If they are left in the image then they make the job of brain extraction and registration more difficult and lead to an increase in the failure rate. Cropping helps with this as long as it is more robust than the brain extraction and the registration steps. Typically cropping is done either by hand (by looking at the image and cropping in a viewing tool, or with a separate command) or with a simple automatic tool. If an automatic tool is used, then it is advisable to check the output visually, to confirm that no parts of the brain were removed erroneously.

SUMMARY

■ Raw data from the scanner are converted into some image format, often DICOM, and this is then converted into a format suitable for neuroimaging analysis (e.g., NIfTI).

■ QC (quality control) should always be applied to the images (e.g., visually), in order to check for artifacts and ensure that the scanning session followed the correct protocol.

■ Reorienting and cropping the images at the initial stage can often increase the robustness of subsequent analysis steps.

3.2 Structural pipeline

All neuroimaging studies, with very few exceptions, require structural images, as these are needed if you are to view the subject's anatomy and to be able to determine the anatomical locations of the results obtained through other modalities. Structural images are also used for the analysis of anatomical changes, and so there are two objectives for structural pipelines: (i) to provide necessary information to support other analyses, such as diffusion or functional analyses; and (ii) to analyze the anatomy. These two objectives share some common steps, but other steps are specific to one objective or the other. In this section we will discuss both types of steps; and, since a number of them are common across different types of analysis, this section will be the longest in the chapter.

3.2.1 Brain extraction

The most common initial stage in a structural analysis is to remove the nonbrain structures from the image or to create a *brain mask* (i.e., a binary image where voxels outside the brain contain a value of 0 and voxels inside contain a value of 1)—or both; see Figure 3.4. This is

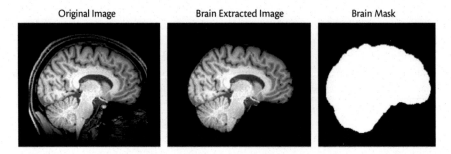

| Original Image | Brain Extracted Image | Brain Mask |

Figure 3.4: Illustration of brain extraction: original image (left), brain-extracted image (middle), and corresponding binary brain mask (right). Voxels inside the white area of the brain mask contain a value of 1 and all other voxels contain a value of 0.

useful because it allows subsequent analysis stages to avoid wasting time analyzing parts of the image that are of no interest; more importantly, it also stops these other nonbrain parts from adversely affecting the results. For instance, registration methods can be distracted by differences in nonbrain structures (e.g., fatty tissue in the scalp), and this can make the registration result less accurate or can even cause it to fail completely (i.e., it can produce a result with large, unacceptable, errors). Hence brain extraction is a useful process so long as it is robust and does not itself fail: this is a general principle in all analysis pipelines—that each stage in the pipeline brings with it a chance of failure and that nonrobust methods should be avoided, or at least monitored with great care.

All analysis pipelines require a brain mask in order to know which voxels are located inside the brain, but brain extraction is not always run as a separate process to generate a mask. Some tools have brain extraction built into them, or will refine the brain extraction from an initial rough estimate. Hence brain extraction is not compulsory, but a pipeline does need to generate a brain mask at some stage. More information on brain extraction can be found in Chapter 4.

3.2.2 Registration

The Group Analysis Box explains how registration is an essential component of all group analysis pipelines, for between-subject alignment. However, the type of registration used to align images from the same subject (with the same modality or different modalities) is different from the type used to align different subjects. For example, there is a type of registration called rigid-body registration (explained in Chapter 5) that can accurately align images from the same subject but is not sufficient to accurately align images from different subjects. As a result, you need to be familiar with different options for registration, both when doing your own analysis and when reading about other people's analyses.

Registration can also be used to quantify anatomical shape and volume, and hence to quantitatively analyze the anatomy. This process is based on registrations of individuals to a group template, where the crucial information about anatomy is obtained directly from the spatial transformations themselves rather than from other images that are transformed. For instance, if the location of the boundary of the hippocampus is known for the template (and digital atlases provide this kind of information), then the spatial transformation tells you where this boundary will be located in an individual subject's image. The spatial transformations contain geometric information about how each voxel is moved, and from that the amount of contraction or expansion of the structures or regions of interest can be calculated. This information can be used to calculate regional or total volumes of structures and represents one of the ways of quantifying anatomical differences.

More details about registration and its use in analysis pipelines can be found in Chapter 5.

3.2.3 Tissue-type segmentation

There are two main types of segmentation: tissue-type segmentation and structural segmentation. Both assign labels to different locations in an individual image on the basis of the anatomical content at that location. For tissue-type segmentation, the labels are normally gray matter, white matter, cerebrospinal fluid (CSF), or a mixture of these. For structural segmentation, the labels correspond to more specific anatomical structures, such as the hippocampus or the cerebral cortex, which will be covered in the next sections (3.2.4 and 3.2.5).

In tissue-type segmentation, most of the information about the tissue is derived from the intensities present in the image. This intensity information is usually taken from a single T_1-weighted image, but can be taken from a set of different modalities (which are already aligned). Either way, it is the intensity values that primarily determine whether a voxel contains white matter, gray matter, CSF, or some mixture. However, the problem is not as simple as setting some intensity thresholds; for example, labeling all voxels over some threshold as being white matter (e.g., in a T_1-weighted image where white matter is the brightest) does a very bad job at segmentation, regardless of how carefully a threshold is chosen. This is because there are two main complicating factors: noise and bias field.

Noise in MR images causes some voxels that actually contain white matter to have lower intensities and be confused with gray matter, and vice versa. So the intensity at a single voxel is not enough to reliably determine the tissue type at that voxel. If there were very little noise and no artifacts, then intensity alone would be enough; but unfortunately this is not the case. A common approach used to overcome this limitation is to use neighborhood information in addition to the intensity information. This method is based on the idea that a voxel of one tissue (e.g., white matter) is always near other voxels of white matter, as the tissue in the brain is connected and does not look like a set of isolated voxels. This is particularly useful, because the noise does not share this characteristic—a particularly high value of noise is unlikely to sit next to another, similarly high value; it is actually more likely to be isolated and surrounded by different, smaller values. Hence the connectedness or smoothness of the biological tissue is quite different from that of the noise, and this can be used to fix segmentation errors that were made on the basis of intensity alone. For instance, if the intensity of a voxel matches that of white matter but all voxels surrounding this voxel have intensities matching gray matter, then it is more likely that this voxel actually contains gray matter and that noise has caused the intensity to be abnormal. Mathematically, this is often done using a Markov random field (you do not need to know anything about how this works), which requires a parameter that weights how important this neighborhood information is by comparison to the intensity information from that voxel. This parameter—which is sometimes called the MRF (Markov random field) parameter or the beta parameter—determines how well the segmentation method performs; and, although a default value is often provided, it is good practice to try different values on your own data in order to see which value works best. The reason for doing this is that the default parameter may work well for a particular range of spatial resolutions and noise levels (or, more importantly, contrast-to-noise ratios), but your images may not be in that range, especially given the fact that MRI acquisition techniques and hardware continue to improve over time.

The other major confound in tissue-type segmentation is the bias field, caused by RF inhomogeneities. This confound results in parts of the image being brighter or darker than they should be, depending on variations in the strength of the RF fields (both transmit and receive fields; see Figure 2.6). As the intensity information is crucial for determining the tissue type, uncorrected bias fields produce large areas of incorrect segmentation (e.g., white matter classified as gray matter in "darker" areas of a T_1-weighted image). However, estimating and correcting bias fields is difficult to do in isolation, as it is hard to separate out intensity differences due to different tissues from intensity differences due to the bias field. Consequently, the correction for bias field is often directly incorporated into the tissue-type segmentation method, so that the latter simultaneously (or iteratively) estimates both the tissue-type segmentation in each voxel and the bias field. Since the bias field is relatively smooth (it changes slowly with position) but the tissue boundaries are sharp, these can be separated successfully through automated methods. An adjustable parameter often exists that specifies the amount of smoothness expected in the bias field (which is less smooth when using higher field scanners or head coil arrays that contain more coils). Note that, although this type of combined segmentation and bias-field correction method is common, it is not the only possible approach; separate bias-field correction methods also exist.

In the description so far we have only considered a voxel containing one type of tissue. In practice, many voxels contain a mixture of tissues; and tissue-type segmentation methods explicitly model this situation by using *partial volume models*. This procedure allows the segmentation method to estimate the proportion of each tissue within each voxel (e.g., a voxel may contain 80 percent gray matter and 20 percent white matter). The results, in the form of *partial volume estimates* (PVEs), are then saved as separate maps—for instance, one image for all the white matter PVEs, so that each voxel contains a value between 0 and 1 that represents the amount of white matter in that voxel (see bottom row of Figure 3.5). It is also possible to get a *hard segmentation*, where each voxel is assigned a discrete label—normally an integer (e.g., 1 for

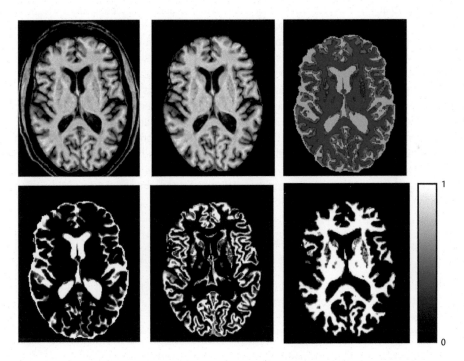

Figure 3.5: Illustration of tissue-type segmentation: original image (top left); brain-extracted and bias-field corrected (top middle); hard segmentation—CSF/GM/WM displayed as green/red/blue (top right); partial volume estimates (PVEs) in bottom row—CSF, GM, WM (left to right), with grayscale representing the partial volume fraction (0 to 1).

CSF, 2 for gray matter, and 3 for white matter: see top right of Figure 3.5). Hard-segmentation labels may be based on a model without partial volume or might represent the tissue type with the highest partial volume in that voxel. Both outputs (PVEs and hard segmentations or labels) have their uses, though when it comes to quantifying the volume of tissue PVEs have an advantage, as they represent mixtures of tissues more accurately.

An application of note that uses volume measurement is the analysis of whole-brain volume, which is of great interest in neurodegeneration, where it is used to quantify brain atrophy. This application is often based on tissue-type segmentation methods and can be analyzed at a group level by using nonimaging statistical packages, since the whole-brain volume is simply a single number per subject. It is also possible to perform voxelwise analyses of tissue volume, but this is typically done by using *voxel-based morphometry* (VBM) methods (see section 3.2.6), as these apply additional processes in order to gain extra sensitivity and statistical power.

So far we have described a common form of tissue-type segmentation method (illustrated further in the Example Box "Tissue-type segmentation"), but other methods exist—from subtle variants on this method to completely different approaches. Two variants that are worth mentioning here are methods that use prior tissue maps and methods that combine segmentation with registration. *Prior maps* are images of where various tissues are most likely to exist in the brain (e.g., gray matter is located predominantly around the edge of the brain and in a set of deep gray matter structures). These images store, in each voxel, a value that represents the (prior) probability of a given tissue being found at that location, and these priors are registered to the individual subject in order to provide extra information for the segmentation method. The trade-off when using prior maps is that, if the individual subject you are segmenting does not fit with the demographics of the population used for generating the prior map, then its use can bias your results. Conversely, not using prior maps can increase the chances of generating biologically implausible segmentations if the noise or the artifacts are strong enough.

The other variant worth noting is the combination of segmentation and registration. Such methods simultaneously perform registration to a template and/or prior maps as well as segmentation of the tissues, using the segmentation information to help the registration, and vice versa. The choice of what method to use will depend on how your subjects match the demographics associated with any prior maps, what methods are available in the software package that you use, and your assessment of the relative performance of the available options, which can be done during your piloting phase.

Example Box: **Tissue-type segmentation**

On the primer website you will find a structural image and instructions on how to run tissue-type segmentation to create partial volume estimates, a hard segmentation, and a bias-field-corrected image.

Tissue-type segmentation methods are usually limited to the dominant types of tissues (white matter, gray matter, and CSF) and do not model other tissues and structures, such as blood vessels or lesions. The number of distinct tissues modeled can often be changed by the user, which in principle allows the user to segment pathological tissues such as white matter lesions.

However, in practice tissue-type segmentation methods often rely on estimations of intensity distributions (histograms) for the different tissue types, and pathologies with a relatively small total volume are difficult to estimate in this way. Consequently, tissue-type segmentation results are often poor for focal pathologies, and alternative methods have been developed that are specifically tailored to that purpose (see Box 3.2). Specific segmentation methods also exist for particular anatomical structures, such as deep gray matter structures and the cortex. These methods are discussed next.

Box 3.2: Segmentation of pathological tissue

Specific segmentation methods are usually required for segmenting specific types of pathological tissue. For example, different methods exist for the segmentation of stroke lesions, age-related white matter hyperintensities, or cancerous tumors. Each case has its own distinctive characteristics and so methods tend to be specific to particular pathologies (e.g., for white matter hyperintensities, see Figure 3.6, but not for stroke lesions) and to particular imaging modalities (e.g., FLAIR or SWI), and often do not generalize well. Such methods often employ training data (manually defined labels) in a set of separate images of the pathology of interest, so that the method can learn to identify the characteristics of that pathology. When the characteristics are similar in different cases (e.g., white matter lesions in multiple sclerosis and age-related white matter hyperintensities), then segmentation tools can generalize to some degree, though pathology-specific methods often still have an advantage (e.g., by being able to use information about the most common locations for the pathologies).

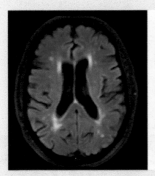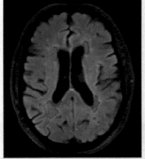

Figure 3.6: Illustration of the segmentation of white matter pathologies (age-related white matter hyperintensities in this case) using a method tailored for this purpose: original FLAIR image (left) and segmentation results in red (right).

3.2.4 Deep gray matter structure segmentation and shape modeling

The segmentation of deep gray matter structures (such as the hippocampus, thalamus or putamen) requires more information than just voxel intensities and neighborhood relationships. It requires some form of anatomical knowledge about where the structures are and what shapes they have. This information is often specified through a set of manually labeled images (see Figure 3.7) and can be used to build an explicit model of structural shape and appearance, or can be used with registration-based methods (see Chapter 5). Like all methods based on information derived from a separate set of individual subjects (e.g., methods using average templates), this one, too, should be used with caution for individual subjects who do not fit with the demographics of that set.

A variety of methods exist for modeling structures on the basis of voxels or on the basis of boundary meshes (i.e., sets of points, or *vertices*, on the boundary that are connected together like a net: see Figure 3.7). Either way, these methods use the information from the labeled images to determine what parts of the image correspond to the structure being segmented (e.g., the thalamus) and often have to deal with complicated and variable image contrasts across the boundary of the structure. For example, the lateral edge of the thalamus is difficult to determine from a T_1-weighted image and needs to use previous information about the expected shape of the thalamus (information that was provided by the labeled images) or information from other modalities.

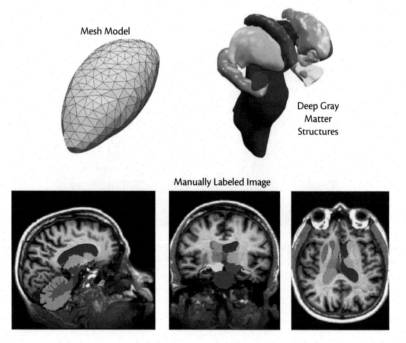

Mesh Model

Deep Gray Matter Structures

Manually Labeled Image

Figure 3.7: Illustration of a boundary mesh of a structure (top left), a set of structures (top right), and a manually labeled image (bottom row).

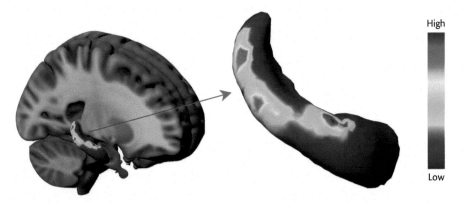

High

Low

Figure 3.8: Illustration of a vertexwise shape analysis of the hippocampus. The result (zoomed on the right) shows areas where the boundary position, and hence the shape, differ between two groups (controls and patients). Results are colored according to the statistics (as indicated by the colorbar); non-significant areas are colored in dark blue (bottom of the colorbar).

The output from these structural segmentation methods is in the form of a boundary mesh (set of coordinates), or a labeled image, or both (see the Example Box "Deep gray matter structure segmentation"). Boundary meshes have the theoretical advantage of being able to represent the position of boundaries more accurately, since the coordinates are not constrained by the image or voxel grid. However, in practice, true accuracy depends on many things. The labeled images, on the other hand, are more directly useful in many cases; for example, in defining regions of interest (ROIs) for other analyses such as seeding diffusion tractography.

In addition to specifying ROIs, the output from structural segmentation can be used directly, to investigate anatomical differences. This can be done either by measuring the volume of the structure in each individual and then doing group analyses on these volume measures, or by investigating differences in shape or boundary position. The volumetric analyses are simply performed by using standard (nonimaging) statistical tools, since there is a single number per subject. However, the shape analysis requires additional analysis steps, which are meant to calculate the statistics at each location (*vertexwise analysis*), or other shape representations (e.g., spherical harmonics). In either case, maps of areas that differ either between groups or in relation to a covariate of interest are generated and can be displayed (see Figure 3.8). This last step usually involves doing an image-based statistical test at the group level and therefore typically requires registration of the structures and the use of the GLM.

Example Box: **Deep gray matter structure segmentation**

On the primer website you will find a set of structural images from a single subject and instructions on how to segment some deep gray matter structures, such as the thalamus. Two tools will be discussed for this: one that uses only a single T_1-weighted image and one that uses a set of images to perform multimodal segmentation. In each case the outputs consist of volumetric and surface representations of the structures being segmented.

3.2.5 Cortical-surface modeling

Segmentation of the highly folded cortical surface is an even more challenging task and requires highly specialized tools; a well established and commonly used tool for this is the FreeSurfer package (see Further Reading). This segmentation is performed by fitting both inner and outer gray matter cortical surfaces (boundary meshes). In fact it is beneficial to fit the surfaces instead of working with voxels, as the former method is generally more accurate and also provides direct measurements of the geometry, such as cortical thickness and curvature (see Chapter 7, which covers cortical-surface analysis in more detail).

Many steps are involved in fitting the cortical surfaces. These steps are initially based on tissue-type segmentation and registration, but are followed by a lot of extra processing designed to ensure correct topology and to compensate for any errors in segmentation and registration. Since the cortex is relatively thin and highly folded, with some sulci containing only a very small amount of CSF, cortical-surface modeling is more sensitive to spatial resolution, CNR, and artifacts than many other methods. Therefore, if you want to do cortical-surface modeling, it is important to acquire high-quality structural images. Typically, T_1-weighted images alone are used, but use of additional modalities, such as T_2-weighted images, is advantageous and becoming more common; for example, this is what is done in the Human Connectome Project (HCP).

The output from cortical-surface modeling can be used directly, to quantify and analyze anatomical differences, especially cortical thickness, but is also useful in supporting analyses of other modalities. These include group-level analyses of data projected onto the surface (e.g., functional data) and registered through surface-based registration methods, which have advantages in enforcing gray matter to gray matter correspondences. More details on cortical-surface analysis and registration can be found in Chapter 7.

When working with cortical surfaces, it is possible, just as it is for surfaces of deep gray matter structures, to run, with the GLM, statistical analyses where data from each boundary point (vertex)—rather than from each voxel—are processed separately. This style of *vertexwise analysis* leads to results that are calculated on the surface and can be viewed directly on such surfaces (see the bottom right of Figure 3.9).

There are also two other varieties of surfaces that are normally available: inflated surfaces and flattened surfaces. These surfaces maintain a one-to-one relationship with the original (native) surfaces (i.e., for every point on the original surface there is a corresponding point on each of the other surfaces) but are deformed to allow for better visualization. The deformation acts in much the same way as taking a crumpled paper bag and blowing air into it: the bag will inflate and the overall surface will become smoother. This is the inflated surface. To continue the analogy, you could then flatten the bag by making some cuts down its side and by pressing it out flat on a table. This is the flattened surface. Figure 3.9 illustrates these surfaces. Their advantage is that they allow you to visualize everything that is on the surface at once; you will be able to see all locations, from the top of the gyri to the bottom of the sulci, and everything in between. This is different from looking at a folded 3D rendering of the native surface, where things are hidden in the depths of the sulci, or at a set of 2D cross-sections from a volumetric image, where it is hard to visualize how areas are connected between slices.

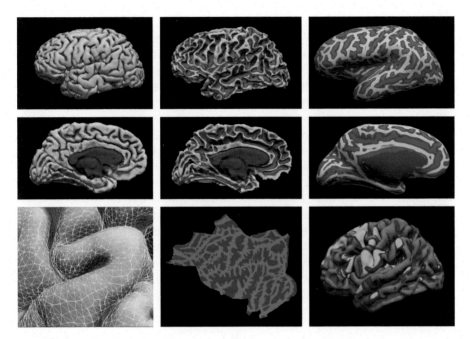

Figure 3.9: Illustration of cortical surfaces of the left hemisphere. First row is the lateral view. Second row is the medial view: outer gray matter, or pial, surface (left); inner gray matter, or white, surface (center); inflated surface (right). Third row shows zoomed inset with mesh representation: vertices, edges, and triangles (left); a flattened surface (center); and the statistical result of a vertexwise cortical thickness analysis (significant differences are shown in blue).

Allowing you to view data on surfaces is one way in which cortical-surface modeling is helpful in supporting analyses of other modalities. However, it is also possible to perform analyses more directly on the surface; and functional analyses benefit particularly from this method, since it allows more biological constraints to be applied in the processing (e.g., smoothing on the surface to avoid mixing signals between gray and white matter voxels) and vertexwise GLMs to reduce the degree of multiple comparison correction needed (see section 3.4 for more information on fMRI processing).

More details about cortical-surface modeling and its use in analysis can be found in Chapter 7.

3.2.6 Voxel-based morphometry

Another widely used tool for examining anatomical differences is *voxel-based morphometry* (VBM). This tool aims to find differences in the local amount of gray matter, either between groups or in relation to a covariate of interest—for example disability, disease severity, or neuropsychological test scores. The analysis that VBM performs is done in a voxelwise manner, and so it produces maps (3D images) of differences in local gray matter volume over the whole brain. There are many steps involved, but fundamentally VBM is based on combining tissue-type segmentation with nonlinear registration (flexible registration suitable for aligning images with different anatomical folding patterns; see Chapter 5) and accounting for imperfections in both.

The basic idea behind the most common form of VBM (we say "most common," because there are a number of variations) is to register each individual image to a template and to measure, in all voxels containing gray matter, the expansion or contraction of the local volume that is needed for the alignment. This is then combined with the local estimate of the gray matter volume from a tissue-type segmentation (see Figure 3.10). If the registration was perfect at aligning images, then the images obtained after the spatial transformation was applied would look virtually identical, and so all the useful information about the differences would be contained in the spatial transformation itself. That is why the local geometric expansion and contraction (known as the *Jacobian* or *Jacobian determinant*) is calculated from the spatial transformation. However, if the registration is not perfect (and it never is), then differences still exist in the intensities after spatial transformation, and this is what the segmentation captures (information related to intensity and contrast differences). Therefore combining this information—effectively multiplying the segmentation volume proportions by the volumetric expansion or contraction (a process called *modulation*)—takes into account both geometric and intensity information and accounts for some imperfections in the registration.

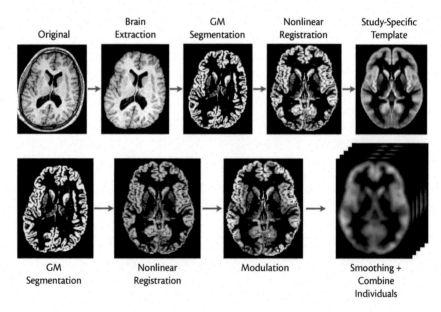

Figure 3.10: Illustration of the VBM processing pipeline (FSL version). First row: original image; brain extracted image; gray matter segmented image; image registered to a standard template; study-specific template (this is the average over some or all of the subjects in the study, each image going through the process depicted in this row, prior to averaging). Second row: the gray matter segmented images are then registered to the study-specific template; local gray matter volume in the common, template space (obtained with a modulation based on local volume expansion/contraction); smoothed local gray matter volume (one 3D image per subject, all combined together into a 4D image and ready for voxelwise analysis).

Another crucial element in VBM is smoothing. This smoothing or blurring of the segmentation proportions, after modulation by the expansion or contraction factor, achieves three things: it helps compensate for alignment errors still further; it makes the distribution of the noise more Gaussian; and it improves statistical sensitivity. The last point is important: smoothing effectively pools information from the local neighborhood, since it is just a weighted average over that neighborhood (see section 3.4.5 on spatial smoothing), and this reduces the noise and thus enhances any differences that are locally consistent. This effect is useful because we expect anatomical differences to be locally consistent, as they affect a region or part of an anatomical structure and not just a voxel here or there. However, smoothing also makes the quantity that is being tested hard to define biologically. Prior to smoothing we had an estimate of the gray matter volume in a voxel, but after smoothing that estimate becomes a weighted average of this over a local area. This value is therefore sensitive to changes in cortical thickness, local folding pattern, surface area and myelination, as well as registration and segmentation errors; hence care is needed in order to interpret the results correctly. These challenges of interpretation are part of a trade-off to gain statistical power, which is often worthwhile. In addition, the amount of smoothing is arbitrary, and this is one of the things that a user needs to choose on the basis of literature, spatial resolution, and the expected size of the regions that are changing. Best practice in VBM is difficult to find, but looking at papers and software documentation can be helpful, with commonly used values being in the range of 7–12 mm for FWHM; see definition in section 3.4.5.

One other thing to note about many varieties of VBM is that the registrations are based on the segmentations (either just gray matter or gray matter and white matter) rather than the original images. This makes the registration insensitive to artifacts and pathologies outside the gray matter, so long as they do not affect the segmentation. Furthermore, methods often use a study-specific template that is created by averaging the gray matter segmentations from the group(s) under study, after they are initialized with a registration to a standard template. Use of such study-specific templates is very helpful for groups with substantial pathology, which is often the case in anatomical studies for clinical research.

3.2.7 Other structural analysis tools

Additional tools for analyzing structural images also exist, beyond what we have covered in this section. For instance, quantification of atrophy is another type of structural analysis that is commonly performed. This, together with lesion and structure segmentation, is often used in studying neurodegenerative diseases such as multiple sclerosis (MS) and Alzheimer's disease (AD). These analyses are commonly performed with *longitudinal* data, where each subject has two or more images taken, one at a baseline and others at specific follow-up times—for example, a baseline scan and a six-month follow-up scan. This procedure is particularly common in atrophy studies, in order to measure the within-subject change in brain volume. There is a whole range of analysis methods that are specifically tailored to longitudinal imaging studies. Although it is also possible to use more general approaches (often referred to as *cross-sectional* methods—which are methods developed for groups without longitudinal data), there are substantial benefits to using the specially tailored tools. For instance, longitudinal methods can take advantage of the fact that the baseline and follow-up images from a single subject share the same anatomy with relatively minor neurodegenerative changes, by comparison with the much larger differences in anatomy between individuals.

More details about the commonly used structural analysis methods of brain extraction, registration, and cortical-surface modeling can be found in Chapters 4, 5, and 7 respectively.

SUMMARY

- Brain extraction is useful for increasing the robustness of registration and other steps in the analysis pipeline.

- At some point in any pipeline a brain mask must be generated, although this is not always done at the beginning, together with brain extraction.

- Registration is a crucial part of all group analyses and plays a significant role in other types of structural analysis as well.

- Tissue-type segmentation aims to quantify the amount of different tissues (e.g., gray matter, white matter, and CSF) with partial volume estimates.

- Segmentation of lesions or other focal pathologies is usually done with separate, specific tools.

- Deep gray matter structure segmentation can be used for determining volume and shape differences in particular structures (e.g., hippocampus) as well as for defining regions of interest (ROIs) for use in other analysis pipelines.

- Cortical-surface modeling is a sophisticated technique and requires high-quality T_1-weighted images or an equivalent. It provides ways of making anatomical measurements, such as of cortical thickness. It also yields surface representations that are useful for the visualization and analysis of other data, such as fMRI.

- Voxel-based morphometry (VBM) typically combines tissue-type segmentation and registration as well as smoothing, in order to measure local gray matter volume and perform statistical tests that look for differences between groups or relationships with covariates of interest.

FURTHER READING

- Helms, G. (2016). Segmentation of human brain using structural MRI. *Magnetic Resonance Materials in Physics, Biology and Medicine, 29*(2), 111–124.
  - *Paper that gives an overview of the methods for tissue-type and structural segmentation, including many freely available methods.*
- Ridgway, G. R., Henley, S. M., Rohrer, J. D., Scahill, R. I., Warren, J. D., & Fox, N. C. (2008). Ten simple rules for reporting voxel-based morphometry studies. *Neuroimage, 40*(4), 1429–1435.
  - *Paper describing ways of running and reporting VBM analyses.*

- Ashburner, J., & Friston, K. J. (2000). Voxel-based morphometry: The methods. *Neuroimage*, 11(6), 805–821.
  - *Original paper on the VBM method.*
- Fischl, B. (2012). FreeSurfer. *Neuroimage, 62(2)*, 774–781.
  - *General paper giving an overview and history of the FreeSurfer software package (surfer.nmr. mgh.harvard.edu), which is used in surface-based analyses.*

3.3 Diffusion pipeline

The type of processing pipeline used for dMRI is very different from that used for structural MRI, which is due to the fact that there are many individual 3D volumes (images) in a dMRI dataset (a brief overview of the pipeline was presented in section 2.3.5). Furthermore, the fast imaging sequence (EPI) used to collect diffusion images and the strong, rapidly changing diffusion-encoding gradients that are employed, induce several substantial artifacts in diffusion images. As a consequence, many of the preprocessing stages in diffusion imaging aim to correct for these distortions.

3.3.1 Eddy-current correction

The eddy currents that are induced by the diffusion-encoding gradients cause large-scale geometric distortions in the images (as described in section 2.3.4 and illustrated in Figure 2.15). If these distortions are not corrected, a given voxel location will correspond to different anatomical points in different images (since the eddy currents vary with the diffusion encoding directions and hence will be different for each diffusion-weighted volume). The distortions are often modeled by linear transformations—such as scalings, skews (also known as shears), and translations (see Chapter 5 and Figures 5.1 and 5.2 for definitions of these terms). This model is an approximation of the true distortion, but a reasonably accurate one. Due to the linear nature of the transformations, registration-based solutions are common, although they need to be insensitive to the intensity changes between the images caused by the diffusion contrast. This, combined with the relatively low spatial resolution (by comparison to that of structural MRI), makes it challenging to get high accuracy from standard registration methods. However, more sophisticated methods also exist that use information from all the diffusion images and combine eddy-current correction with B_0-distortion correction or with motion correction or with both (see the Example Box "Correcting for distortions and artifacts in diffusion images").

3.3.2 B_0-distortion correction

Inhomogeneities in the B_0 field affect the local frequency of the hydrogen nuclei; this leads to errors in spatial location, and thus to geometric distortion. This distortion is much more localized than the distortions introduced by eddy currents and is not dependent on the diffusion-encoding directions. It mainly affects the inferior frontal and inferior temporal lobes, since these are the parts of the brain closest to the air-filled sinuses and air cells in the skull. As the distortion is highly dependent on the individual subject's anatomy and even on how clear that subject's sinuses were, correcting it requires extra, subject-specific information; the distortion is typically not well corrected by registration alone. This extra information comes either from a fieldmap acquisition (see Box 3.3) or from some phase-encode reversed $b = 0$ pairs (blip-up–blip-down scans). Both are quick to acquire (they take anywhere from 20 seconds to a couple of minutes) but make a huge difference to the ability to accurately correct distortions. This, in turn, improves the anatomical accuracy of the results, which is important for anatomical precision, especially in tractography. In dMRI studies it is often more convenient to acquire the extra $b = 0$ pairs, as some $b = 0$ scans need to be acquired anyway. Either $b = 0$ pairs or fieldmap images can then be used to correct the B_0 distortions in the diffusion images (and remember that B_0 is different from $b = 0$) by either registration-based methods (more details in Chapter 5) or specific methods that combine this correction with motion correction, with eddy-current correction, or with both.

Box 3.3: Fieldmap acquisitions

There are, currently, two main ways to acquire information about subject-specific B_0 inhomogeneities that can be used to correct the associated distortions. One is based on acquiring two undistorted gradient-echo images with different parameters (echo times) and then using the phase information to calculate the B_0 field at each voxel; this is the more traditional form of fieldmap and we will call it a gradient-echo fieldmap. The other involves acquiring two distorted images by using spin-echo EPI (same as the $b = 0$ diffusion images), but with opposite phase-encode directions; this is sometimes called either a blip-up–blip-down acquisition or a phase-encode reversed acquisition.

A gradient-echo fieldmap relies on the relationship between the B_0 field and the phase of the acquired signal, since the frequency of the signal is defined by the rate of change of phase, which is proportional to the B_0 field. Therefore, for each voxel, the difference between the phase in the two images is proportional to the B_0 field (in that voxel), multiplied by the difference in the echo times.

A phase-encode reversed acquisition relies on the distortion being equal and opposite in the two images and then uses a registration-based method to calculate the undistorted midpoint, given that the distortion occurs along the phase-encode direction. The amount that the registration must shift each voxel to the midpoint is equal to the distortion, and from this the B_0 field can also be calculated.

Either form of acquisition can be used to determine the B_0 field at each voxel, and the choice of which method to use is based on what is available on the scanner, the acquisition time, and how well available analysis methods work. It takes one to two minutes to acquire a gradient-echo fieldmap, as high resolution is not needed, while phase-encode reversed fieldmap images can be acquired in less than a minute. Both fieldmaps provide a good way to correct for B_0-distortions; more details can be found in Chapter 6.

3.3.3 Motion correction

There is always some movement of the head during any scan; and even small motions can cause problems. Movements that are smaller than a voxel in size (subvoxel motions) are problematic because of partial volume changes. For example, at the edge of the cortex a voxel may contain 50 percent gray matter and 50 percent white matter, but that could easily change to 100 percent gray matter or 100 percent white matter by a shift of only half a voxel. However, we are often trying to analyze signal changes that themselves can be quite small, so even movements of 10 percent or 1 percent of a voxel can introduce changes of similar magnitude in the image intensity; hence it is important to correct for these effects.

One method for correcting motion is to use a special acquisition technique called *prospective motion correction*, which in turn uses modified MRI sequences or customized hardware (or both) to measure the motion in real time and to correct for it during the scanning. This can be particularly valuable when scanning subjects that are likely to move substantially in the scanner. The accuracy of these methods varies with the specific technique and installation, and the methods often remove large motions well but do not fully correct for smaller motions.

Another method for correcting motion consists of a step in the analysis that is called *(retrospective) motion correction* and is run on the images after they have been acquired. This step estimates the amount of head motion between the different 3D images in a 4D acquisition (such as used for dMRI) and corrects for it by realigning each image in the series to a consistent orientation and location. This is achieved through registration methods and can be used on its own or in combination with prospective motion correction methods, to further improve the accuracy. More details about motion correction will be discussed in Chapter 6.

3.3.4 Combined corrections

Unfortunately the different types of distortions—due to eddy currents, B_0 inhomogeneities, and head motion—all interact, and hence correcting for each one individually will not fully correct for all the distortions. In addition, there are slice-by-motion effects (see sections 3.4.3 and 6.1.2). The order in which the individual tools are applied can help to get better corrections, depending on the relative strengths of the distortions, but all serial combinations (i.e., applying one after another) are limited and the best solution is to have a tool that combines the corrections together, simultaneously. Such methods are starting to become available and have been shown to provide considerable extra benefit, although individual tools and serial corrections are still the ones most commonly used.

Example Box: **Correcting for distortions and artifacts in diffusion images**

On the primer website you will find instructions on how different artifact correction methods are applied in diffusion analysis; and you will be able to view the results. This will demonstrate the ability of these methods to correct the artifacts; it will also emphasize the importance of acquiring data that support these methods, such as phase-encoding reversed b = 0 pairs or fieldmaps, and of having diffusion-encoding directions distributed over a full sphere.

3.3.5 Diffusion tensor fitting

The diffusion tensor is a simple mathematical model for the relationship between the direction and the amount of diffusion. It assumes that the diffusion in different directions can be modeled using a spatial Gaussian probability, often visualized by an ellipsoid, and this is a reasonably accurate description of the expected diffusion of the water molecules when a single fiber bundle is present in the voxel (see Figure 3.11). The orientation of the long axis of the ellipsoid provides an estimate of the direction of the fiber, and the relative width (along the other axes) provides information about how hindered or free the diffusion is. Width changes can reflect more CSF, less dense packing, large diameter axons, sparse or poor myelination, or more than one fiber crossing or kissing within the voxel.

Fitting the diffusion tensor to the intensity data, which is done separately for each voxel, provides quantitative estimates that can be related to this ellipsoid (see Box 3.4)—that is, the orientation of the long axis, the length of the long axis, and the lengths of the other two axes. These quantities are also known as the principal eigenvector (orientation of the long axis) and eigenvalues (the lengths along the three main axes of the ellipsoid). From these, a

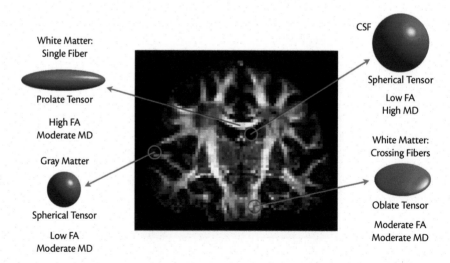

Figure 3.11: Diffusion tensor ellipsoids in different tissues: the background image is an FA image where white matter is bright for single fibers (corresponding to an elongated, or prolate, tensor) and darker in areas of crossing fibers (corresponding to an oblate or disc-like tensor). Gray matter and CSF have equal diffusion in all directions (corresponding to spherical tensors), hence they look identically dark on an FA image but can be distinguished on an MD image (see Figure 3.12).

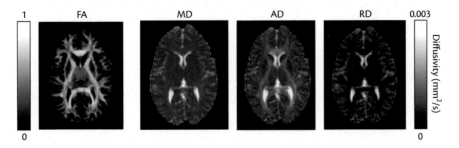

Figure 3.12: Illustration of quantitative diffusion tensor imaging metrics: FA, MD, AD, RD (left to right). FA most clearly distinguishes white matter from other tissues and highlights variations within white matter, whereas the MD most clearly distinguishes CSF from other tissues. AD and RD show some contrast between all tissues. Units for MD, AD, and RD are mm²/s, while FA is dimensionless (see colorbars).

number of standard diffusion metrics are calculated (see Figure 3.12), the main ones being the following:

- MD (mean diffusivity)—the average of the diffusion over all directions;
- FA (fractional anisotropy)—the variance of the diffusion over the main directions (normalized so that the values lie between 0 and 1, i.e., from very isotropic to very anisotropic);
- AD (axial diffusivity)—the amount of diffusion in the direction of the long axis (which is assumed to match the direction of the fiber bundle);
- RD (radial diffusivity)—the amount of diffusion perpendicular to the long axis;
- MO (mode)—which quantifies the type of shape of the ellipsoid (from -1 for planar to + 1 for tubular). See the Example Box "DTI" for illustrations with real data.

These diffusion metrics provide a description of the diffusion tensor that is often interpreted in terms of the underlying biology: for example, (i) low FA and high MD represent relatively unhindered diffusion, as in the CSF; (ii) low FA and moderate to low MD represent areas with hindered diffusion but not in any particular direction, such as in gray matter; (iii) high FA and moderate MD represent diffusion that is hindered predominantly in one direction, such as in white matter with a single fiber; and (iv) high to moderate FA, with moderate to low MD and a mode near -1 (planar), represents areas such as white matter, where there are crossing fibers or some complicated (but structured) fiber architecture.

Box 3.4: Diffusion tensor model

The diffusion signal is modelled by:

$$S = S_0 \exp\left(-b\, x^T D\, x\right)$$

where
b is the b-value of that image (which depends on aspects relating to the gradient strength and timing, and can take on different values for different images in multi-shell/HARDI acquisitions);

x is a column vector representing the direction of the diffusion encoding gradients (unit vector);

D is the diffusion tensor—a 3 by 3 symmetric matrix summarizing the diffusion behavior of water molecules;

S_0 is the signal intensity in the absence of diffusion.

From the sequence setup we already know the b-values and diffusion-encoding directions, and so it just remains to estimate S_0 and D from the acquired data. As the b = 0 scans can be averaged to give S_0, the diffusion tensor can then be obtained as a linear regression by using a rearranged equation:

$$b\, x^T D\, x = -\log(S / S_0)$$

where the tensor is formulated with the six independent elements of D as the unknowns, in a form:

$$M d = -\log(S / S_0)$$

where M is a matrix (collecting terms from b and x) and d is a vector (six independent elements from D).

From the diffusion tensor we can obtain the eigenvalues and eigenvectors; the principal eigenvector provides information about the direction of the axonal fiber bundle (as long as there is only one); and the mean of the eigenvalues is equal to the mean diffusivity, while a normalized form of the variance of the eigenvalues is equal to the fractional anisotropy.

The tensor metrics are very commonly used in the dMRI literature and provide useful, though indirect, information about the white matter microstructure. For example, changes in microstructure, such as axonal loss, lead to a reduction in diffusion restrictions and less directionality, with the corresponding changes being reduced FA and increased MD. However, other types of change, such as differences in axon diameter, could also lead to potentially similar differences in FA and MD. Thus it is not possible to determine the exact nature of the biological changes from the tensor quantities alone, though some interpretations are possible and they can help support or refute different hypotheses about the biology.

Example Box: DTI

On the primer website you will find a preprocessed diffusion dataset with instructions on how to fit the diffusion tensor and calculate quantities such as FA, MD, and so on. Examples include visualizing and interacting with the resulting images in order to demonstrate the relationship between these quantities and the original diffusion data.

3.3.6 Voxelwise and regional analysis

A group analysis of the diffusion tensor metrics, undertaken in order to investigate differences in tissue microstructure, can be done in a number of ways. The simplest way is to average the values over an ROI that is anatomically consistent across subjects, such as large regions of the white matter. Doing this gives a single value for each subject and these values are then easy to analyze in standard (nonimaging) statistical packages, such as SPSS or R. It is also possible to define ROIs directly from the diffusion data (e.g., by using tractography), but care must be taken not to generate ROIs influenced by the data that are being analyzed. For example, if FA is being analyzed, then FA or something correlated with it should not be used to define an ROI. If such a selection was used, then it would depend on the data themselves, and the statistics will be invalid due to the *circularity* of the selection process (e.g., if a region was selected on the grounds that it contained voxels with large FA values, then the average FA value must also be large, which is a bias).

An alternative method is to perform a voxelwise test, although this requires accurate anatomical alignment in the white matter. However, structural MR images are relatively featureless in the white matter and hence registrations using them alone are often inaccurate in areas of the deep white matter. It can therefore be better to use diffusion information to drive the registrations, as long as this done carefully in order to avoid circularity in the statistics. One method of achieving this is to align the images by using the *skeleton* of the major white matter tracts—that is, the voxels that lie at the center of the tracts, which is estimated by using the ridge of maximum FA within the tract (see Figure 3.13). Although this method uses the FA values to find the skeleton, it will still pick out a skeleton regardless of whether the FA values in a subject are unusually high or low. Hence the skeleton selection does not depend on the relative differences in FA values

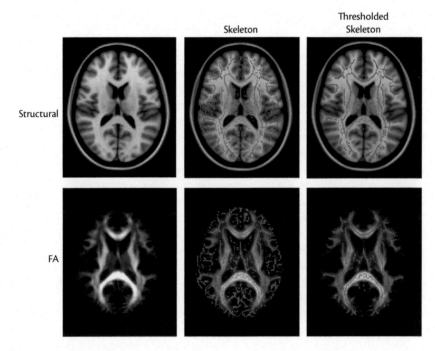

Figure 3.13: Illustration of white matter skeleton (e.g., as used in TBSS). Top row uses a structural image (MNI152) as the background, while the bottom row uses an FA template (FMRIB58) as the background. In each case the left column shows the template on its own, and the other columns show the skeleton from a TBSS analysis (in red) on top of the background image. The full skeleton is shown in the middle column and the skeleton after thresholding (which is designed to eliminate weaker, less reliably estimated tracts) is shown in the right column.

between subjects and, accordingly, does not create any bias related to group or covariate. It is also possible to analyze changes in other metrics besides FA, although FA is still used to define the skeleton. One method commonly used for this form of analysis is the tract-based spatial statistics (TBSS) tool (see the Example Box "TBSS"). Other alternatives for voxelwise analysis also exist, with different approaches to registration (see the references in the Further Reading section).

Example Box: **TBSS**

On the primer website you will find a preprocessed diffusion dataset with instructions on how to run part of a TBSS analysis and how to inspect the outputs, particularly the white matter skeleton and the values of FA that are projected onto that skeleton.

3.3.7 Tractography

Estimating anatomical connectivity requires the use of fiber orientation information obtained from dMRI, either through diffusion tensor models or alternative models. An example of an alternative model is the *ball and stick(s) model*, which represents one or more axonal fiber bundles in addition to an isotropic (free-water) component. This model explicitly accounts for the partial voluming in the signal by having a parameter that represents the proportion of free, isotropic diffusion (the ball) and parameters for the proportion and direction associated with each fiber (perfectly anisotropic diffusion; the sticks). Figure 3.14 illustrates this model for one and two fibers. The model-fitting process can also estimate the number of fibers that are present in each voxel, which is dependent on the quality of the data, since it is more difficult to estimate separate fiber directions with fewer data or with noisy data. This is why it is more important to acquire many directions (e.g., more than 60) when performing tractography, especially when tracing tracts through areas that contain crossing fibers.

Directional information (of the stick or sticks) can then be used in tractography to trace the path of the axonal bundles from voxel to voxel, following these estimated directions. That is, starting at an initial location, the tractography algorithm takes a small step (a voxel, at most) along the locally estimated direction, then uses the directional information in this new location to make another small step, and so on, tracing out a path step by step. The two main varieties of tractography algorithm, *deterministic tractography* and *probabilistic tractography*, are both based on this fundamental idea of local tracing but treat the directional information differently.

In deterministic tractography a single direction is used in each voxel to trace out a single curve (a *streamline*) from each starting point (the *seed point*). The streamlines are further constrained by extra information such as termination, exclusion, and waypoint conditions (see later). Using multiple seed points to create multiple streamlines then allows for a larger white matter tract to be built up and is often used to visualize tractography (see Figure 3.14).

In probabilistic tractography the noise in the signal and the finite amount of data are taken into account in estimating the uncertainty in the directions at each voxel. The tractography algorithm then takes a random sample of the direction at each step, using a distribution based on the local mean direction and its uncertainty. Due to the random nature of this

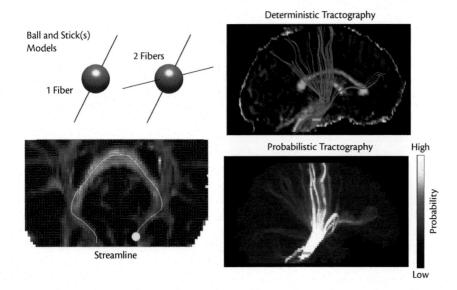

Figure 3.14: Top left: models used to represent the free diffusion (ball) and axonal tracts (sticks). Bottom left: single streamline (yellow) obtained by tracing from a seed point (yellow circle), from voxel to voxel, following the local diffusion direction (red). Top right: deterministic tractography result showing a small number of individual streamlines from selected seed points (shown in green). Bottom right: probabilistic tractography result showing a probability distribution of connectivity from the same seed points (in green).

Right hand figures from "Processing of diffusion MR images of the brain: From crossing fibres to distributed tractography," S. N. Sotiropoulos, PhD thesis, Univ. of Nottingham, 2010.

algorithm, two streamlines started from the same seed point would be different. By repeating this many times and by averaging these randomly sampled streamlines, a probability distribution for the connection from a particular starting point is generated. See Figure 3.14 for examples of both deterministic and probabilistic tractography results.

One consequence of the fact that probabilistic tractography takes into account the local uncertainty in direction is that the further from the seed point the tractography goes, the more these uncertainties accumulate over distance. This can lead to a form of probabilistic bias where short tracts have tighter distributions and higher probabilities than longer tracts, and so it can be difficult to compare probabilities between tracts and to threshold tracts consistently for generating ROIs. In addition, anatomical connectivity estimates (often represented as connectivity matrices between regions) also exhibit this bias.

Both varieties of tractography algorithm also use other information and constraints, such as termination masks (a streamline stops when it reaches any point in a termination mask); waypoint masks (only streamlines that pass through the waypoint mask are kept, others are thrown away); FA limits (to keep streamlines in the white matter); and curvature limits (to stop streamlines backtracking on themselves or switching between unrelated fibers). In order to generate anatomically correct tractography results it is common that some of these constraints and limits need to be customized; this prevents unrelated tracts, which often cross or pass nearby, from being tracked erroneously (see the Example Box "Tractography").

Example Box: **Tractography**

On the primer website you will find a preprocessed diffusion dataset suitable for tractography. The instructions will explain how to run tractography from a seed location of your choosing and will illustrate how exclusion and waypoint masks can help refine tractography results.

Another use of tractography is in performing connectivity-based segmentation. The idea behind this is to segment or parcellate areas of the brain on the basis of where they are more probably connected. A classic example is the parcellation of the thalamic nuclei (see Figure 3.15). This process starts with an ROI (mask) of the whole thalamus, obtained from a structural segmentation, and then takes each voxel of the thalamus in turn as a seed point. From each single voxel seed, probabilistic tractography is performed and the connectivity with a set of target masks in the cortex is calculated. The target masks used are normally large regions, such as the major cortical lobes. Connectivity with a target mask is calculated by summing the probabilities of the tractography result (normally stored in the form of an image) over all the voxels in the target mask. The label that is given to a seed point in the thalamus corresponds to the target mask that had the highest connectivity value, or maximum probability. In this way each point in the thalamus is given a label on the basis of its connectivity. This provides information that is completely complementary to that obtained from structural images, where typically there are no discernible features within the thalamus (see Figure 3.15a). Connectivity-based segmentations can be applied to any structures in the brain, provided that the tractography and ROI delineation are accurate.

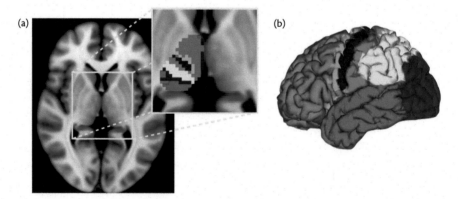

Figure 3.15: Connectivity-based segmentation of the thalamus: a structural image with the zoomed insert showing the parcellated left thalamus (panel a), where each voxel is labeled based on the cortical area (shown in panel b) that has the highest probability of connection with that voxel (with corresponding colors).

SUMMARY

- There are a number of preprocessing steps in the dMRI pipeline that can be used to correct for a range of artifacts such as eddy-current distortion, distortion due to B_0 inhomogeneities, and also head motion.

- Combined correction of all distortions has some advantages, due to the fact that they all interact, but serial correction is most common and can still work well.

- The diffusion tensor model can be fit to data to create surrogate measures of the white matter microstructure, such as FA, MD, and so on. This model is a simple approximation of the underlying diffusion signal and anatomy, and is very widely used.

- Voxelwise analysis of microstructural measures is complicated by the difficulty of aligning white matter anatomy tracts, since these do not show up on standard T_1-weighted structural images. Calculation of the white matter skeleton (the center of the tracts) is one approach used to perform alignment and voxelwise analysis of dMRI.

- Tractography is used to trace out long-range anatomical connections through the white matter tracts. It typically comes in two varieties: deterministic and probabilistic.

- Connectivity obtained from probabilistic tractography can be used to create a connectivity-based segmentation (or parcellation) of regions (e.g., the thalamus).

FURTHER READING

- Jones, D. K. (ed.) (2010). *Diffusion MRI*. Oxford University Press.
  - *A comprehensive textbook with many individual chapters, written by experts in the field and with variable amounts of technical detail.*

- Johansen-Berg, H., & Behrens, T. E. (eds.). (2013). *Diffusion MRI: From Quantitative Measurement to in vivo Neuroanatomy*. Academic Press.
  - *A comprehensive textbook with many individual chapters, written by experts in the field and with variable amounts of technical detail.*

- Le Bihan, D., & Johansen-Berg, H. (2012). Diffusion MRI at 25: Exploring brain tissue structure and function. *Neuroimage*, 61(2), 324–341.
  - *General overview paper on dMRI.*

- Smith, S. M., Jenkinson, M., Johansen-Berg, H., Rueckert, D., Nichols, T. E., Mackay, C. E., et al. (2006). Tract-based spatial statistics: Voxelwise analysis of multi-subject diffusion data. *Neuroimage*, 31(4), 1487–1505.
  - *Original paper describing TBSS—the skeleton-based voxelwise analysis of diffusion quantities, such as FA.*

- Johansen-Berg, H., & Rushworth, M. F. (2009). Using diffusion imaging to study human connectional anatomy. *Annual Review of Neuroscience*, 32, 75–94.
  - *A critical review of diffusion tractography and its application to the study of connectivity.*

- Behrens, T. E., Johansen-Berg, H., Woolrich, M. W., Smith, S. M., Wheeler-Kingshott, C. A., Boulby, P. A., et al. (2003). Non-invasive mapping of connections between human thalamus and cortex using diffusion imaging. *Nature neuroscience*, 6(7), 750–757.
  - *Original paper describing the use of tractography for in vivo parcellation of the thalamus.*
- Thesen, S., Heid, O., Mueller, E., & Schad, L. R. (2000). Prospective acquisition correction for head motion with image-based tracking for real-time fMRI. *Magnetic Resonance in Medicine*, 44(3), 457–465.
  - *Paper describing a variety of prospective motion correction methods.*

3.4 Functional pipeline (task and resting state fMRI)

The processing for fMRI is similar to the processing for dMRI, since they both acquire many 3D images and both typically use the EPI sequence. Consequently, the functional pipeline also starts with a set of preprocessing stages designed to correct for distortions, remove other artifacts, and improve the signal-to-noise ratio (SNR). These preprocessing stages are largely the same for task fMRI and for resting state fMRI, so we will present them in a general manner first and describe the more specific parts of the task and resting state pipelines afterwards. In this section the standard volumetric version of the pipeline for fMRI will be discussed, although surface-based analysis methods are increasingly being used. More information on surface-based methods can be found in Chapter 7.

3.4.1 B_0-distortion correction

Inhomogeneities in the B_0 field cause distortions for fMRI in the same way as for dMRI, since both fMRI and dMRI use the EPI sequence. However, the use of gradient-echo acquisitions for fMRI means that there is signal loss in regions with B_0 inhomogeneity, as well as distortions. The signal loss is a necessary consequence of making the image intensities sensitive to the BOLD effect (deoxyhemoglobin concentration), since the same physical mechanism is at work: a reduction in signal intensity in the presence of B_0 field inhomogeneities. In one case the source of the B_0 inhomogeneities is related to blood oxygenation, whereas in the other case the source is mainly due to the air-filled sinuses and air cells in the skull. Inhomogeneities due to these sinuses and air cells are much larger than those due to the BOLD effect, hence the signal loss is more substantial in the inferior frontal and inferior temporal regions of the brain.

Correction for the geometric distortion caused by B_0 inhomogeneities in fMRI can be applied in the processing pipeline just as in dMRI, and usually requires extra acquisitions that can measure the subject-specific B_0 distortions—that is, either specific gradient-echo fieldmap image(s) or spin-echo phase-encode reversed b = 0 pairs (blip-up–blip-down pairs).

One thing to be careful of, when acquiring fieldmaps or b = 0 pairs, is that the scanner does not *re-shim* at any point in between these and the main fMRI acquisition. Otherwise the B_0 field will change (which is what shimming does) and, if that happens, then the information needed to correct the distortions in the fMRI scans is no longer accurate, depending on how different the new shim is. Such re-shims can be triggered by changes in the field of view (FOV) of the scan or by other factors, so you need to be alert when scanning and try to prevent them from happening. Problems with re-shimming also occur in dMRI scans, though this is less likely to happen if b = 0 pairs with the same resolution and voxel size are being acquired as part of a dMRI scan. If a re-shim does occur (in either fMRI or dMRI), then it is necessary to acquire a new fieldmap (or b = 0 pairs) to measure the new B_0 field.

Either type of acquisition, fieldmap or b = 0 pairs, should give accurate corrections of geometric distortion, provided that the images are of good quality. Both types of images are quick to acquire (they take between 20 seconds and a couple of minutes), and accurate distortion correction makes a huge difference to the alignment between subjects' datasets and, importantly, to the statistical power of the study. Therefore it is important to acquire these images in every fMRI study if you are using standard pipelines. Some fieldmap-free distortion correction approaches also exist, but they are less commonly available and typically more reliant on having fMRI data with higher resolution and contrast-to-noise ratio (CNR). More information on both forms of fieldmaps and their application in distortion correction can be found in Chapter 6.

Correcting distortion involves applying a spatial transformation to the image ("moving" the voxel within the image) and hence is related to registration. In fact, the analysis tools for correcting this distortion in fMRI are typically based on registration (see section 3.4.8 and Chapter 6), and differ from some of the options available for correction in dMRI, due to the signal loss in fMRI. This signal loss cannot be corrected or reversed in the preprocessing or analysis, as signal that is lost during the acquisition is really lost and can never be recovered. This is why it is important to modify your acquisition methods if you want to do fMRI studies that include the inferior frontal or inferior temporal areas. There are several options available in the acquisitions to restore signal in these areas, though there is normally a trade-off to be made in some way (increased distortions elsewhere, reduced temporal resolution, reduced SNR, etc.).

3.4.2 Motion correction

Head movement in the scanner, and the associated motion-induced changes in the images, are an even bigger problem in fMRI than in dMRI. This is largely because the changes in the signal due to the BOLD effect are quite weak (around 1 percent), whereas the changes in signal intensity that can be induced by motion are much larger, even for very small motions (e.g., a 10 percent intensity change can be induced by a movement as small as 10 percent of a voxel, due to partial volume changes, which could be a movement of 0.3 mm or less). Furthermore, it is more likely that the timing of the motion could match the timing of key features of the acquisition—particularly with task stimuli and stimulus-correlated motion—and this can be mistaken for neuronally induced signal, which may lead to false activations. This is why, when getting subjects to do a task, it is worth thinking about whether the task will cause the subject to move, either voluntarily or involuntarily.

In the same way as for dMRI, prospective motion correction (during the acquisition) and registration-based, retrospective motion correction (during the analysis) can be performed separately or together. Whether prospective motion correction is used or not, it is advisable to also apply the registration-based methods, which estimate the changes in orientation and position from the images and then realign them. The registration-based methods can achieve subvoxel accuracies, but unfortunately this does not eliminate all the effects of motion, as there are also some interactions with the physics of the acquisition that cause other changes in intensity (e.g., spin-history effects, varying B_0 distortions—see Box 3.5 if you are interested in more details). In fMRI there are also additional stages in the pipeline that are introduced to remove or clean up such signals, for example regressing-out motion parameters (estimates of translation and rotation) from the data, outlier detection and correction, and more general artifact removal methods (e.g., ICA-based cleanup). More details on motion correction and related methods can be found in section 6.1.

Box 3.5: Motion artifacts

There are many changes induced in the MRI signal as a result of motion. The most obvious change is spatial displacement (movement) in the image, but there are also changes in the signal intensity that spatial realignment or transformation does not compensate for. There are many causes of such changes; all are based on MR physics and two of them are specifically worth mentioning: spin history and varying B_0 distortions.

Spin history effects are caused when hydrogen nuclei (spins) move between different slices of the image. When this happens, the timing of the RF (excitation) pulses received by these nuclei departs from the regular pattern in the original slice and, as a consequence, their magnetization (and hence signal intensity) alters, purely due to the motion.

In addition, changes in orientation alter both the magnitude of the B_0 inhomogeneities (this is due to the varying angle between the B_0 field and the head) and the direction of the phase-encode axis with respect to the anatomy. Hence both the amount of the distortion and its direction change as the head moves.

For typical head movements, these effects are not large, but they can be problematic in comparison to the small changes in signals induced by diffusion or function.

3.4.3 Slice timing corrections

One acquisition detail that we skipped over in Chapter 2 was that many MRI acquisition methods, including EPI, acquire images a slice at a time (or possibly several slices at a time, if they use simultaneous multi-slice accelerations, e.g., multiband). The order in which slices are acquired is an acquisition option for most sequences on the scanner and it is common to see

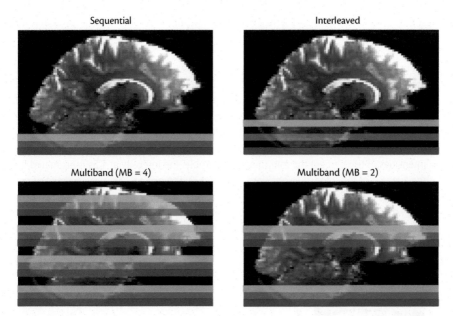

Figure 3.16: Illustration of different slice acquisition orders. For purposes of simplification, only the first three slices (or slice groups) acquired are shown here—the first in red, the second in blue, the third in green: (a) sequential (bottom-up) option; (b) interleaved (bottom-up) option; (c) multiband (MB = 4) option; (d) multiband (MB = 2) option. Multiband acquires more than one slice at a time, the number being given by the multiband factor, MB. For the interleaved option all odd-numbered slices (1, 3, 5, 7, etc.) are acquired first and the even slices (2, 4, 6, 8, etc.) are acquired afterwards. Equivalent top-down versions of all of these options also exist.

sequential, interleaved, or grouped orders (groups for simultaneous multi-slice accelerations), going either bottom up or top down; see Figure 3.16. There are some trade-offs involved in these choices, often relating to MR physics effects at the fringes where overlap exists between slices. However, all of these acquisitions are quite common in practice.

The fact that slices are not acquired all at once means that the time at which the dynamic BOLD signal is captured is not the same in different slices. It is therefore important to match the timing of any model or comparison data (e.g., timeseries from a remote voxel or region) with the timing of the data in the voxel being analyzed. There are two main options to correct for this mismatch in timing: shifting the data (called *slice-timing correction*) and shifting the model.

Slice-timing correction is a method of shifting the data to make them as if they were all collected at a fixed set of times, which are the same across the whole image. This involves choosing a reference timing, which is normally set to be halfway through the acquisition of each image, as this minimizes the average amount of shifting required. Once the reference timing is known, the data at each voxel are shifted in time according to the difference in their acquisition times (set by the slice they are in) and the reference times. An example of this is given in the Example Box "Slice timing effects and corrections."

Example Box: **Slice timing effects and corrections**

Let us consider a specific example of slice timing. If a volume takes 3 seconds to acquire, the reference timings would be at 1.5s, 4.5s, 7.5s, etc., but a voxel in the first slice would have acquisition times of 0s, 3s, 6s, etc. Performing slice-timing correction would create a set of intensities for that voxel that was shifted in time, to estimate what the intensities would have been in that voxel if the acquisition times were 1.5s, 4.5s, and so on. A simple way to do this for our example voxel would be to just average each pair of intensities in time, to get the midpoint: for example, the intensity at 1.5s is estimated by the average of the intensities acquired at 0s and 3s; the one at 4.5s is the average of the ones acquired at 3s and 6s, and so on. This is an example of linear interpolation, which is one way of performing slice-timing correction, although it is more common to use sinc interpolation, which is based on some nice mathematical properties. Either way, it is an

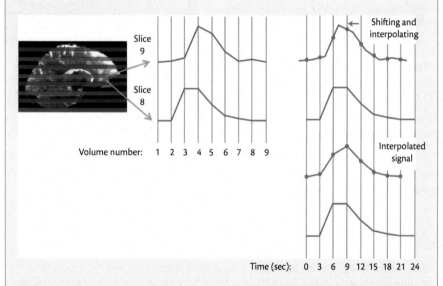

Figure 3.17: Illustration of slice-timing correction for an interleaved slice acquisition with TR = 3 seconds. Left: slice 8 for this example is chosen, arbitrarily, as the reference slice (the first acquisition in this slice defines t = 0). The true acquisition times in slice 9 precede slice 8 by nearly 1.5 (as odd slices are acquired before even slices). Middle: timeseries from a voxel in each slice, aligned so that each vertical green line represents data belonging to one 3D volume (e.g., in volume 3 the BOLD signal has not risen much when slice 9 is acquired, but slice 8 is acquired later, when the signal is higher). Note the obvious differences in the peak times, whereas the underlying activations happen at the same time. Right: a slice-timing correction is applied to shift the data in slice 9, by interpolation, in order to match the acquisition timing of slice 8 (the intermediate shift is illustrated at the top, the final result at the bottom). The green vertical lines now represent time, since the aim of the correction is to align all data to a common timing (the timing of slice 8). Note that the peak times are now much more similar but the shape of the timeseries in slice 9 has changed a little. Linear interpolation is used in this example, though sinc or spline are more commonly applied in practice.

interpolation process that is used to perform slice-timing correction, and it creates an approximation of what the intensities would have been if the acquisition time had not varied with the slice. Another example is shown in Figure 3.17 for an interleaved slice acquisition.

The alternative to shifting the data is to adjust the timing of the model so as to fit the actual acquisition timings. In task fMRI this is possible to do via the predicted responses that are used in the GLM, whereas in resting state fMRI the analysis uses the timeseries from other locations to define relationships, and therefore there is no external model that can be adjusted. Hence, for resting state data, the only option is to use slice-timing correction of the data to account for this effect, although this option is not always applied (especially in data with relatively high temporal resolution, e.g., TR < 2s), since the strongest resting state signals are very slowly changing (they have low frequency) and thus the effect of these timing changes is relatively small. For task fMRI there is also another alternative, which is to let the GLM itself estimate the timing differences, by introducing extra regressors (called *temporal derivatives*) that can effectively shift the model forwards or backwards in time, as needed, in order to get the best match. An advantage of this approach is that it can also compensate for other timing changes, such as those related to differences in the timing of the hemodynamic response. This is useful, as it is known that the hemodynamics have variations in timing that are similar in magnitude to the slice timing changes and exist between different brain regions, between different physiological states (e.g., caffeine levels), and between different subjects. However, estimating these timings can be inaccurate and the relative merits of this method versus slice-timing correction of the data directly are still debated; the results will vary with the different types of acquisitions and SNR levels.

3.4.4 Combined corrections

All of these processes—that is, B_0 distortions, head motion, and slice timing—actually interact with each other. It is not necessary for you to understand all the details about this, certainly not at this stage, but some examples might help you appreciate the nature of the problem. For example, when the head is moved, the relative orientation of the sinuses and air cells with the main B_0 field change, so the B_0 inhomogeneities in these areas change, and the distortion due to them also changes as the phase-encode direction (which is the direction along which all the B_0 distortions occur) will be oriented differently with respect to the head. Furthermore, if the head rotates during the acquisition of a volume, then the slices will no longer be perfectly parallel to each other; hence simple motion correction methods, which assume that the motion happens instantaneously and that slices stay parallel, become inaccurate to some degree (see Figure 3.18). The only way of accurately correcting for all of these effects is to have tools that simultaneously model and correct for them, and this is why combined corrections have an advantage over serial combinations (that is, one after the other), as the latter are only an approximation of the true combined correction. At present it is still common to apply individual corrections in a serial way (e.g., to do motion correction, then distortion correction, then slice-timing correction), but combined correction methods are starting to become available. Note

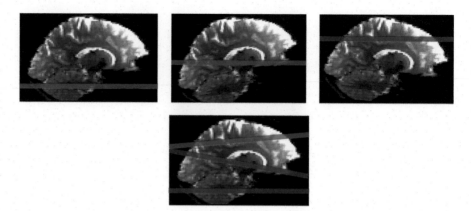

Figure 3.18: Illustration of the interaction of slice timing and motion. Top row shows the acquisition of three separate slices, from the point of view of the scanner, with changes in head orientation between the acquisitions (these changes are due to motion). Bottom row shows the same three slices from the point of view of brain anatomy. Rigid-body motion correction cannot realign these different slices correctly, as they are no longer parallel with each other and an acquired image built from such slices (not shown) would have significant anatomical distortions. For illustration purposes this example uses extremely large motions, which are not commonly seen in practice; hence the typical inaccuracies introduced by assuming parallel slices are often very small.

that, although serial corrections are an approximation, they are often a good approximation, so analyses done with them are both common and acceptable.

3.4.5 Spatial smoothing

A common step in the fMRI analysis pipeline, usually after distortion, motion, and slice-timing correction, is *spatial smoothing* (also known as *spatial filtering*). This involves blurring the fMRI data by calculating a locally weighted average of the intensities around each voxel, done separately at each point in time (see Figure 3.19). This may seem a very odd thing for us to do to data, given that we would like to have higher spatial resolution in our fMRI and this is actually making the effective resolution worse. However, there are two reasons for this step: (i) it improves SNR; and (ii) it allows us to use a method called Gaussian random field (GRF) theory in the later statistics. Of these, the first reason is the strongest in most cases.

Smoothing, which is implemented as a local weighted average (see Figure 3.19), is able to improve the SNR because averaging the noise will reduce its amplitude, whereas averaging the signal maintains the same value. This is helpful as long as the neighboring voxels (or vertices, if smoothing on the surface—see Chapter 7) contain signal of interest. Averaging with a voxel that contains no signal will reduce the SNR rather than increase it, since it will reduce the size of the signal even more than it reduces the noise. Therefore it is important not to smooth too much, and it is safer to use small amounts of smoothing.

The "amount" of smoothing that is done is a choice you must make when running an analysis. It is specified by the *full width at half maximum* (FWHM) in millimeters, which sets the size of the Gaussian used to calculate the weights for the local averaging (see Figure 3.19).

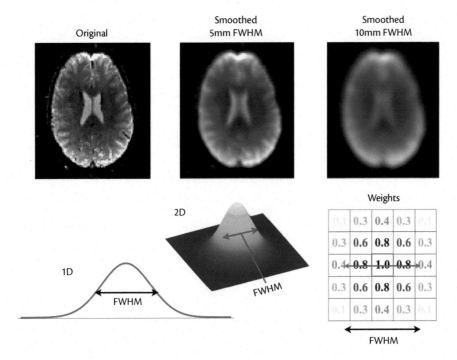

Figure 3.19: Illustration of spatial smoothing and weights. Top row: original image (left); smoothed image with FWHM = 5 mm (middle); smoothed image with FWHM = 10 mm (right). Bottom row: illustration of the FWHM for a Gaussian (i.e., the width at half the maximum height): 1D cross-section of a Gaussian (left); 2D Gaussian (middle); 2D cross-section of the weights associated with a discrete 3D Gaussian (right). In the discrete case the FWHM can be seen as the distance between where the weights would equal 0.5, if interpolated. In practice the smoothing is implemented discretely, by using these discrete weights to calculate a weighted average of the intensities of neighboring voxels.

If the SNR is very low or only large regions of activity are of interest, then using larger values for the FWHM can be beneficial for statistical power; but it comes at the expense of being insensitive to smaller regions of activity. As a consequence, small values of FWHM (e.g., 1.5–2 times the voxel size) are often preferred in order to get some SNR benefit without losing the ability to find small regions of activity.

The second reason for applying spatial smoothing is to be able to use GRF theory in the later statistics as a method of *multiple comparison correction*. Some smoothness in the data is essential for this method to work well, as GRF theory is based on an assumption that requires a minimum amount of smoothness. Partly due to this, and partly due to older low SNR acquisitions, larger amounts of smoothing used to be applied in fMRI analysis, whereas it is now becoming more common to use small amounts of smoothing or to skip this entirely. Since GRF is not the only method of doing multiple comparison correction, it is not necessary to use smoothing in order to perform this correction (although some form of multiple comparison correction must be done in order to have valid statistics). As smoothing also reduces the effective spatial resolution, limiting the ability to precisely localize the activations or functional networks of interest, smoothing is not always desirable and hence is not always applied. Whether to use smoothing or not is a decision you must make when doing the analysis, and this decision will depend on factors such as the data quality, the amount of statistical power required, and the desired spatial precision of the results.

3.4.6 Temporal filtering and physiological noise removal

Preprocessing steps aim to remove artifacts and artifactual signals wherever possible, and one way in which these can be distinguished from the neuronal signals of interest in fMRI is by their frequencies. Temporal filtering is a method that removes or suppresses signals on the basis of their frequencies. Since the neuronal signals of interest usually have frequencies in a relatively well-defined range, it is possible to separate and remove some of the artifactual signals that are outside of this range, for example, slow drifts.

Non-neuronal signals that are commonly found in fMRI data include scanner-related drifts and physiological effects. The drifts are very slowly changing signals that are often induced by hardware imperfections, such as changes in signal related to the heating of components within the scanner. Physiological effects arise from the subject and are mainly induced by cardiac and respiratory processes. For instance, cardiac pulsations and related pressure changes in the CSF cause some structures, such as the brainstem, to move. There are also inflow effects of blood during the cardiac cycle, as well as changes in oxygenation caused by the respiratory cycle, especially when the subject changes their breathing pattern (e.g., through changes in speed, or by going from shallow to deep breathing). In addition, respiration changes the amount of air in the chest cavity, and this can change the B_0 field throughout the torso and the head (including within the brain), producing geometric distortions that appear as spatial shifts of the head in the image.

Although the cardiac and respiratory cycles have quite well-defined frequencies (around 1Hz and 0.3Hz respectively), these frequencies are not well defined in typical fMRI data due to a phenomenon known as *aliasing*. This arises from the fact that we do not sample the signal particularly quickly (by comparison with breathing or heart rates), and only get a measurement at each voxel every few seconds. In order to avoid aliasing, it is necessary to get at least two samples per period of the time-varying process of interest, and that would mean having samples every 0.5s or more often, to avoid aliasing of the cardiac frequencies. It is very rare to use such a small repetition time (TR: time between volumes in fMRI or samples in the timeseries), as it reduces the SNR, although modern accelerated imaging methods now make it more feasible. If the requirement to avoiding aliasing is not met, the signal can appear to have a different frequency in the sampled data (see the Example Box "Aliasing of physiological signals").

Example Box: Aliasing of physiological signals

Imagine that we have fMRI data with a TR of 3 seconds and the subject's respiratory cycle is 2.95 seconds long. In this case, between each sample there is just over one full respiratory cycle, and is seen as a very small change per period, since we effectively move very slowly through the respiratory cycle—0.05 seconds difference in each period (see Figure 3.20); therefore

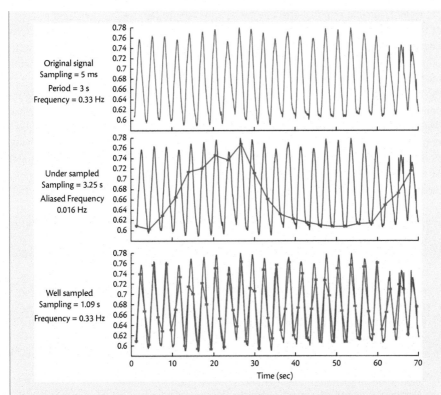

Figure 3.20: Illustration of aliasing. Upper panel: blue plot is a respiratory trace recorded with high temporal sampling (5 ms). Middle panel: undersampled version in red, showing how the aliased frequency is much lower due to the sampling period (3.25 s) being quite similar to the respiratory period (3 s). Lower panel: red plot is a version sampled at 1.09 s, which does not induce any aliasing (it is well sampled, meaning at least two samples per period).

this appears as a low frequency. The process can also go the other way and make signals seem to have relatively high frequencies instead (by comparison to the sampling frequency). Consequently, physiological signals can have frequencies in the fMRI data that appear at the high or low end of the sampled frequency range, or anywhere in between, depending on the extent of aliasing. This aliasing is in turn dependent on the relationship between the data sampling frequency (1/TR) and the real physiological frequencies.

Aliasing limits the ability of temporal filtering to cleanly remove these physiological signals and there are alternative methods for removing such signals; for instance, approaches such as retrospective image correction (RETROICOR) or physiological noise modeling (PNM). These methods require separate physiological recordings to be made during the scanning session— normally measurements from a pulse oximeter and respiratory bellows. The physiological measurements are then processed in order to generate predictive models of the MRI signal that would be induced. This usually involves the creation of a set of regressors in the GLM (see section 3.4.9 and the online appendix titled *Short Introduction to the General Linear*

Model for Neuroimaging) that are fit to the data in order to remove this signal, either as part of the statistical processing (which has some extra advantages in accounting naturally for degrees of freedom and for correlations with any stimulus-based regressors) or as a separate preprocessing stage. A set of regressors is needed in order to adjust for unknown parameters relating to the relative timing and nature of these effects in the brain by comparison to the peripheral recordings. These methods are hugely beneficial for studies investigating the brainstem, the spinal cord, or other inferior areas of the brain, as this is where both the cardiac and the respiratory signals (or physiological noise) are the worst. The benefits in the rest of the brain are much smaller, and these methods are not often applied in general task fMRI studies, although they do have some advantages, even in higher cortical areas. An example of the this method applied to real data is given in the Example Box "Physiological noise modeling."

Example Box: **Physiological noise modeling**

On the primer website you will find an fMRI dataset and a set of physiological recordings (pulse oximeter and respiratory bellows) along with instructions on how to process these data in order to make a set of regressors for modeling the physiological noise. These regressors are then fit to the fMRI data and the results are visualized to show where the cardiac and respiratory signals are present.

There is also another type of method for removing physiological noise, which is actually a general method of artifact removal: *ICA-based denoising*. This involves running ICA (independent component analysis) on the fMRI data, which decomposes the data into a set of sources or components (much like in principal component analysis or factor analysis). Each component consists of a spatial map (reflecting which voxels are associated with the component and how strongly) and a timecourse (reflecting how the signal changes over time for this component). If a component can be classified as being artifactual, physiological noise, or clearly not related to the neuronal signals of interest, then this component can be removed from the data, effectively "denoising" them. This classification needs to be done for each component, and there can be tens to hundreds of components, depending on the amount and quality of the data. Manual classification has traditionally been applied, but accurate automatic classification methods are now available and are increasingly being used. The automatic methods often require a training dataset where manual classification has been done, and so skills in manual classification are still required. Physiological noise is usually recognizable in components by the characteristic spatial patterns rather than by the timecourses, as aliasing stops the timecourses from containing predictable, recognizable frequencies. These methods are very commonly applied in resting state fMRI studies, due to the importance of removing confounding signals (see Figure 3.21 for an example of ICA components and classifications). More information on this processing and resting state analysis can be found in the Example Box "Independent component classification" and in the primer titled *Introduction to Resting State fMRI Functional Connectivity.*

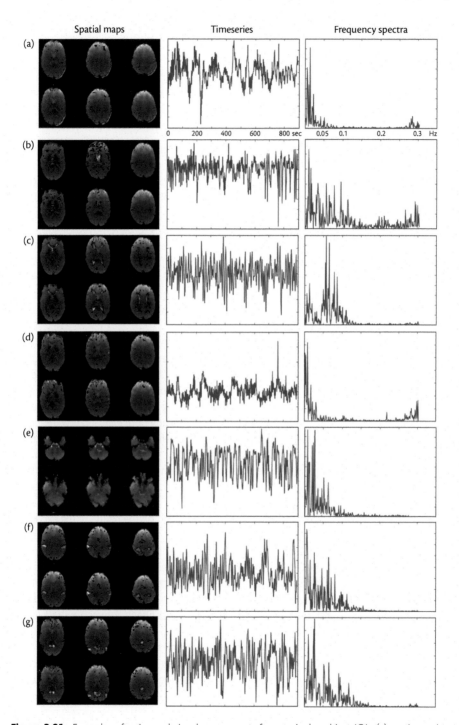

Figure 3.21: Examples of noise and signal components from a single-subject ICA: (a) motion noise component; (b) CSF noise component; (c) white matter noise component; (d) susceptibility motion noise component; (e) cardiac noise component; (f) motor signal component; (g) default mode network (DMN) signal component.

> *Example Box:* **Independent component classification**
>
> On the primer website you will find a resting state fMRI dataset and an example of an output from ICA that includes neuronal components, physiological noise components, and artifacts.

Physiological noise removal and ICA-based denoising are becoming increasingly common, but they are not always applied. *Temporal filtering*, on the other hand, is applied in almost all studies. It predominantly removes slow drifts (which can often be very large), although it is also capable of removing some artifacts, physiological noise, and other unstructured noise signals, depending on the degree of aliasing.

Temporal filtering works by selecting a set of frequencies to be removed or suppressed (i.e., reduce but not necessarily remove), while others are left as they were. Consequently, it is necessary to define which frequencies to leave and which to remove or suppress. However, due to aliasing, many artifactual and noisy signals will have frequencies that overlap with the neuronal (BOLD) signals of interest, and thus temporal filtering cannot remove all the noise, even when it was originally outside the frequency range of the predicted BOLD signals.

There are three main types of temporal filter that can be applied, and these are described by the frequencies they pass through, leaving them unchanged. They are *lowpass, highpass*, and *bandpass* filters (see Figure 3.22). Highpass filters let high frequencies pass and remove or suppress low frequencies. This type of filter is useful for removing the slow drifts in the signal. Lowpass filters work in the opposite way, removing or suppressing high frequencies. Bandpass filters combine the two by removing or suppressing both high and low frequencies but letting through frequencies in between. The precise definition of a high or low frequency depends on the user, who needs to set a cutoff frequency (or two, in the case of a bandpass filter) that divides the frequency range into low (below cutoff) and high (above cutoff). The frequency can also be specified as a cutoff period rather than as a frequency, since period = 1/frequency.

The type of filter to choose and the cutoff(s) for it depend on the nature of the experiment and on the data. For instance, in task fMRI the range of the frequencies of interest depends on stimulus timings, but it is also important to preserve enough high frequency information to measure the noise characteristics. Consequently, highpass filtering is almost always done, in order to remove slow drifts, but lowpass or bandpass are less commonly used. Tools exist to calculate appropriate cutoff frequencies (or periods), so that you avoid having filters that throw away useful signals. For resting state fMRI, a bandpass filter is sometimes used; and it is set to retain only the frequencies of the strongest neuronal signal fluctuations (e.g., 0.01–0.1 Hz). However, recent work has shown that there are useful resting state fluctuations in the higher frequencies, which suggests that highpass filtering may be more advantageous by virtue of retaining high-frequency information (depending on the relative SNR and on the overall quality of the data). These are good examples of the sort of decisions and trade-offs that need to be made when doing fMRI analysis.

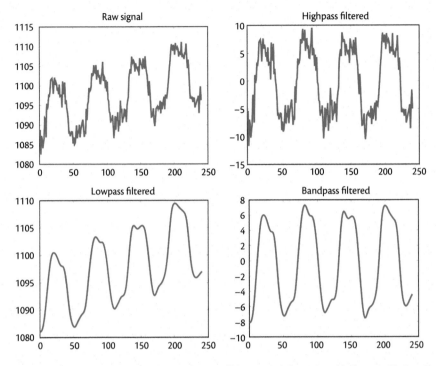

Figure 3.22: Examples of different types of temporal filtering. Top left: raw signal before any filtering. Top right: signal after highpass filtering, where the low frequencies (slow drifts) have been removed. Bottom left: signal after lowpass filtering, where the high frequencies have been removed. Bottom right: signal after bandpass filtering, which is a combination of highpass and lowpass filtering where both high and low frequencies are removed but the frequencies of interest are retained.

3.4.7 Intensity normalization

Another preprocessing step in fMRI is *intensity normalization*. There are two different types of it: through-time normalization and between-subject normalization. In the through-time version, the normalization aims to make the mean intensity over time constant, whereas in the between-subject version it aims to make the mean intensity over the entire 4D data from each subject consistent. The through-time version is a necessary step in the analysis of PET data (and early fMRI analyses followed the same steps as PET analyses), where the radioactive tracer decays over time, and hence the signal reduces throughout the experiment and the through-time intensity normalization restores it to a constant level over time, to make the analysis easier. However, modern MRI scanners produce very stable intensities (subject to some slow intensity drift, which is easily removed by temporal filtering), and so this form of intensity normalization is not needed. In fact it is not recommended for MRI, as it has the potential both to reduce the size of some changes of interest and to induce spurious changes. For example, the mean intensity over the brain can be influenced by large areas of activity, and applying through-time normalization will reduce changes in the truly active areas but will induce opposite changes in areas that were not active. Hence through-time intensity normalization is best avoided in MRI.

The between-subject version of intensity normalization, also called *grand mean scaling* or 4D normalization, is applied in all fMRI analysis pipelines, as it provides a way to compensate for a variety of changes between subjects that otherwise would reduce our statistical power. It rescales the entirety of a subject's dataset (multiplying each subject's data by a single number), so that the mean intensity, taken over all brain voxels and all points in time, is equal to some chosen, fixed value (e.g., 10,000). This is very different from through-time intensity normalization or other corrections like global signal regression, as the whole 4D dataset is just multiplied by a single value. The effect is that the overall mean (across all voxels and timepoints) is then consistent across all subjects, which compensates for a range of confounding factors, such as the arbitrary scaling of the intensities by the MRI scanner. The result is a reduction in between-subject (or between-session) variance, which improves statistical power at the group level. Unusually, this is a simple step in the analysis pipeline, which is always performed behind the scenes and does not require any choice of parameters or other user input.

3.4.8 Registration

As we discussed in the Group Analysis Box, registration is crucial for all group analyses, because it makes sure that the information at a voxel location corresponds to the same point in the anatomy for every subject. There is also a registration step that is needed within subject, namely to align the functional images to the structural image of that subject. Although this registration is always done, the resampling of the functional data can either happen at the beginning (transforming all the original images so that they align with a structural image or with a standard template) or after the statistics (transforming the statistical results so that they align with a structural image or with a standard template). The transformations involved are the same (i.e., the same amount of rotation, translation, etc.), but pipelines end up being a little different initially—often larger file sizes when doing registration first, but less interpolation of statistical values afterwards, versus simpler or direct overlays with the functional images (to see relationships with signal loss areas and distortions) when doing registration later. Either way leads to very similar results at the group level, and this is normally a decision made by the software developers and not something that you will have control over. However, it is good to be aware that such different approaches exist, especially when moving between software packages.

One important aspect of functional to structural registration that you do have control over is the use of fieldmaps to correct for distortion, as discussed in section 3.4.1. These are very important for improving the accuracy of the registration, which increases the statistical power in the group analysis. A complication of B_0-distortion in fMRI is the presence of signal loss. Although signal cannot be restored in the analysis, it is important for the correction methods to identify the signal loss areas; otherwise they can lead to very poor registrations. This is because registration methods expect that image structures will match well after alignment, but areas where there is signal loss in the fMRI will never match well with anatomical areas in the structural images, as the structural images do not suffer from noticeable signal loss. Signal loss is compensated for by masking out these areas from the registration, and therefore effectively ignoring them, in order to prevent them from biasing the registration. Even if the analysis is to be done on the cortical surface (see Chapter 7) and registrations between subjects are done on the surface, the registration of fMRI data to an individual structural image (needed in order to get the fMRI data on to the surface) will still be volumetric; hence this step is of vital importance. More details on the registration methods used for B_0-distortion correction can be found in section 6.2.

3.4.9 Task fMRI statistical analysis

The material up to this point has covered fMRI preprocessing, which is largely the same for both task and resting state fMRI. In this section we will move on to analysis that is specific to task fMRI and will give a very broad overview of the standard approach to statistical analysis. More information on the GLM and statistics can be found in the online appendix titled *Short Introduction to the General Linear Model for Neuroimaging*.

For task-fMRI, the GLM that models the relationship between the measured time-varying MRI signals and the response induced by the stimuli is known as the *first-level* model. Such a model is applied in each separate run or session (a run being one continuous acquisition, performed within a single session on the MRI scanner; in principle there can be several runs within each session). This first-level model is all that is required for a single-subject analysis, which shows how brain activity relates to the statistical hypothesis for that single subject only (see Figure 3.23). However, the vast majority of research studies scan a set of subjects (possibly with multiple runs or sessions per subject) in order to look for what is common across a group or population. A *group-level* analysis (also known as a *second-level* or *higher-level* analysis in this case) is used to combine first-level estimates of activation across subjects. This group-level analysis is also performed with the GLM.

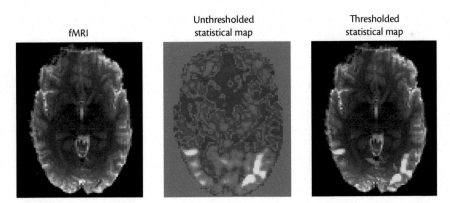

| fMRI | Unthresholded statistical map | Thresholded statistical map |

Figure 3.23: Illustration of a first-level analysis result. The image on the left shows a slice from one fMRI volume in the 4D series. An unthresholded statistical map (positive values in red–yellow and negative in blue) is shown in the middle and corresponds to a parameter map from the GLM (see Figure 3.24), while the thresholded statistical map is shown on the right. In the thresholded map only voxels where the statistical value was above the threshold (as determined by inference with multiple comparison correction) are shown in color, on top of the background image (in this case, the fMRI volume on the left). Note that, for group-level analysis, it is the unthresholded values that are fed up into the group-level GLM.

The first-level analysis works within the subject, on data from a single session, by analyzing changes in intensity with time. Using the GLM we can attempt to describe the timecourse in every voxel by a weighted sum of regressors (or EVs) whose weights we seek to determine from the data. Predicted responses to the stimulation (what the MRI signal is expected to look like if activity was present), are constructed using a model that incorporates the timing of the stimuli and the known properties of the hemodynamics—that is, the HRF (hemodynamic response function). The results of fitting the data with the GLM are estimates of the effect size for each regressor (the magnitude of the part of the signal that matches the predicted response) as well as estimates of the magnitude of the unexplained part of the signal—the *residual noise*. This information can be used immediately, to create maps (3D images) of statistically significant results after multiple comparison correction (see Figure 3.23); or the information can be passed up to the group-level analysis (see Figure 3.24 and the Group Analysis Box).

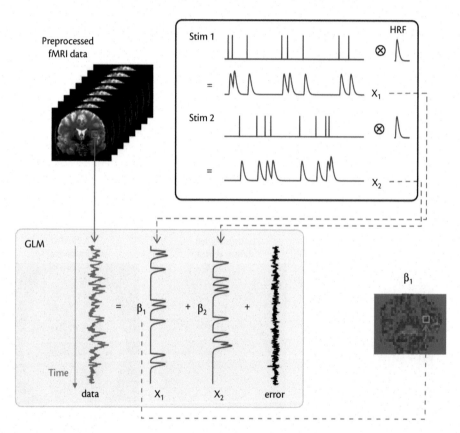

Figure 3.24: Illustration of a single-subject task fMRI analysis. Top left shows a set of fMRI volumes from a single subject, after preprocessing. Top right shows two stimulus timings (Stim1 and Stim2) corresponding to different types of stimulus, which are convolved with the HRF to form separate predicted responses (x_1 and x_2). Bottom left illustrates the GLM analysis that models the timeseries from each voxel separately. The timeseries is modeled by scaled versions of the set of predicted responses (and any additional covariates— none shown here), plus an error term. The scaling parameters (β_1 and β_2, also called "effect sizes") are determined by the GLM for each voxel and form the main outputs, as they indicate how strong the predicted responses were at each voxel; they are stored as maps (images) of effect size, and these can be further analyzed at the group level (across subjects; see the Group Analysis Box).

For task fMRI, the group-level analysis explicitly combines information from the first-level analyses (see the Example Box "Task fMRI data"), including the variations within each subject (the *within-subject* differences, which are related to measurement noise), with information about the differences between subjects (the *between-subject* differences, which are related to physiological and biological variation). The combination of the two sources of variability, within-subject and between-subject differences, makes a *mixed effects* analysis, which can test hypotheses that relate to the population as a whole. More specifically, a mixed-effects analysis can test hypotheses about the population that these subjects came from. For example, is it true that a positive activity in area X, in response to stimulus Y, would occur for any individual drawn from population Z? This contrasts with a *fixed-effects* analysis, which, by neglecting between-subject variation, can only test hypotheses about the specific set of individuals in the study. A mixed-effects analysis helps prevent individuals in the study with unusually strong (or weak) activations from biasing the results, since by including a measure of the variability between the subjects we take account of how consistent the results are likely to be across individuals in the wider population.

The values used as inputs for the group-level analysis, which are taken from the first-level analyses, are usually the estimated effect sizes and the noise (or, more precisely, the estimated variances of the effect sizes), but different software methods can use slightly different sets of quantities. These values are then analyzed again using a GLM, but this time the model is set up for a group-level analysis, each regressor (EV) modeling an effect across subjects (see the Group Analysis Box).

Example Box: **Task fMRI data**

On the primer website you will find an example task fMRI dataset, along with analysis results, that you can to explore if you wish to get some experience of what the data are like, what effect the preprocessing stages have, and how well the model fits. Full instructions on how to navigate through the different images and outputs are all given on the website.

3.4.10 Resting state fMRI statistical analysis

Following on from the preprocessing discussed previously, resting state pipelines often apply some extra preprocessing for more stringent denoising, and especially for removing potential motion-induced signals. This is because in resting state there is no external reference signal, and hence removing common confound signals (e.g., due to motion or other physiological processes or artifacts) from distant brain regions is crucial for preventing erroneous estimates of connectivity. After this additional denoising, a number of different analyses can be performed to investigate functional connectivity. Two commonly used examples of resting state analyses are seed-based correlation analysis and ICA.

In seed-based correlation analysis a timeseries is extracted from a region of interest and then correlated with the timeseries at all other voxels. This results in a map that shows the strength of the correlation of each part of the brain with the seed region (as was illustrated in Figure 2.20). A drawback of this method is that it is sensitive to the definition of the seed region, although it is a simple method to use.

Spatial maps   Timeseries   Frequency spectra

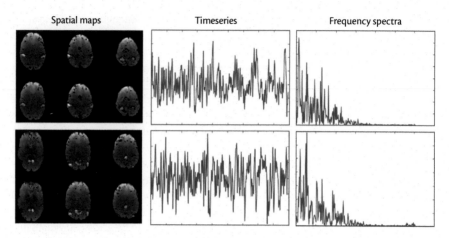

Figure 3.25: Illustration of two ICA components that represent neuronal networks of interest from a single subject: motor signal component, top row; default mode network (DMN), bottom row. The left column shows the thresholded spatial map (colored on top of a grayscale functional image). The middle column shows the timecourses of the components. The right column shows the power spectra of the timecourses.

In ICA, the dataset is decomposed into a set of sources or components, each one containing a spatial map and a timecourse. Components may be related either to neuronal signals or to artifacts. Values in the spatial map represent the amount of that component's timecourse that is present in the data from each voxel. If the component was neuronal in origin, then voxels with high values in the spatial map would be part of the network, since they would share a relatively large amount of that component's timecourse (see Figure 3.25). This is how ICA is used in decomposing the data into a set of resting state networks—see the Example Box "Resting state fMRI networks."

Example Box: **Resting state fMRI networks**

On the primer website you will find an example of a result from ICA that was run on a resting state fMRI dataset from a single subject. This example shows a set of components that include not only the interesting neuronal networks but also some artifacts, in order to help you see what ICA finds in the data.

One method for resting state statistical analysis at the group level is the dual-regression approach. This approach starts with a group-level spatial map of a network (e.g., derived from a group-level ICA) and then refines this spatial map to create subject-specific versions of it. These subject-specific spatial maps can then be analyzed using a GLM-based group-level statistical analysis, in the same way that effect sizes are analyzed in task fMRI. This allows for tests to be performed in order to see if there are differences in the local shape or strength of the network between, for example, patients and healthy controls.

An alternative to the voxelwise analysis of resting state data is the analysis of *network matrices*. These matrices store values that represent the strength of the connectivity (edges) between brain regions (nodes), with the size of the matrix being the number of regions by the number of regions. The matrices can be used in various ways; for example, by comparing edges directly, in group-level analyses, or by using graph theory or related techniques such as dynamic causal modeling (DCM). A drawback of these methods is their sensitivity to the definition of the specific nodes (regions) used, and even to which regions to include. However, the analysis of connectivity networks is of great interest and is an active area of research in neuroimaging.

Resting state fMRI is currently one of the most popular areas of MRI neuroimaging research, because it offers new ways of investigating normal and abnormal brain function as well as allowing functional imaging to be performed in subjects who cannot understand or perform tasks. Results in this field have shown that subtle differences in brain function can be detected, and it is hoped that these differences can inform models of healthy brain function, form the basis of biomarkers for disease, and lead to new understandings of disease mechanisms. We do not yet have a good understanding of neuronal networks and functional connectivity results from a biological or a psychological perspective, but the interpretation of the meaning of these networks is progressing, although much work still remains to be done; for more details see the primer titled *Introduction to Resting State fMRI Functional Connectivity*.

SUMMARY

- As in the dMRI pipeline, the first stages of the fMRI pipeline are devoted to the correction and compensation of artifacts (e.g., distortion and signal loss due to B_0-inhomogeneities, motion, slice-timing effects).

- Many artifacts interact and combined corrections, again, have advantages, although they are still not commonly available. Serial corrections offer an approximation to combined corrections that can be quite accurate for a lot of data (e.g., where the motion is not too severe).

- Spatial smoothing (or spatial filtering) is an optional step that can be used to increase SNR, but with a penalty of lowering the effective spatial resolution.

- Temporal filtering is most often used to remove low frequency drifts.

- Physiological noise cannot be removed with simple temporal filtering unless the temporal resolution is very high (TR < 0.5 s). Alternative physiological noise removal techniques exist; they are based either on separately acquired physiological measurements or on the use of data-driven methods, such as ICA, on the images directly.

- Intensity normalization between subjects is commonly applied by scaling all the data from one subject by a single value, in order to keep the overall mean value (across the brain and all points in time) consistent between subjects. Other forms of intensity normalization are not usually applied in fMRI.

- Task-based fMRI analysis applies a first-level GLM to the individual subject's data and then passes estimates up to a higher-level (group-level) GLM for group analysis.

■ Resting state fMRI can be analyzed in several ways: through seed-based correlations; through voxelwise, spatial network decompositions (with ICA); or through node-based network/graph analysis. These are applied after additional preprocessing, in order to stringently remove confounding signals (structured noise) that could affect estimates of connectivity between remote areas of the brain.

FURTHER READING

■ Bijsterbosch, J., Smith, S., & Beckmann, C. (2017). *Introduction to Resting State fMRI Functional Connectivity* (Oxford Neuroimaging Primers). Oxford University Press.
  ▪ *This primer provides an introduction to the acquisition, analysis, and interpretation of resting state fMRI.*

■ Huettel, S. A., Song, A. W., & McCarthy, G. (2014). *Functional magnetic resonance imaging* (3rd ed.). Sinauer Associates.
  ▪ *This is an accessible, introductory-level textbook, with more of a focus on the physics of acquisition as well as on functional physiology and task fMRI studies.*

■ Poldrack, R. A., Mumford, J. A., and Nichols, T. E. (2011). *Handbook of Functional MRI Data Analysis.* Cambridge University Press.
  ▪ *Generally accessible textbook, with many sections on preprocessing and statistics (including multiple comparisons correction) that are relevant to both task and resting state fMRI.*

■ Bandettini, P. A. (2012). Twenty years of functional MRI: The science and the stories. *NeuroImage, 62*(2), 575–588.
  ▪ *Paper introducing a special issue that covers many aspects of functional MRI acquisition and analysis.*

■ Amaro, E., Jr., & Barker, G. J. (2006). Study design in fMRI: Basic principles. *Brain and Cognition, 60*(3), 220–232.
  ▪ *General paper describing experimental design for task fMRI.*

■ Friston, K. J. (2011). Functional and effective connectivity: A review. *Brain Connectivity, 1*(1), 13–36.
  ▪ *A good review of the differences between functional and effective connectivity.*

■ Friston, K. J., Holmes, A. P., Worsley, K. J., Poline, J. P., Frith, C. D., & Frackowiak, R. S. (1994). Statistical parametric maps in functional imaging: A general linear approach. *Human Brain Mapping, 2*(4), 189–210.
  ▪ *An early paper describing the GLM approach to voxelwise fMRI.*

■ Birn, R. M. (2012). The role of physiological noise in resting-state functional connectivity. *NeuroImage, 62*(2), 864–870.
  ▪ *A review paper on physiological noise influences and removal from resting state fMRI data.*

■ Poldrack, R. A., Fletcher, P. C., Henson, R. N., Worsley, K. J., Brett, M., & Nichols, T. E. (2008). Guidelines for reporting an fMRI study. *NeuroImage, 40*(2), 409–414.
  ▪ *A paper that provides guidelines for reporting fMRI analysis results, with suggestions for best practice in analysis.*

- Cole, D. M., Smith, S. M., & Beckmann, C.F. (2010). Advances and pitfalls in the analysis and interpretation of resting-state FMRI data. *Frontiers in Systems Neuroscience*, 4, 8.
  - *This review paper provides summaries of many of the methods described in this chapter.*
- Beckmann, C.F. (2012). Modelling with independent components. *NeuroImage*, 62(2), 891–901.
  - *Review paper of ICA in neuroimaging.*

3.5 Perfusion pipeline

The perfusion pipeline is generally quite similar to the fMRI pipeline. As in BOLD fMRI, a set of images is acquired that are of a relatively low resolution by comparison to structural images and need some further processing to extract the information of interest. While for ASL we might perform a GLM analysis similar to that used in task fMRI to measure an effect size in response to a stimulus, it is more common to analyze perfusion data using a nonlinear kinetic model in order to extract quantitative (or semi-quantitative) measures of perfusion. The very different ways in which the two perfusion methods we met in Chapter 2 work lead to quite different issues of analysis. Thus, while the overall pipeline might look similar, some of the choices at each stage are different and we will consider them separately.

3.5.1 Arterial spin labeling

ASL can be used in a very similar way to the task-based BOLD experiments discussed in section 2.4.5, and its analysis can be done in an analogous way to that outlined in section 3.4.9. However, ASL is more often used to generate separate perfusion images from a subject under different conditions, including simply "at rest," or to compare different groups of individuals. We will consider this type of study here, with the note that all the preprocessing discussed here is pretty much identical to the preprocessing for a task-based design. More details of ASL analysis can be found in the primer titled *Introduction to Perfusion Quantification using Arterial Spin Labelling*.

Preprocessing

It is not unusual for ASL to use an EPI sequence, just as diffusion or fMRI methods do. Thus B_0-distortion is present in the ASL data and the same correction methods considered in section 3.4.1 are applicable. The correction typically requires either blip-up-blip-down pairs or a separate fieldmap acquisition. For the former, it is generally only the calibration image that is repeated, in the same way that the b = 0 images are repeated in diffusion. In practice, few studies have adopted this form of correction for ASL data to date, but this correction is likely to become more common as the tools for it become more widespread.

There is a further form of distortion correction that is sometimes used in ASL in addition to B_0-distortion. This is specifically associated with 3D ASL imaging sequences and seeks to address the blurring effect of the increased acquisition time for a full 3D image compared to a 2D slice, as discussed in section 2.5.1. The blurring occurs predominantly in one direction in the images, normally inferior–superior, and can be improved by using *deblurring*–a process that is very similar to the sharpening you might apply to a photo in your favorite photo editing package. The trade-off with this correction is that it amplifies the noise; thus some combination of a segmented acquisition (which reduces this effect) and deblurring is often preferable.

As in fMRI, motion is a problem for ASL, since we are interested in measuring a small signal change associated with the delivery of labeled blood-water. Motion artifacts can be quite prominent in ASL perfusion images because the first step in creating a perfusion-weighted image is the subtraction of adjacent label–control pairs. Motion will cause a mismatch between adjacent images across the whole of the brain and will thus appear in the perfusion image as artifactual signal. These artifacts will be more obvious in areas of high contrast between neighboring voxels, for example around the edge of the brain. This is why there are advantages to reducing both the static signal magnitude (i.e., the signal arising from the brain tissue, as opposed to the labeled blood-water) and the tissue contrast in the raw ASL images as much as possible. This is why background suppression is recommended.

It is possible to use registration-based methods to attempt to correct for motion between ASL images, applying such methods to the raw data before subtraction, in order to reduce the artifacts that arise from subtraction. The challenge in this approach is that, especially if we are using background suppression, the contrast in these images is poor and thus registration might not be robust or accurate. Additionally, the differences in contrast between pairs of images due to the labeled blood-water might get interpreted by the registration as motion; and the registration could then try to "correct" for it. Thus motion correction is not always applied to ASL data, and it is up to the experimenter to judge whether this might make things better or worse.

Slice timing is an issue for ASL when combined with EPI because the post-labeling delay (PLD) is greater for slices that are acquired later (normally the superior slices). This is relatively easy to correct as part of the quantification process, by accounting for the actual PLD of each slice within the kinetic model; hence other forms of slice timing correction used for fMRI are not normally applied to ASL. Spatial and temporal filtering are not routinely used with ASL data; the already low resolution of ASL means that people prefer to avoid further spatial filtering, except perhaps when combining perfusion images in a group study. Temporal filtering is often not needed for ASL, since the subtraction scheme employed removes the influence of slow drifts, which are a problem for BOLD fMRI.

Registration is also a common step for ASL data, both when the perfusion images are to be used in group studies and when some quantification processes are applied to an individual subject, for instance defining the location of the ventricles in order to use them as a reference for calibration. The process for ASL is largely the same as for BOLD fMRI (see Chapter 6), since both start with low-resolution data. In practice it is the perfusion-weighted image (after subtraction of label–control pairs) that has the best tissue contrast and should be used as a basis for registration, the raw data deliberately having minimal tissue contrast in order to control for motion artifacts.

Perfusion quantification

As we noted in section 2.5, the fundamental step used to generate a perfusion-weighted image from ASL is subtraction of the label and control images. If perfusion weighting is all that is

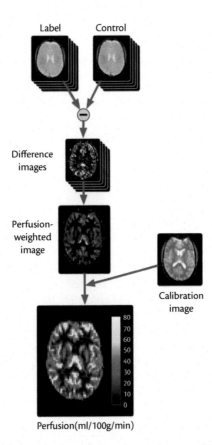

Label   Control

Difference
images

Perfusion-
weighted
image

Calibration
image

80
70
60
50
40
30
20
10
0

Perfusion(ml/100g/min)

Figure 3.26: The process of analysis of ASL data starts with subtracting all label–control pairs in order to create difference images. These can be averaged to produce a perfusion-weighted image. Subsequent kinetic modeling and calibration ultimately provide an image of absolute perfusion.

required, then the analysis can stop there. However, the appeal of ASL is in allowing you to get quantitative perfusion measurements in every voxel. The process for that follows three steps (see Figure 3.26):

- subtraction—the same as for the perfusion-weighted image;

- kinetic modeling—in which a (nonlinear) model is used to account for the relationship between the measured signal and the rate of labeled blood-water delivery, and therefore perfusion. This step includes correction for the decay of the label with time due to relaxation;

- calibration—normally a separate (proton density) image is used to estimate the relationship between signal intensity as measured by the scanner and the "concentration" of the labeled blood-water. Strictly speaking it is a measure of the magnetization of labeled blood-water that we want, as the tracer we use in ASL has been created by manipulating the magnetization of the water in blood.

The kinetic modeling step varies depending upon the form of the ASL data (e.g., pcASL versus pASL). It can be as simple as solving a mathematical equation in every voxel that includes known values of various parameters, as defined by the sequence or taken from the literature. However, for multiple postlabelling delay data, this process involves more complicated model-fitting techniques, with the bonus that other measures apart from perfusion can also be estimated at the same time. The calibration process can be as simple as dividing the perfusion-weighted image in each voxel by the value of the proton density-weighted image at the same voxel, but it might involve a process that seeks to estimate signal across all the voxels in a specific brain region, normally CSF or white matter, in order to get a less noisy calibration value.

Partial volume correction

As noted in section 2.5.1, partial volume effects (PVEs) have a substantial influence on perfusion images. The result is that the perfusion value in any given voxel will be modulated by the proportion of tissue within that voxel. The combination of low perfusion in white matter and the low SNR of ASL means that most applications of ASL focus on gray matter perfusion. However, at a typical ASL spatial resolution, very few voxels in the image contain pure gray matter, or even a high proportion of it (see Figure 3.27). This has an important implication for the analysis of perfusion data, where we want to report mean perfusion over all the gray matter in the brain or within a defined ROI: the value will depend upon what voxels are counted as representative of gray matter (the gray matter mask). Figure 3.27 illustrates this, showing the dependence of the calculated mean whole-brain gray matter perfusion value on the threshold applied to the gray matter partial volume in order to define the gray matter mask.

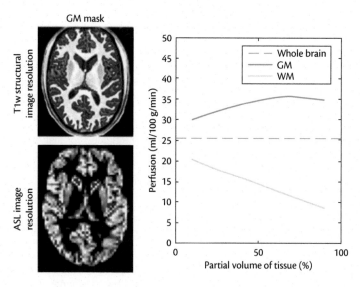

Figure 3.27: At a typical ASL resolution there are very few "pure" gray matter voxels. This is illustrated on the left by the comparison of a gray matter mask (blue voxels) based on a threshold of 90% gray matter partial volume using a T_1-weighted image of 1 mm resolution (top) and using an ASL-like resolution of 3 mm (bottom). On the right are shown mean whole-brain gray and white matter perfusion values from an ASL perfusion image, plotted as a function of the threshold used to define the tissue ROI.

Partial volume effects also have implications when you are trying to examine subtle changes in perfusion between groups of individuals—or even within the same individual, when subjected to some sort of intervention (e.g., a pharmacological study). Even if the alignment of the individuals to the template were perfect, the PVE would mean that corresponding voxels in different individuals still contain different proportions of gray matter, adding extra unwanted variability to the perfusion measurements and reducing the statistical power for detecting differences. Methods now exist to correct for PVE that have been developed specifically for ASL perfusion data, and they all make assumptions about either the relationship between gray matter and white matter perfusion or the spatial homogeneity of the perfusion maps. Correction for PVE is still an area of active research, but there is growing evidence that this is a process you should try on your data to examine whether PVE correction is important for your study.

Group analysis

Like BOLD fMRI task-based studies, the analysis of group effects from ASL perfusion data typically employs the GLM. Unlike in BOLD, where an effect size image from each subject is used as input for the group analysis, here it is perfusion images that are used. These images also have to be transformed into a common template space by using registration (see Chapters 5 and 6). An important question that the experimenter has to resolve is whether to use the quantitative perfusion maps from each subject directly or whether to "intensity" normalize each individual (e.g., the most common normalization involves division by the mean gray matter perfusion value in each subject). The former procedure would seem to be ideal, since it makes it possible to examine the absolute change in perfusion associated with any effect that is detected; it also allows for large-scale or even global changes in perfusion to be detected. However, it is well established that there is a lot of natural between-subject variability in perfusion, and this can reduce the statistical power for detecting subtle and localized differences or changes in it. Therefore it can be helpful to take the approach of intensity normalization, which is the only option in cases where calibration, for whatever reason, cannot be done.

3.5.2 Dynamic susceptibility contrast

Preprocessing

DSC typically acquires images by using an EPI sequence and thus suffers from the same B_0-distortions discussed in section 3.4.1. As a consequence, the same distortion correction methods can also be employed. Since it is normal to collect a number of images before the contrast agent reaches the brain (it is common to start scanning some time prior to injection), this is a good time to collect a blip-up–blip-down pair or other fieldmap acquisition. Motion correction is normally applied using registration-based methods and in theory should be more robust than BOLD or ASL, because DSC can normally be acquired at a higher resolution and the images contain better tissue contrast, both of which assist in the registration process. However, the contrast in the images varies over time, as the contrast agent passes through the vasculature and this can be problematic for registration-based motion correction, which can misinterpret the contrast changes as motion and try to "correct" for it.

Correction for differences in slice timing may be important for DSC, but the need for it depends somewhat on the subsequent quantification and on whether the quantification method can itself correct for timing effects. The good tissue contrast and resolution of DSC data lends itself to registration, and therefore DSC perfusion data work well for group studies. However, the experimental design is less flexible, since it is only possible to give a subject a single dose of contrast agent and this dose passes through the brain's vasculature too quickly to allow any further manipulation of the subject during the acquisition.

Perfusion quantification

The main analysis options open to the experimenter who uses DSC come at the quantification stage. There are numerous different ways to interpret the timeseries response seen in the DSC images, associated with the passage of the contrast agent. As noted in section 2.5.2, the DSC timeseries in a voxel starts at a baseline value, reduces during the passage of the contrast agent, and then returns to the baseline value; these changes are the result of the indirect effect of the contrast agent on the magnetic properties of the tissue. Thus a fundamental step in the analysis, which is almost always used, is the conversion of the observed signal change to a relative measure of contrast agent concentration. The relationship used for this conversion is an approximation and breaks down at very high concentrations, but the step is still widely used. Once the concentration versus time curve is available in each voxel, it is possible to extract a range of semi-quantitative metrics (e.g., area under the curve, time to peak). These capture features of the curve that in turn can be related to perfusion but are not direct measures of it. A problem with these metrics is that they can vary between individuals even when the perfusion does not, if the delivery of contrast agent in the arterial blood is different between subjects. These metrics are most commonly used for clinical purposes and are less suitable for neuroimaging research studies.

Robust, quantitative measurements of perfusion (or related parameters) from DSC require a measurement of the *arterial input function* (AIF). This is the concentration-versus-time signal of the contrast agent, as delivered by the arterial blood, to the voxel. In practice it is impossible to measure this signal for each voxel, but a good substitute is to measure it in a large artery. A lot of research effort has gone into accurate extraction of the AIF directly from DSC imaging data in order to overcome errors associated with arteries only partially filling a voxel (thus arterial signals are mixed with perfusion signals) and nonlinearities in signal response due to high concentrations of contrast agent. Different software tools may have their own automated methods for the extraction of AIF or may ask you to make your own manual selection. With a measurement of the AIF it is possible to derive a number of quantitative measures—the simplest being the cerebral blood volume (CBV), which is calculated from the ratio of the areas under the AIF and the concentration-versus-time curve in the voxel. Having an AIF also allows correction for timing differences between voxels (differences related to slice timing, but also differences in the time of arrival of the contrast agent in different areas of the brain). This permits quantitative timing metrics to be calculated, such as Tmax—the time to maximum signal. Finally, it is possible to combine the AIF and concentration-versus-time curve, using a process called deconvolution, in order to extract a relative measure of perfusion in the voxel.

Unlike in ASL, it is less common to see DSC studies reporting absolute perfusion. While it is possible to get a relative measure of perfusion by using deconvolution, the calibration process needed to get absolute perfusion is more challenging. Generally the correspondence between

DSC signal magnitude and the actual concentration of contrast agent is unknown, largely because the contrast agent has become mixed with the blood in the subject and thus its concentration is unknown. Other imaging methods, such as PET, have used arterial blood sampling to overcome this limitation, but this is not justifiable in many neuroimaging research studies.

One thing to be alert to when examining DSC perfusion data is that some of the measures that are regularly used, and certainly the interpretation of the metrics, often depend upon the fact that the contrast agent remains within the vasculature and does not accumulate in the tissue. This is generally true of the brain; but in some pathologies—particularly in tumours—this is not the case. The situation can become quite complex, as the contrast agent not only remains for longer, but also has a different magnetic effect on the measured signal once it is out of the blood and distributed in the extracellular space. Special care or analysis techniques are required in this situation if you are to get consistent, quantitative, and interpretable measurements.

SUMMARY

- Correction for distortion and motion is generally performed for perfusion imaging by using much the same methods as in BOLD fMRI.
- Particular artifacts can arise from ASL, for example artifacts due to motion and the label-control subtraction process.
- Motion correction of perfusion data using registration methods can be imperfect due to the changing contrast in the perfusion image timecourse.
- A perfusion-weighted image can be generated from ASL using label-control subtraction and averaging over the timecourse.
- Full perfusion quantification using ASL also requires kinetic model inversion (model fitting for multi-PLD ASL) and calibration.
- From DSC perfusion a wide range of semi-quantitative metrics, based on contrast arrival and passage through the microvasculature, can be simply derived.
- With an arterial input function (AIF), DSC data can be converted into a measure of arterial blood volume and mean transit time. With "deconvolution," a perfusion-weighted image can be obtained.
- Partial volume effects are noticeable in perfusion images due to the differences in perfusion between CSF, gray matter, and white matter. These are most problematic in ASL, which typically has a lower resolution than DSC perfusion.

FURTHER READING

- Chappell, M., MacIntosh, B., & Okell, T. (2017). *Introduction to Perfusion Quantification Using Arterial Spin Labelling* (Oxford Neuroimaging Primers). Oxford University Press.
  - *This primer provides an introduction to the acquisition and analysis of ASL perfusion MRI.*

■ Alsop, D. C., Detre, J. A., Golay, X., Günther, M., Hendrikse, J., Hernandez-Garcia, L., et al. (2015). Recommended implementation of arterial spin-labeled perfusion MRI for clinical applications: A consensus of the ISMRM perfusion study group and the European consortium for ASL in dementia. *Magnetic Resonance in Medicine*, 73(1), 102–116.

  ▪ *This ASL "white paper" or consensus paper (recommended reading in the previous chapter) gives a very good summary of the various ASL methods available and provides recommendations for a simple ASL protocol for routine clinical applications.*

■ Willats, L., & Calamante, F. (2012). The 39 steps: Evading error and deciphering the secrets for accurate dynamic susceptibility contrast MRI. *NMR in Biomedicine*, 26(8), 913–931.

  ▪ *This paper provides an overview of DSC analysis methods.*

■ Welker, K., Boxerman, J., Kalnin, A., Kaufmann, T., Shiroishi, M., Wintermark, M., American Society of Functional Neuroradiolgy, & MR Perfusion Standards and Practice Subcommittee of the ASFNR Clinical Practice Committee. (2015). ASFNR recommendations for clinical performance of MR dynamic susceptibility contrast perfusion imaging of the brain. *American Journal of Neuroradiology*, 36(6), E42–52.

  ▪ *This paper, although aimed primarily at clinical applications, summarizes consensus recommendations on acquisition and analysis of DSC perfusion MRI.*

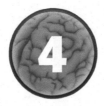

Brain Extraction

The purpose of *brain extraction* or *skull stripping* is to enable the analysis to focus on what we are interested in: the brain. By removing parts of the image relating to other structures, such as nose, ears, jaw, and so on, we reduce the chances of these nonbrain structures causing problems in some analysis steps. Furthermore, even when they do not cause problems, we avoid wasting time analyzing irrelevant portions of the image. Nonbrain structures are often most prominent in structural images, but we apply some form of brain extraction to functional and diffusion data too. In this chapter we will describe brain extraction, when it is used, how it relates to masking, what level of accuracy is required, and how to deal with difficulties. As this is the first chapter devoted to a single stage of the analysis pipeline, it will also outline some general principles that are true of most other analysis stages, such as evaluation of outputs, optimizing parameters, and troubleshooting.

One common problem that both cropping and brain extraction help avoid is registration failure caused by a mismatch in the coverage of the images (i.e., when one image contains a lot of structures outside the brain, such as the neck, and the other does not). This happens frequently when registering to the MNI template, as it has a very tight field of view (FOV)—that is, it is tightly cropped—whereas a lot of structural T_1-weighted images extend well below the brain and include the neck and sometimes the shoulders (see Figure 4.1). Although registration methods will sometimes work fine on these data as they are, applying reorientation, cropping (see section 3.1), and also brain extraction is often very helpful and increases the *robustness* of the whole analysis pipeline.

This rest of this chapter will present details about brain extraction. The aim is not to explain the details of how the method works but to enable you (a) to make the right choices about when and how best to use the method and (b) to understand what its limitations are.

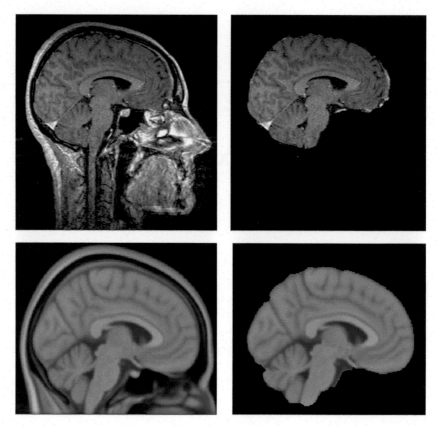

Figure 4.1: Illustration of brain extraction. Top row shows an image with a large coverage, going well down into the neck, both before (left) and after (right) brain extraction. The bottom row shows the MNI152 template before (left) and after (right) brain extraction. Note how the FOV of the image is much tighter with respect to the brain for the MNI152 template. We would generally recommend cropping as well as brain extraction for the image in the top row, so that the FOV better matched the MNI152.

4.1 When it is needed

In general, brain extraction is one of the very first steps in most analysis pipelines. Steps that often come before brain extraction include axis reorientation and cropping (see section 3.1), though these are not always needed or may be automatically done at the reconstruction or file conversion stages. Brain extraction, in some software tools, can also be subsumed within other steps (e.g., registration and segmentation). Here we will discuss the simpler variety, where brain extraction is a separate step near the start of the pipeline; but be aware that brain extraction or the generation of a brain mask occurs at some point in every analysis pipeline.

As brain extraction occurs very early in typical analysis pipelines, it is important for it to be highly robust and generic, so that it may work with a very wide range of image acquisitions and cope with common, expected artifacts. However, it is still possible for it to fail (see Figure 4.2), and it may need parameter settings to be tuned in order to produce acceptable results. Therefore it is very important for you to *look at your data*—and in this case we are talking about the data *after* the brain extraction is run—in order to assess whether the extraction has failed or not. This is an example of the general principle that you should be checking that each stage in your analysis has run correctly. Visual inspection is the most straightforward way to do this; it is able to detect the widest range of problems, as all sorts of things can go wrong, from algorithmic failures (e.g., some of the surrounding nonbrain tissues was not removed) to user error (e.g., the wrong image was used as input) and computer failure (e.g., the output is blank or corrupted). Depending on your application, this kind of check might just require a quick look to see that the extraction has not removed substantial portions of brain tissue or left behind large areas of nonbrain tissue. Alternatively, your application might require very accurate results, for example if the image would be subsequently used to quantify the volume of brain tissue. In that case much more careful scrutiny will be required in order to determine that no brain tissue was removed and that no nonbrain tissue of similar intensity to brain tissue is left; leaving cerebrospinal fluid (CSF) is normally fine. See the troubleshooting section (4.5) for information on what to do if something does go wrong and requires fixing.

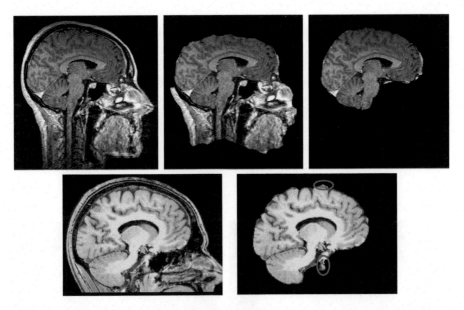

Figure 4.2: Illustration of brain extraction errors. The top row uses the same image as in Figure 4.1: original (left); obviously erroneous brain extraction (middle); good brain extraction (right). The bottom row shows a subtler example of brain extraction errors (right); by comparison to the original (left). These small errors are unlikely to affect rigid-body or affine registration but could be problematic for some between-subject registration methods and even more problematic for quantifying absolute tissue volumes using segmentation.

4.2 Skull stripping versus cortical modeling

There is a big difference between skull stripping (brain extraction) and cortical (surface) modeling. Skull stripping only aims to remove the main nonbrain structures and does not try to represent the fine detail of the cortical folds. Modeling the fine detail of the gray matter surface and separating the latter from the surrounding CSF is what cortical (surface) modeling aims to achieve. This is a much more difficult task and requires sophisticated analysis pipelines (see Chapter 7). What we are talking about here for brain extraction is much simpler (see Figure 4.3).

One consequence of not modeling all the fine details is that typically some of the CSF outside the brain will be left in the output image, although some of it will be removed. For the purposes of registration or segmentation, this is absolutely fine, but if you want to obtain a measure of *total intracranial volume* (TIV) it is not. Other methods exist to measure TIV or provide equivalent measurements (see section 4.4) for the purposes of "correcting for head-size," which is commonly done in many analyses. For example, it is known that the size of subcortical structures scales with the size of the head, so it is desirable to remove this head-size effect in order to more clearly study the relationship between subcortical structures and other variables of interest (such as disease duration).

In addition to the arbitrary amount of extracerebral CSF that is removed, there are also difficult areas that require arbitrary cutoffs; that is, the method must choose what to keep in the "brain" and what to remove. The two main areas where this applies are the optic nerves and the brainstem or spinal cord. Most brain extraction methods aim to exclude the eyes, but these are connected to the optic nerves that go directly into the brain, and hence they need to be cut off at some arbitrary point. This is worth keeping in mind when interpreting the results of anatomical studies, and you should be mindful of the fact that changes could be driven by the arbitrary amount of optic nerve that is excluded, as it can vary between subjects. Similarly, the brainstem and spinal cord are seamlessly connected, and a brain extraction method will make a cutoff at some point (see Figure 4.1).

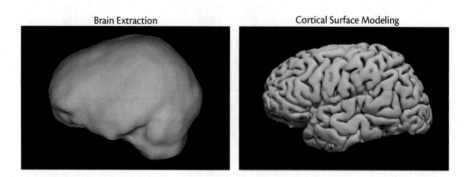

Brain Extraction   Cortical Surface Modeling

Figure 4.3: Example of the boundary surface used in brain extraction (left) versus the one used in cortical surface modeling (right). Note that the cerebellum is included in the brain-extracted case but not in the cortical surface model.

The scalp (including fatty tissue and muscle) is normally further from the brain in most subjects and is usually removed successfully. However, there are other tissues and structures that we do not want to be included in the brain extracted images and yet they are often present to some degree, such as bone marrow (in the skull), meninges (and other membranes), draining veins, and sinuses (spaces containing blood). Some of these tissues and structures are extremely difficult to differentiate from brain tissue on the basis of intensity in the structural images and also come very close to the surface of the brain (see Figure 4.4). One technique that can help distinguish these tissues is to apply *fat suppression* (also known as *fat saturation*) when acquiring the images, in order to reduce the intensity of signals from tissues containing fat (see Figure 4.4). Even partial fat suppression, which is sometimes easier to achieve, can be helpful; but either way it needs to be done at the acquisition stage, since it cannot normally be applied retrospectively.

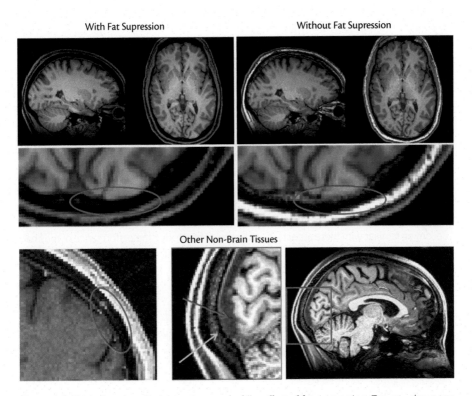

Figure 4.4: Examples of nonbrain structures and of the effect of fat suppression. Top row shows two slices from an image with (left) and without (right) fat suppression applied. The second row shows a zoomed-in portion from the axial images in the top row, illustrating how nonbrain material such as marrow is near to the brain and sometimes has a very similar intensity when no fat suppression is applied, which makes it difficult for brain extraction or segmentation methods to distinguish between these tissues. The bottom row shows further examples of membranes (left), marrow, and sagittal sinus (right, with zoomed portion in the middle; the blue arrow shows marrow and the red arrow shows blood in the sagittal sinus).

As already mentioned, the level of accuracy that is necessary for brain extraction depends on the application. For within-subject registration purposes, it is sufficient to remove the majority of the nonbrain tissues and tolerate small errors, such as nonbrain tissues left behind (e.g., some small portions of marrow or meninges and most of the sagittal sinus, all of which are common); the bottom row of Figure 4.2 shows an example of some of these kinds of errors. Even removing small amounts of brain tissue can be tolerated, provided that this operation does not exclude it from later analyses (see section 4.3). However, if your aim is to quantify the amount of brain tissue, then many of these errors would not be acceptable, especially the removal of true brain tissue. Whether leaving portions of nonbrain tissue behind matters for tissue quantification depends on whether the later segmentation stage (which defines the tissues) might mistake the nonbrain tissue for brain tissue or not. For CSF this is not a problem, but for tissues with intensities that are similar to those of gray matter or white matter it usually is. Thus extra care is needed when looking at the brain extraction results and when optimizing the method for this application. That being said, small brain extraction errors are relatively common, and some subsequent analysis tools or steps are explicitly written in such a way that they can correct for minor errors (e.g., some between-subject registration methods or atrophy calculation tools). You should find out if this is the case for the specific tools you will be using, as that will determine how accurate your brain extraction needs to be.

The specific way that a brain extraction method can be optimized depends on the individual tool being used (see the Example Box "Brain extraction"), but this optimization illustrates the common principle that all nontrivial analysis methods involve choices and have adjustable parameters. This is because they must be applied to a wide range of subjects (e.g., of different ages and species), pathologies, and acquisitions containing various artifacts. Default settings are usually provided, but it is good practice for brain extraction, or any other analysis step, to explore how changing some of the main parameters affects the results, especially the first time you use a tool or when you use it on different data. Occasionally you may find a tool where you do not have access to any parameter settings, but that is the exception rather than the rule. Becoming familiar with these aspects of analysis and monitoring the performance of the analysis methods as you go will reward you in the long run and will lead to better results.

Example Box: **Brain extraction**

On the primer website there are instructions on how to run brain extraction, visualize the outputs, explore different parameter choices, and critically examine the results.

4.3 Brain masks

The standard output from a brain extraction is an image where all the nonbrain voxels have had their intensity set to zero and the remaining (brain) voxels are left with their original intensity. This results in an image that looks like a brain surrounded by black (see Figure 4.1). Another output is a *binary mask* (or just a *mask*) that represents the valid brain voxels; that is, an image containing an intensity value of 1 at all voxels inside the brain and a value of 0 outside (see Figure 3.4). This can be obtained by *binarizing* the brain-extracted image (setting nonzero values to 1), or it can be a separate output created by the brain extraction method.

Binary masks are very common and useful in analysis pipelines, and not just for brain extraction. They can be used to define the regions where voxelwise operations should be performed (e.g., filtering or statistical tests) or the *regions of interest* (ROIs) for quantifying values of interest (mean diffusivity, functional activity, etc.) or for measuring volumes (e.g., of structures like the hippocampus). You will find binary masks generated and used in many analysis steps.

Whole-brain (binary) masks can also be used to generate a brain-extracted image from the original image, if needed. This is done by simply multiplying the original image with the mask (voxel by corresponding voxel). That is, each voxel intensity in the original image is multiplied either by 1 (if it is "in" the mask) or by 0 (if it is outside). This is useful because you can apply this mask to brain-extract another image and you can rely on it having exactly the same geometry and volume. Knowing that the brain extraction is consistent between images (i.e., has the same geometry and volume) is important, as this ensures that valid data are present in the same voxels and that all images can be treated equally.

Before you can apply one mask to another image you need to make sure that the two images are well aligned. Sometimes this is already the case (e.g., some acquisitions produce pairs of images that are naturally aligned, such as certain sequences for T_2-weighted and PD images) or has been done for you beforehand, but most often a good alignment requires you to register the images together first (more details in Chapter 5). This ensures that voxels represent consistent anatomical locations in each image and therefore the same anatomical structures will be masked out in each case. Applying a brain mask to an image that was created using another image and with appropriate registration is a common method of getting good quality and consistent brain extractions in different images. This method can be very useful when one of the images works well with a brain extraction tool (e.g., it has good resolution and brain-to-nonbrain contrast), but the other one does not (e.g., this is often true for fieldmap or calibration images; see the Example Box "Brain masks"). These same principles also apply to working with other masks—not just with whole-brain masks.

Finally, it is worth pointing out that, even when working with analysis pipelines that do not explicitly run a separate brain extraction stage, a brain mask will be used at some point in the pipeline. It is still strongly advisable to check, visually, that the brain masking that is done in any pipeline is sufficiently accurate for your purposes. You should also keep in mind any imperfections in the brain masks when interpreting the results, to ensure that the erroneous results that might have been generated by these imperfections (e.g., changes in gray matter near the optic nerves) are not just blindly accepted as valid biological findings. If in doubt, it is best to dig deeper into the analysis to see where the results came from, to check with more experienced colleagues, or to report such potential limitations in publications and presentations.

Example Box: **Brain masks**

On the primer website there are instructions for how to create brain masks and apply them to different images.

4.4 Skull estimation

In many neuroimaging studies it is only the brain that is of interest. However, in some cases the skull is also of interest; and estimating the skull is an optional extra stage that some brain extraction methods can perform. This is a difficult problem because of the lack of water or fat in bone: as a result, bone has a very low signal in MRI (except when we are using very specialized and uncommon sequences, such as ultrashort TE methods), although bone marrow usually produces a clear signal. Hence it is normally very difficult to distinguish between skull (which often contains very small amounts of marrow) and other dark areas, such as air in various sinuses, or areas of fatty tissue if fat suppression is applied. Bias fields (the result of RF inhomogeneities) where image intensities become brighter or darker than they should (see Figure 4.5) often cause additional challenges, as the intensities can become quite dark in the superior or inferior parts of the brain (or in both); and this is even more so for the nonbrain tissues. As a consequence, it is often extremely difficult to get accurate estimates in the inferior and superior regions. Thus skull estimation is not generally recommended for getting accurate total intracranial volume (TIV) measurements.

When the aim of getting a skull estimation is to derive a measure of head size that can be used for the "correction" of head size in statistical analyses (i.e., to remove confounds related to

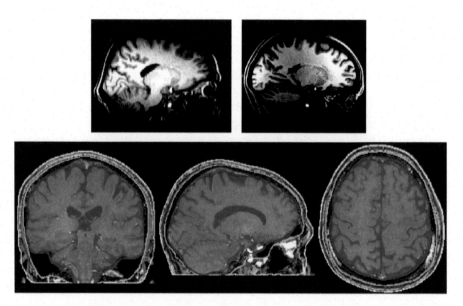

Figure 4.5: Examples of images with different bias fields (top row), where estimating the superior and/or inferior portions of the skull/scalp is even harder than estimating the edge of the brain tissue. Thus the estimation of nonbrain structures, when it is an available option in the software, requires good-quality images, but from such images it is possible to obtain estimates of various surfaces for the brain (red), inner skull (blue), outer skull (green), and outer scalp (yellow), as shown in the example in the bottom row (using an acquisition with minimal bias field).

the size of the head, for instance when studying groups with members of different heights or ethnicities), a reasonable degree of local inaccuracy can be tolerated. This is because the result will be reduced to a single number that only needs to be strongly correlated with head size in order to achieve the desired statistical correction, and so precise a TIV is not required in this scenario. If the aim of getting the skull estimate is to use it for EEG or MEG modeling, where knowing the geometry of the skull is useful for calculating source locations, then inaccuracies in the estimation matter a lot more. In this case it would be important to optimize the method for accuracy and to use images with fewer artifacts. This can be sufficient to give good skull estimates—at least in the superior portion of the head, as the uncertainties related to the proportion of air and bone in the air-filled sinuses in the inferior portions remain a problem, but are less important in this application.

A third possible application of estimating the skull is in longitudinal studies, where there is brain atrophy (e.g., due to neurodegeneration), so that the brain size is changing but the skull should not (for adults). Skull size is then used to normalize the images to account for any small inaccuracies in the volumetric calibration of the scanner, which can change by fractions of a percentage over months and is one of the things that MRI service engineers recalibrate on site visits. In longitudinal studies the pair of scans (baseline and follow-up) for each individual are usually spaced months or even years apart, and so correcting for these volumetric calibrations is important if you want to get accurate measurements of the small changes in brain volume (which are often only fractions of a percentage). Skull measurements or some alternative calibrations are essential in these applications, as the brain is changing size and cannot itself be used to compensate for the miscalibrations.

Another option for estimating the skull or for getting a value suitable for head-size correction is to use registration methods (see Chapter 5). However, since the nonbrain tissue intensities can vary substantially between different types of image acquisitions (due to changes in sequences, parameters, fat suppression, etc.), this can be difficult without a template image that is well matched to the precise acquisition sequence being used. Even so, registration-based methods may struggle if there is pathology such as neurodegeneration present in the image of interest but not in the template (or templates).

4.5 Difficulties and troubleshooting

Brain extraction does not work infallibly all the time, due to the wide range of acquisitions, pathologies, and artifacts—and this is true for all analysis steps. Therefore it is important to check the output to see if the result is good enough for the current application (e.g., for within-subject registration purposes the brain extraction can contain small errors, whereas for tissue quantification it usually needs to be much more accurate). If things do go wrong, then there are usually a number of parameters that can be tuned in the method itself, additional or different preprocessing steps that can be run, or even alternative brain extraction methods that can be used instead.

For instance, bias field is often a cause of problems in brain extraction. If the bias field is strong in the image and the errors appear to be plausibly related to this fact (e.g., there is brain material missing in or near the areas where the bias field has made the image darker than normal), then applying extra preprocessing steps to reduce the bias field is likely to help. Such bias field correction methods either exist as standalone methods or are built into other methods, such as tissue-type segmentation (which usually estimates simultaneously both the segmentation and the bias field). Sometimes these methods require the image to be already brain-extracted, which then generates a chicken-or-egg problem: Which one should be applied first? But often an approximate brain extraction, even with errors, is enough to elicit an approximate bias field correction, which is enough to improve the next brain extraction. This kind of iterative approach is commonly used in analysis methodology, and you should be aware of it and apply it when necessary.

From this example you can get a sense of the range of different options you may try when troubleshooting; and you can see that troubleshooting often is a trial-and-error process. It is worth becoming familiar with the main user-adjustable options provided by different methods and to seek guidance from experienced colleagues, documentation, and any discussion or help forums associated with the software. It is also worth becoming familiar with other alternatives (e.g., registration-based approaches to brain extraction) that are often available within the same software package, although it is useful to consider alternative software packages too, if you are having a lot of difficulties. For brain extraction there is also the ultimate fall-back position of manually editing the results, which is laborious but sometimes necessary, in very tricky cases or when very accurate results are needed. Although usually this can be avoided, there is no theoretical problem with manual editing apart from the amount of time and effort it requires and the lack of repeatability. However, manual fixes are not available for many other analysis steps, so optimizing parameters, employing different preprocessing steps, or using alternative algorithms are generally useful skills to learn. See the Example Box "Troubleshooting brain extraction" for some practice in this area.

Example Box: **Troubleshooting brain extraction**

On the primer website there are some examples of difficult cases of brain extraction and instructions on various options for improving the results. In addition, some alternative approaches for brain extraction will also be presented.

SUMMARY

- Brain extraction is a very useful but not an essential step in most analysis pipelines. It typically improves the robustness of subsequent operations by removing the influence of nonbrain structures.

- Brain extraction does not aim to model the detail of the cortical folds (as cortical/surface modeling does); rather it aims to remove the bulk of the nonbrain material. This involves some arbitrary cutoffs in the brainstem and optic nerves.

- Visual inspection of the results should be performed, as no methods are 100 percent robust.

- Small errors are relatively unimportant for some applications (e.g., initialization for within-subject registration) but can be very important for others (e.g., quantifying the volume of gray matter).

- A brain mask is necessary in any analysis pipeline and would often be created by the brain extraction at the beginning, but may be refined later (e.g., through cortical surface modeling) or created in some other way.

- Some brain extraction methods can also estimate skull and scalp surfaces, which are useful for calibration in longitudinal studies or for EEG/MEG head modeling.

FURTHER READING

- Smith, S. M. (2002). Fast robust automated brain extraction. *Human Brain Mapping*, 17(3), 143–155.
  - *This is the original paper for the FSL brain extraction tool (BET), which is at a fairly detailed, technical level.*
- Iglesias, J. E., Liu, C. Y., Thompson, P. M., & Tu, Z. (2011). Robust brain extraction across datasets and comparison with publicly available methods. *IEEE Transactions on Medical Imaging*, 30(9), 1617–1634.
  - *This paper compares a range of available brain extraction methods and demonstrates the difference that cropping can make. There are also a number of other comparison papers in the literature.*

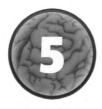

Registration

Alignment, or registration, of images is a crucial step in the analysis pipeline for all types of imaging, especially for group studies. This is because the position of the subject's head, the field of view of the image, and the resolution of the imaging data typically vary between different acquisitions, between different volumes within one acquisition, and between images of different subjects. The purpose of registration (also sometimes called *spatial normalization* or *spatial alignment*) is to take two images and align them with each other so that subsequent analysis steps can extract data from consistent anatomical locations across different images of the same subject, or even of different subjects. The images involved might be completely different acquisitions (e.g., a structural image and a functional image), the same type of acquisition (e.g., two T_1-weighted images) or even 3D volumes (images) from the same 4D dataset.

The basic principles of registration are the same in all cases, although the specific options that give the most accurate (or valid) registrations change depending on the particular circumstance. Knowing how to choose the best parameters or options is the key thing you need to learn about registration. This chapter will explain the main principles behind registration—spatial transformations, cost functions, and resampling—each one of which is associated with a choice that needs to be made when doing your own analysis. The practical application of these choices, how to make them, and how they interact are topics explored in a series of case studies in section 5.4 and supported through online examples. Finally, other applications involving registration—such as standard spaces, atlases, and atlas-based segmentation—are presented at the end of the chapter.

5.1 Spatial transformations

Since registration is all about aligning the anatomy between different images, the most fundamental element in it is the one that describes how registration can transform the image in space. In this context, spatially transforming an image involves changes such as rotating the brain or shifting it within the image, or more substantial alterations, such as changing the size and shape of the ventricles and cortical folds. It is necessary for the user to specify the type of allowable transformations, since different ones are valid or advantageous in different contexts. By specifically choosing certain types of transformations we can provide appropriate constraints that not only help the registration method get more accurate results but also ensure that the results are physically plausible and biologically appropriate for that situation. For example, two scans of the same person in the same session will only differ by the position and orientation (translation and rotation: see Figure 5.1) of the brain, whereas scans of completely different people can vary enormously, due to the large variability in anatomy. A great deal of flexibility in the allowable transformations is required in the second situation to accommodate this large variability and to achieve accurate alignment, although some transformations (e.g., ones that would involve

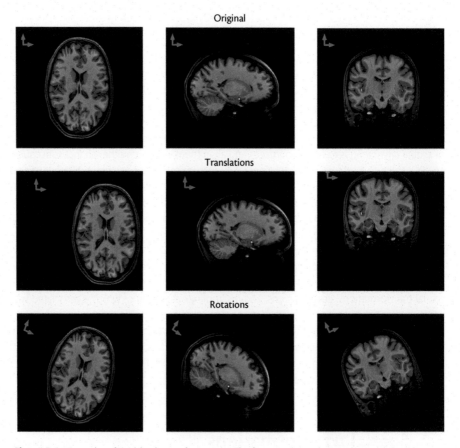

Figure 5.1: Examples of rigid-body transformations. The first row shows three orthogonal slices from the original brain image (before any transformation). The middle row shows examples after translation (shifting) of the brain along the x (left–right), y (posterior–anterior), and z (inferior–superior) axes respectively. The last row shows examples after rotation about the z, x, and y axes respectively. These three translations and three rotations are all independent and, together, make up the six degrees of freedom of a 3D rigid-body transformation.

breaking up a brain structure into several pieces) would not be considered plausible and so should not be allowed. The next sections describe the main types of spatial transformations that are used to specify the appropriate constraints for registration.

5.1.1 Linear transformations

The first major category of spatial transformations is that of linear transformations. These are the most limited, but also the most appropriate ones for cases where the anatomy of the brain is not changing. For example, two images taken in the same session will show the same anatomy, but the subject's head might have moved in between the acquisitions. This movement (of the brain) can only consist of translations (shifts) and rotations. Such a transformation is described as a *rigid-body transformation*, which is one type of linear transformation (the other common type is the *affine transformation*, which will be presented later).

The example of different images of the same subject taken in the same session is extremely common, and a rigid-body transformation is used most often in this situation. Furthermore, this is not just a convenient transformation in this situation but it is the *most appropriate* one, since allowing more flexibility in the transformation would permit the registration to change the geometry of the brain, and hence the depiction of the anatomy, in ways that are just not physically or biologically plausible in this situation. Such implausible or nonphysical changes could occur if the appropriate constraint is not used, since the registration method can be influenced by noise or artifacts rather than by the anatomical content. This is an example of the general principle that, for registration, more flexibility is not normally beneficial, and we need to have the right constraints by choosing the appropriate type of spatial transformation.

Rigid-body transformations

The previous example has already introduced *rigid-body transformations*, which consist only of rotations and translations. In 3D there are three independent rotations (one about each axis) and three independent translations (one along each axis), as shown in Figure 5.1, and a combination of these six independent constituents can fully describe how an object (like the head or the brain) can move in 3D without changing size or shape. This is the crucial constraint that rigid-body transformations impose: no changes in size or shape.

Another naming convention that you will come across in linear transformations is based on their *degrees of freedom* (DOF), and in 3D the rigid-body transformation is a 6-DOF transformation (three independent rotations and three independent translations). This is only true for 3D; in 2D a rigid-body transform has 3 DOF (i.e., one rotation and two translations) and in general the number of DOF is not unique and can be ambiguous (e.g., 3 DOF can also describe a translation-only transformation in 3D), although the DOF are commonly reported. Each DOF corresponds to some numerical parameter that is needed in order to specify the transformation, but the kind of parameter depends on the implementation or software used; for example, to specify a rigid-body transformation in 3D, there are several ways to define the three rotation angles and the three translation values that we need (see Box 5.1 if you are interested in more details about the conventions used for specifying parameters).

Box 5.1: Transformation parameters, coordinates, and conventions

Spatial transformations map a location in one image to a location in another image, and these mappings are specified mathematically, in terms of functions that map the coordinates. A transformation is specified by a set of parameters and a definition of the coordinate conventions. For example, a 3D rigid-body transformation is specified by three rotation angles and three translation parameters, which in turn can be used to calculate a matrix that maps coordinates from one image to coordinates in another.

A 2D rigid-body transformation is described by the matrix:

$$\begin{bmatrix} \cos(\theta) & -\sin(\theta) & T_x \\ \sin(\theta) & \cos(\theta) & T_y \\ 0 & 0 & 1 \end{bmatrix}$$

where θ is the angle of rotation and T_x and T_y are the translation values. Together these three parameters constitute the 3 DOFs of this transformation. Note that here we represent the transformation with a 3 × 3 matrix rather than a 2 × 2 matrix (rotation) and a separate 2 × 1 vector (translations), as the single 3 × 3 matrix is a convenient way to encapsulate everything together and to allow simpler expressions for the concatenation and inversion of transformations. It operates on a 3 × 1 vector, which takes the form $[x\ y\ 1]^T$—that is, the typical coordinate values, with a 1 tacked on the end—and these are called *homogeneous coordinates*. When multiplying these coordinates by these matrices, the bottom row of the matrix ensures that the last element of the homogeneous coordinate vector always remains equal to 1. The same principle operates in 3D, where the homogeneous coordinates are $[x\ y\ z\ 1]^T$ and the matrices are 4 × 4.

Unfortunately there is no unique way to specify transformations, and even simple transformations such as a rotation can be specified using different units (e.g., degrees or radians), a different center of rotation, or different orders of rotations about the three axes. For example, a 90° rotation about the x axis followed by a 90° rotation about the y axis is completely different from a 90° rotation about the y axis followed by a 90° rotation about the x axis. Hence both the rotation angles and the order of rotation is important, which involves arbitrary choices even for this way of representing rotations. Other ways of representing rotations also exist and include angle-axis and quaternion representations. Similarly, the center of rotation (the coordinate that is unchanged by the rotation) is an arbitrary choice, as combining rotations and translations has the same effect as shifting the center of rotation, so any choice of a center can be made if it is appropriately compensated by the translations. The key point here is that parameters are not unique and cannot usually be compared across different software packages, as each package typically uses a different representation.

Coordinate conventions also vary substantially, on the basis of different choices made in different software packages. For instance, the units can be different (mm or voxels), the location of the origin can be different (e.g., center or corner of image), or even the definition or naming of the axes can be different (e.g., what might be x,y,z for one software package might be treated as y,x,z in another). Transformation matrices and warp fields are tied to coordinate conventions and hence are also not the same across different software packages.

The conventions for transformation parameters become most apparent when plotting them for motion correction (see section 6.1) or when using them for motion artifact correction. Although the values (and even the units) can differ between software packages, the crucial information about when substantial motion occurs and how this can be used to identify and remove motion artifacts is conveyed well by any of the conventions. Thus one convention is not really "better" than another, but it is useful to know that these differences exist and that certain information is not compatible between different software packages without appropriate conversions.

The rigid-body constraint of no changes in size or shape means that this transformation is the most appropriate one to use in situations where the anatomy is the same. Such situations include different images of the same subject from within the same session, as well as different 3D volumes within a 4D acquisition (e.g., functional or diffusion MRI) and cases where the images are of the same subject but come from different scanning sessions. The last case can cover split sessions, where a structural image might be acquired on one day and another image (e.g., ASL) on another day. However, in longitudinal studies with much larger time periods between the sessions (months, or even years) some detectable changes in anatomy are expected, and so a rigid-body registration (i.e., a registration using a rigid-body transformation) is not sufficient for a highly accurate registration, although it can provide a good approximate initial alignment.

As this longitudinal example illustrates, sometimes rigid-body registrations are performed in order to get an approximate alignment, which might be refined by further registration steps or might be used in conjunction with other analysis methods (e.g., some atrophy quantification tools use a rigid-body initialization and then detect any additional shifts in boundary locations). It is not just longitudinal cases where this is useful either, as rigid-body initialization is also used for more sophisticated registration methods, such as those that incorporate distortion corrections for EPI-based acquisitions (functional, diffusion, perfusion, etc.), or where individual slices are allowed to change separately, or where both B_0 and eddy-current distortions are taken into account (more details in Chapter 6).

In summary, rigid-body transformations are the most appropriate transformation for *within-subject registrations*, especially when the anatomy has not changed. They are also useful for initializing more sophisticated methods that account for additional changes in anatomy or for geometric distortions.

Affine transformations

The other type of linear transformation that is commonly used is the *affine transformation*, which has 12 DOF in 3D. These DOFs consist of 6 DOF from a rigid-body transformation (three rotations and three translations) as well as three scalings and three shears or skews (see Figure 5.2). These additional constituents allow the shape and size of the objects in the image to change, though in quite limited ways. Although these additional types of transformation do not correspond to what a single subject's brain is physically able to do when the head moves,

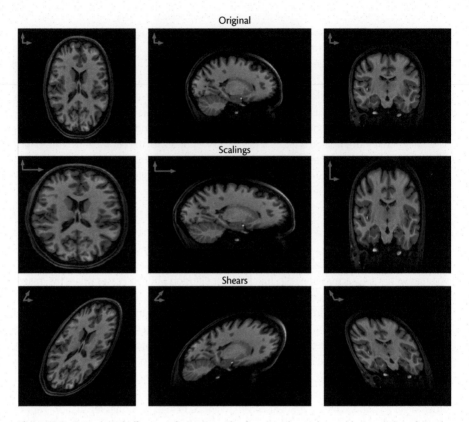

Figure 5.2: Examples of affine transformations. The first row shows three orthogonal slices from the original brain image (before any transformation). The middle row shows examples after scaling of the brain along the x (left–right), y (posterior–anterior), and z (inferior–superior) axes respectively. The last row shows examples after skew (shear) in the x–y, y–z, and x–z planes respectively. Note that the skews are different from rotations in that each point only moves horizontally (in these example images) rather than rotating about a point. These three scales and three skews, together with the 6 DOF from the rigid-body transformation (three rotations and three translations), make up the 12 DOF of a 3D affine transformation.

affine transformations do have two common uses: (i) to correct for eddy-current distortions; and (ii) to initialize more flexible transformations.

Eddy-current distortions, as discussed in sections 2.3.4 and 3.3.1, are reasonably well approximated by scalings, shears, and translations. As a consequence, registrations based on affine transformations are able, in principle, to correct both for these distortions and for rigid-body head motion. This is because combining together any set of affine transformations is just another affine transformation, and so shears, scalings, rotations, and translations, taken together, are capable of capturing the linear effects of eddy-current distortion combined with head motion. In fact affine transformations include all types of linear transformations (e.g., rigid-body is technically a subset of affine), while any other form of transformation is nonlinear. One useful property to know about linear transformations is that they apply equally to the whole image and cannot do different things in different parts of the image; for instance, if you want to scale one part of the image with a linear transformation, then you must scale the whole image by the same amount. Nonlinear transformations are more flexible and do not have to follow this constraint.

The other common use of affine transformations is to initialize the more flexible, nonlinear transformations. This is done so that a good approximation of the position, orientation, and size of the brain can be established, minimizing the amount of additional transformation that the following step needs to do. The reason why this is important is that it makes the combined registration (affine, then nonlinear) more *robust*. This initialization is normally used in the situation where the two images being registered have different anatomies, and hence the affine transformation is not able to align the fine details of the anatomy particularly well, since it is very unlikely that the anatomies only differ by a scale-and-shear transformation carried out in a homogenous manner across the brain. However, the affine transformation is able to get the general brain outline and position of ventricles roughly right, which is very helpful.

In summary, affine transformations (with 12 DOF) are typically used for eddy-current distortion corrections and for initializing nonlinear transformations. Even though the alignment from an affine transformation is only approximate for between-subject registration, it is an extremely useful and common step to apply, since it leads to significant improvements in robustness and accuracy in the following nonlinear step.

5.1.2 Nonlinear transformations

When there is a substantial difference in anatomy (e.g., different folding patterns), or any form of local geometric change (e.g., large pathology or surgery), then it is necessary to move beyond linear transformations. Only *nonlinear transformations* are able to accurately align images where these local differences exist. Any transformation with more than 12 DOF is technically a nonlinear transformation (also called a *warp*), but the ones most commonly used in neuroimaging have a lot more flexibility and typically have thousands to millions of DOF. For nonlinear transformations, the parameters usually describe local geometric changes, such as vectors associated with grid points in the image, which indicate how that point and its neighbors are displaced.

Being able to change the geometry locally enables the transformation to align anatomical structures from different subjects, which is absolutely necessary given the highly folded nature of the cortex and the amount of individual variability. Changing the geometry locally is also essential for being able to align images of a single subject before and after anatomical changes due to pathology, surgery, ageing, or development. However, there are still constraints that need to be applied to prevent these transformations from producing physically or biologically implausible results.

The strongest constraint, which is applied in almost all nonlinear registration methods, is to ensure that the *topology* of the image does not change. This means that an individual structure cannot be split up into separate structures and cannot disappear. Also, structures not present in an image cannot be created by the transformation, although the shape of a structure can change greatly, as must happen for the folded cortex. In mathematical terminology, the constrained transformation is a *diffeomorphism*, or we can say that the transformation is *diffeomorphic*. You may come across these terms, but the mathematical details do not need to be understood—the key thing to know is that these transformations preserve the topology.

In addition to the topological constraint, nonlinear transformations are also *regularized* to some degree. This, roughly speaking, is a way of making the transformation smoother or of limiting how much the geometry can change. As the *regularization* increases, the resulting transformations are smoother and any changes are spread over a wider region (they are less local), involving less change in shape. Regularization allows a trade-off between matching image features more precisely and being robust to noise and artifacts. If very little regularization is used, then a high DOF transformation is capable of local and fine detailed changes in geometry; but there is also more potential for it to be influenced by artifacts and noise in the images. When a large amount of regularization is used, the transformation is more robust to noise and artifacts but cannot represent the fine details of the geometrical changes as well (see Figure 5.3). The optimal amount of regularization depends on resolution, SNR, CNR, artifacts, and type of acquisition (e.g., T_1-weighted structural, diffusion, etc.).

Some registration methods attempt to determine the optimal amount of regularization from the images being registered, but the majority have one or more user-adjustable parameters to set the regularization, along with some standard default values. These defaults may apply well to common situations (e.g., for registering 1mm T_1-weighted images to a standard template like the MNI152), and in those cases it is not necessary to change the defaults. However, in other situations it is useful for you to try different values in order to gain an understanding of how much the result is affected by regularization and whether for your particular case there is a better setting, especially if you have less common types of images (unusual resolutions, fetal images, different species, etc.). One particular example is registering images from two individual subjects directly rather than registering an individual subject to a template, as is more common. For registration between two individuals, less regularization can often help improve the accuracy of the fine details in the alignment, although the result still depends on image quality. In general, low-quality images (whether the poor quality is due to resolution, SNR, or CNR) require higher amounts of regularization.

Nonlinear transformations can be represented in a number of ways. One of those representations is through control-point grids, where degrees of freedom (parameters) are associated with the control points. In this case the number of DOFs is proportional to the number of control points and inversely proportional to the spacing between them. Number of DOFs and regularization are closely related, with fewer DOFs being capable of less local changes, just as when higher regularization is used. This offers another way to effectively control the regularization or smoothness of transformations; and it is a parameter that you should also investigate, especially if you are working with unusual images.

In general, nonlinear registrations are most commonly used to register individual subject T_1-weighted images to a T_1-weighted template, such as the MNI152. This is a step in the analysis pipeline for group studies in all types of neuroimaging, as it is essential for obtaining a correspondence between anatomical locations in different individuals. To be more robust, it is preceded by an affine registration, which is designed to get a closer initialization, and this corrects for differences in overall position, rotation, and scale (further details in section 5.4 and online examples). Another common application is to register images from two individual subjects (or two time points for one subject) in order to transfer information from one to the other, as in multi-atlas-based segmentation methods,

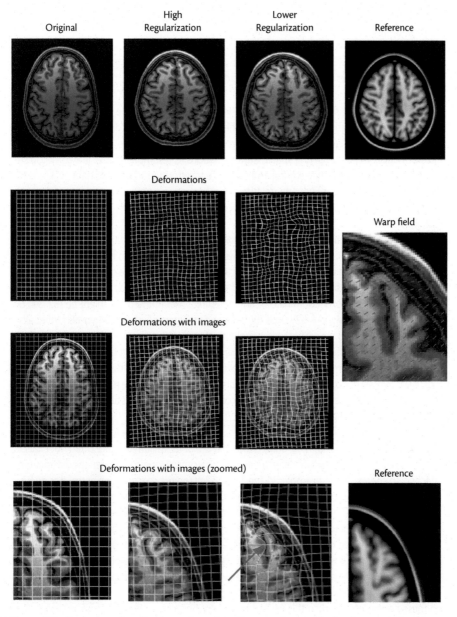

Figure 5.3: Illustration of nonlinear transformations. First row shows one slice from a structural image of a single individual before (left) and after (middle) nonlinear registration to the MNI152 template (right). The two middle cases represent registrations using nonlinear transformations with high regularization (left middle) and lower regularization (right middle). The second row shows the transformations in terms of how they distort a regular grid that is initially aligned with the individual image. It can be seen that the grid is more distorted and less smooth in the case of lower regularization. The third row shows the same as the second row, but with the images from the first row underneath the grid. The fourth row shows a zoomed-in version of the top-right portion of the third row, with a corresponding portion of the template (without grid) on the right. It can be seen from these images how one sulcus in particular is reoriented to match the template (red arrow), which results from stronger, more local deformations that are visible in the transformation with lower regularization. The image in the middle of the right-hand column represents the transformation with lower regularization but with vectors (without arrows) used to display the transformation.

in building group-specific templates, or in investigating changes in anatomy. More details of these applications will be given in later sections.

5.1.3 Coordinate and transformation conventions

The outputs of a registration method are the aligned image or the spatial transformation that achieved this alignment (or both). It is the transformation that contains the most crucial information, as the aligned image can be regenerated easily from the original image and the transformation. In fact, applying spatial transformations to resample images is a common step in many pipelines, and hence storing and using the transformations is important.

Spatial transformations encode relationships between locations or coordinates in the images. There are actually two main types of coordinates: *voxel coordinates* and *world* (or mm) *coordinates*.

Voxel coordinates specify the location of a voxel within a particular image and have no units or fixed points of anatomical reference—they always just give the offset from the corner of the image. That is, the corner of the image is the origin, and then the voxel coordinate counts how many voxels along each axis a voxel location is: for example, the corner of the image may have a voxel coordinate of (0, 0, 0) while the voxel coordinate of an interesting voxel in the brain might be (52, 94, 66), which means that this voxel is 52 voxels further along the image's first axis, 94 voxels further along the second axis, and 66 voxels further along the third axis. Unfortunately there are many different conventions for coordinates and different software tools will use different conventions and names; for example, the origin might be (1, 1, 1) and not (0, 0, 0) and the axes of the image might be called x,y,z or i,j,k. We will not concern ourselves with this level of detail here. The main thing to understand is that a voxel coordinate is relative to the corner of the image and that it is always in whole numbers (integers), counting along the axes of the image.

World coordinates, in contrast, have units of millimeters and therefore can take floating point values, such as (102.3, 75.8, 66.0)—note that the units, millimeters, are often not explicitly written. They may or may not refer to a fixed anatomical origin or have special meanings attached to the axes. For example, in the MNI152 standard space coordinates, the origin at (0, 0, 0) is the location of the anterior commissure (a well-defined anatomical feature) and the axes are x = left–right, y = posterior–anterior, z = inferior–superior (see section 5.5 for more information on standard space and standard coordinates). However, other images may have world coordinates that relate to the space inside the scanner and not to the anatomy.

The key point here is that a location in the image can be described by either a voxel coordinate or a world coordinate and that these may have different conventions associated with them. Viewing tools may show you one or both sets of coordinates. Spatial transformations are based on these coordinates, and so this variety of conventions also applies to transformations. Both coordinates and transformations are typically tied to a particular software package and are difficult to translate between packages.

Linear transformations, given that they have very few DOF, are normally stored in small text files that may be shaped into a matrix or listed as individual parameters. These normally contain 12 numbers for 12 DOF, although a four-by-four matrix with a last row set to "0, 0, 0, 1" is also common (the exact format varies with the software: see Box 5.1 if you are interested in more details). However, nonlinear transformations require too many DOF to be stored in text files, so they are typically stored as images (called *warp fields* or *deformation fields*), where the values in the voxels represent the transformation. One common format for this (though many other formats exist) is to store a vector at each voxel. The interpretation of this format is then relatively simple, as each vector describes how that voxel is displaced by the spatial transformation. This process can then be visualized (much like visualizing the directions from a diffusion analysis), to indicate how different locations in the image are warped by showing the vectors directly, or by showing their effect on a grid (see Figure 5.3).

The most important point here is that you should be able to identify which outputs are the transformations and to make sure that you keep them, as they represent the most crucial information from a registration. They are also often combined together and applied to other images at later stages in pipelines, and so they play an important role. See the Example Box "Spatial Transformations" for examples of this using real data.

Example Box: Spatial Transformations

On the primer website there are some examples of datasets demonstrating registrations that use spatial transformations with different DOFs and instructions on how to view and apply the transformations.

5.2 Cost functions

Once the appropriate type of spatial transformation has been selected, a registration method needs to be able to determine the parameters that result in the best alignment of the images— for example, the values of the rotation angles and translations for a rigid-body registration. In order to do this, the registration algorithm needs a numerical way to measure the goodness of a potential alignment—the *cost function*—which is its way of defining what is "best." The human visual system is extremely good at determining alignment, hence doing this comes very easily to us when assessing images by eye. However, there is no single, universal cost function that works in all cases for registration methods; instead there is a whole range of options and you need to choose the one that is appropriate for your current application.

A cost function assigns a value to a particular alignment, and the smaller the value the better the alignment (similarity functions are the opposite; see Box 5.2 if you are interested). The registration algorithm then searches for the values of the parameters that give the smallest cost value. For example a 30° rotation might have a cost of 0.8 by comparison to a 31° rotation, which has a cost of 0.81, and to a 29° rotation, which has a cost of 0.85, and this makes the 30° rotation the "best" alignment out of these three. This search process is also known as *optimization* and many different approaches exist, which differ in how robust, accurate, and fast they are. However, these are normally hard-coded into the software and you do not have any choice about what method is used. They are usually sensitive to the initialization of the alignment, with poor initialization normally leading to registrations that have very large and obvious misalignments. Initialization is something where you do have some control, and it is the reason why affine registration is used before nonlinear registration and axis reorientation is used before rigid-body or affine registration.

Box 5.2: Similarity functions

There are similarity functions as well as cost functions, and they do precisely the same job but go the opposite way, in that a larger value is "better" for a similarity function. Cost functions and similarity functions are really the same thing, as any cost function can be turned into a similarity function (or vice versa) just through multiplication by -1, and sometimes the terms are used interchangeably. Each registration method will use one type or the other, depending on whether its optimization routine is set to look for the minimum value (cost functions) or for the maximum value (similarity functions), though this level of detail is normally hidden from the user.

There is a variety of cost functions to choose from, and each one makes different assumptions about the images and how they relate to each other. This means that each cost function is applicable in a range of situations. For example, the *sum of squared differences* cost function assumes that the intensities in the images would be identical after an appropriate spatial transform. This would be true for a pair of 3D volumes from the same 4D acquisition (e.g., a pair of images from an fMRI acquisition) but is not true if you are registering a T_1-weighted image and a T_2-weighted image since, for example, the cerebrospinal fluid (CSF) has low intensities in one and high intensities in the other. Therefore registering a T_1-weighted image with a T_2-weighted image requires a different type of cost function—one that is designed to be able to determine when an alignment is good even though the intensities in the images are quite different.

Table 5.1 lists a range of common cost functions, the situations where they are valid, and an example of where they are most often used. This information is what you need to use in order to decide what cost function is an appropriate choice for an individual registration problem—in particular the second column of the table. For example, if you wanted to register two T_1-weighted images together, then any of the cost functions in the table could be used, except maybe the first one (sum of squared differences) if you were not sure that the scaling would be consistent (i.e., they were not acquired in the same session). However, if you have two different MRI modalities (e.g., a T_1-weighted and a FLAIR image), then you definitely cannot use cost functions that only work for pairs of images of the same modality (e.g., sum of squared differences or normalized correlation), but any of the other cost functions could be used. It is generally the case that there are several valid choices for cost functions for a particular situation, but also some cost functions that should not be used. If an incorrect choice of cost function is made, the registration normally fails, with very obvious misalignment. For those interested in the mathematical details behind the cost functions, see Box 5.3.

Table 5.1 A list of some common cost functions and their properties. The most important part of this table is the second column, which indicates under what circumstances a cost function can be used.

Cost Function	Valid for	Example
Sum of squared differences (SSD)–also known as mean square error or least squares	Two images of the *same modality* (and same scaling)	Two 3D images (volumes) from a 4D acquisition (e.g., fMRI)
Normalized correlation	Two images of the *same modality* (but intensities can be scaled and offset)	Two T_1-weighted images, possibly acquired in separate sessions
Correlation ratio	Any two *MRI modalities*	T_1-weighted image and a FLAIR image
Mutual information or normalized mutual information	Any two *images*	T_1-weighted image and a CT image
BBR (Boundary-Based Registration)	Two images, both with some contrast across boundaries of interest (more details in section 6.2.2)	EPI image and a T_1-weighted structural (using the white–gray matter boundary)

Box 5.3: Intensity models for cost functions

Each cost function is related to some model of how the intensities in one image relate to those in the other when they are well aligned. The simplest example of this is for the SSD cost function, which is based on an intensity model where the corresponding intensities would be identical in images that are well aligned. That is, $I_2(x) = I_1(x)$. Other cost functions allow for more complicated relationships, such as $I_2(x) = a.I_1(x) + b$ for normalized correlation or $I_2(x) = f(I_1(x))$ for correlation ratio. In both of these cases the relationship is a mathematical function: a scaling and an offset for normalized correlation and a general function for correlation ratio. The correlation ratio model works in such a way that it considers all possible functions, $f(...)$, and estimates the most likely; that is, you do not have to specify the function. As a consequence, the correlation ratio allows for cases where the intensities are reversed (such as would be true when relating a T_1-weighted and T_2-weighted image) or for more complicated relationships (as might be needed when mapping a FLAIR image showing pathological tissues to a T_1-weighted image where the pathological tissues have the same intensities as healthy tissue).

Even correlation ratio does not capture all the possible relationships between image intensities—such as when the two images distinguish between very different types of tissues—and in that case it is necessary to have an even more flexible intensity model. For example, in CT images air and bone have different intensities; but they are similar in MRI (both near 0), whereas in MRI gray matter and white matter have significantly different intensities, but the intensities are almost the same in CT. In such a case no single-valued function, regardless of which way around it is applied, can split both sets of tissue intensities appropriately. Consequently, a statistical relationship is needed, as specified by a joint probability density: $p(I_1, I_2)$. This probability-based description allows for a single intensity value in one image to be associated with more than one possible intensity in the other image, and vice versa. This is the basis of the mutual information cost functions and is what makes them much more general and flexible.

The other cost function included in the table is BBR (boundary-based registration), which is an example of a cost function that does not use all the intensities in the image. It focuses on the intensities around a defined set of features—boundary points in this case (usually the white matter boundary, extracted from a structural image). The model is that intensity differences are (locally) maximized across the boundary. More details about the BBR method can be found in section 6.2.2.

There are also other cost functions that exist, and different software tools will have different options available. We have only listed cost functions that are based on intensity values, as these are the most commonly used, but you may also come across cost functions based on low-level features in the images (edges, corners, etc.) or landmarks. The important thing to know is what cost functions are available and in what situations they can be used. For example, registration of MRI and computed tomography (CT) images is difficult, because soft tissues have minimal or no contrast in the CT, whereas bone–air interfaces are very strong in the CT but invisible in the MRI. This is why only a few cost functions (e.g., mutual information and its normalized variant) are able to quantify the quality of an alignment between the two images. So you should check what the available cost functions are for the software you are using; and do not rely on the default option always being best.

One thing that we have only touched on so far is what properties of the images effectively drive the registration; that is, what properties most influence the cost function. This is important, as it determines what kinds of images can be used for registration purposes. As mentioned previously, many common cost functions use the intensity information from all the voxels and not just from features (e.g., boundaries or interesting anatomical points) in the image. This allows for images to be registered when not all of the anatomy is distinct (e.g., in a functional image that has lower resolution and tissue contrast), yet it is still necessary to have a reasonable amount of anatomical information in the images. For example, a functional activation map (the output of an fMRI analysis) cannot be *registered* directly to a structural image; that is, it does not contain the right information to drive the registration. This is because the activation map does not contain information about anatomy (such as edges of anatomical structures), and so no cost function will be able to register these two images directly. Instead, the raw functional images must be used for registration, as they contain anatomical information. The functional activation map can then be transformed to be aligned with the structural image by using the transformation derived from the registration of the raw functional image. The key points here are that not all images contain useful information for driving registrations and that cost functions typically rely on anatomical information to drive the registrations between modalities or between subjects. There are some exceptions—for instance, the use of functional maps to drive registrations between subjects in order to align functional areas with surface-based methods, after an initialization that uses information from the anatomical images (see section 7.4)—but these are definitely the exceptions and not the rule.

Some tools may have very restricted cost function options; they may only provide functions suitable for images of the same modality. This is not unusual for nonlinear registration tools, as the most common application of nonlinear registration is between two T_1-weighted structural images (where one is often the MNI152 template). This is not really a limitation, though, since images of different modalities (e.g., functional MRI and a T_1-weighted structural) can be aligned within-subject by using rigid-body registrations, while the between-subject alignments can be done with nonlinear registrations of two T_1-weighted structural images (often via a standard template). In fact, T_1-weighted images are used in most pipelines for between-subject registrations (either directly or to a standard T_1-weighted template), and hence we recommend that T_1-weighted images be acquired in every study. Thus, by combining transformations appropriately, anatomical correspondence can still be established between any images, regardless of modality, provided that an appropriate set of images is acquired in the first place (see the Example Box "Registration"). More details about such multistage registrations will be discussed in section 5.4.

In addition, some tools incorporate models of distortions or artifacts that combine alignment and distortion or artifact correction, and these often appear in the cost function. One example that occurs in structural MRI is that of building in bias-field correction. As we saw in section 2.2.4, the bias field can have a substantial impact on intensity, and this may cause misalignments if differences in intensities between images are not corrected. Such corrections can be done through a separate preprocessing step or simultaneously with the registration, by using registration with a cost function that has a bias-field model incorporated into it.

Example Box: **Registration**

On the primer website there are images and instructions demonstrating how to register images using different combinations of spatial transformations and cost functions.

5.2.1 Cost function weighting

The accuracy and robustness of a registration method depends largely on the cost function and its interaction with the optimization method used, and this is also what determines whether the registration is sensitive to initialization and to errors in brain extraction, or to mismatches in brain structures (e.g., due to substantial pathology). Behind most cost functions there is an assumption about what the intensity relationship is between the images when they are well aligned. If there are parts of the images where there will be a clear mismatch in the relevant intensity information (e.g., poor brain extraction, or artifacts/pathologies that are only visible in one image), then these parts will cause errors in the registration if they are not accounted for in the cost function. In nonlinear registrations, these errors tend to be localized around the area of mismatch; but in linear registrations such mismatches can cause global errors. The extent of any global error will depend on whether the mismatch is strong enough to perturb the matching of the remaining features in the image, which is dependent on the size of the area affected and on how bad the mismatch is in terms of its impact on the cost function value.

When it is known that a mismatch exists in a part of the image, it is possible to apply an appropriate weighting (or masking) operation, within the registration method, so that this area is effectively ignored when the cost function is calculated. This operation is known as cost function weighting or cost function masking and is available in many registration methods. It differs from masking the images directly, as in brain extraction, since masking the images directly sets voxel values to zero and this creates a boundary between the areas where the intensities are nonzero and where they are zero. Most registration methods will try to align such boundaries. After brain extraction, the boundary generally aligns with the edge of the brain, which we want to be aligned, and thus the masking due to brain extraction assists the registration. In some areas the masking is arbitrary, such as where the brainstem is cut off; but, as the arbitrary section of the boundary is relatively small, the overall effect on linear registrations tends to be minimal. However, in general, if large areas or large intensity mismatches (e.g., gross pathologies) are known to exist, it is better to use cost function masking than to create artificial boundaries in the images. For example, in Figure 5.4 a pathology is shown along with a mask. If the mask were applied directly to the image, the image would appear to have a large black hole where the mask is (as applying the mask sets those voxel intensities to zero in the image), and this would not match well with an image where there is no pathology. Instead, making the mask ignore the intensities in this area, by using cost function weighting, will mean that the registration is not influenced by the fact that the pathology is only present in one image.

To use cost function weighting, a mask or a weighting image needs to be created that stores a weight value for each voxel, such that voxels with zero weight are completely ignored and voxels with unit weight are included as usual. It is also possible to "upweight" by using values larger than 1, but this is rarely done. Typically, a binary mask is created so that voxels within the mismatching area have 0 values and all other voxels contain a value of 1 (see Figure 5.4). This mask is then used inside the registration method, along with the usual pair of images to be registered, to determine whether voxels are included in the calculation of the cost function value or not. The intensities in the images at the voxel locations where the mask is 0 have absolutely no effect on the cost function values, and hence no effect on the final registration. This is particularly useful when large pathologies exist in the images (e.g., a tumor, or an area of missing tissue after surgery). In that case the mask is usually created manually: it is drawn on one image with an appropriate viewing/editing tool. Using this mask then stops the cost function from detecting that there is a large mismatch in intensities in that area (e.g., between the image with pathology and a previous image of the same subject without pathology or a standard template, like the MNI152, that has no pathology). The cost function mask will be associated with only one of the input images, as it is drawn using that image's orientation, FOV, and resolution; and the registration method also needs to know this.

Cost function masking is an extremely useful feature when dealing with clinical subjects who have substantial pathologies. If both images in the pair being registered have the same pathology and show it, then no cost function masking is required. However, when one of the images has a visible pathology and the other does not (e.g., the MNI152), using cost function masking makes a substantial difference to the accuracy and robustness of the result. Cost

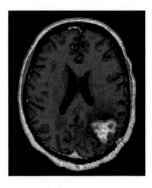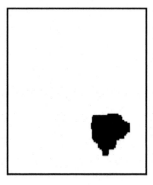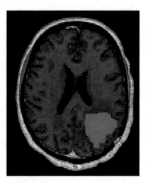

Figure 5.4: Illustration of a cost function mask (weight). The original image (left) contains a pathological lesion; the cost function mask (middle) is created such that voxels in black would have 0 weight and voxels in white would have a weight of 1. The image on the right shows the overlay, where the tissue outside of the zero-weighted (red) area contains no obvious pathologies and is therefore suitable for registration to another image (e.g., a template) that contains no pathologies.

function masking can also be used in other cases, such as when localized artifacts exist (it is used to deal with signal loss in fMRI: see section 6.2) or for areas that are known to be problematic (e.g., are routinely found to contain brain extraction errors).

Using cost function masking to ignore areas of the image is only helpful if the areas are not too large; otherwise too much useful information can be lost and the registration may lack sufficient features to find a good alignment successfully. In particular, the background of the image (the area outside the brain) should be kept by the cost function mask (voxels in this area should contain a value of 1, not of 0), even though it is not included in the brain mask. This is because the boundary between zero and nonzero values in the image, at the edge of the brain, is usually a very helpful feature, and without this information the registrations often fail. Therefore make sure that you include the background voxels in your cost function masks.

Masks do not have to be drawn manually, although that is common. Methods that automatically segment pathological regions can be used to create such masks, although the masks often need inverting if you want to make sure that the pathological region contains values of 0 and the nonpathological regions contain values of 1. An alternative approach is to use cost functions based on *robust statistics*, which automatically determine whether values are unusual and should be treated as outliers, or in some way less important or influential with respect to the cost function. In this way these methods implicitly apply a form of cost function weighting, but without the necessity to provide additional masks or weighting images.

5.3 Resampling and interpolation

So far we have discussed two fundamental options that need to be specified when running registration: the type of spatial transformation allowed and the cost function to be used. These are crucial in determining how well a registration method is able to align the two images being registered. The previous discussion has deliberately avoided some of the practical points about what form the aligned output image takes and which image is aligned to which in the pair. This section will go into details about how the image(s) are transformed (i.e., about applying a spatial transformation, or resampling), which is a key step in any pipeline; and further details will be presented through the case studies in section 5.4.

5.3.1 Image spaces

To understand how resampling is applied, we need to define the concept of image "spaces", as this is a commonly used term and will help us to clarify what is happening in the resampling. The term *resampling* simply means applying a spatial transformation to an image to create a modified version of that image, such as one where the brain is rotated. The transformation is normally applied to one of the images being registered, bringing it into a new image "space," which we will now explain.

Let us start with an example: two images are being registered—the T_1-weighted structural image of an individual subject and the MNI152 template. Each of these images is in a separate *space*: the structural space of that individual image and the MNI space. A space effectively represents a coordinate frame for a brain, the MNI space being a standardized one (e.g., the world coordinate origin of this space is at a fixed anatomical location, namely the anterior commissure), while the structural space of the individual only really relates to the location and orientation of that particular image—in other words a subsequent structural image, say a FLAIR, would have its own space. All images in a particular space share a common coordinate frame and are therefore all aligned with each other. This is useful because we often want to register two images and then transform (or resample) an image from one space to another. In our example we are registering an individual subject's structural image to the MNI152 image, and once this is done we can either transform that individual's structural image into the MNI152 space (creating a version of the structural image that is aligned with all the MNI152 images) or do the opposite and transform an image from the MNI152 space into that individual's structural space. Because the registration determines the alignment of the information in the images and establishes an anatomical correspondence between the spaces, any image transformed to a new space like this is aligned with other images in the new space (though the "alignment" will still contain any inaccuracies due to the registration).

It might help to be even more specific in our example: let us take a mask of the caudate nucleus that exists in the MNI space (and lots of atlases that contain this sort of information are in the MNI space) and transform this into the individual's structural space. This transformation will create a version of the atlas's caudate mask that is aligned with the anatomy of this individual's structural image, allowing us to use it as an ROI for that image (see Figure 5.5). Any images in the same space have their anatomy aligned, by definition, like all the different atlases in the MNI space. However, images in the same space do not have to have the same resolution or FOV, and a good example of this is the MNI template, as there are multiple different versions with different resolutions (e.g., 0.5 mm, 1 mm, 2 mm) and different FOVs. What they have in common is a coordinate system (the world coordinates, or millimeter coordinates), which is used to specify consistent anatomical locations for any image in this space.

In a typical experiment there may be several acquisitions, such as a 3D structural image, a 4D diffusion image, and a 4D functional image. Since there may have been head movement

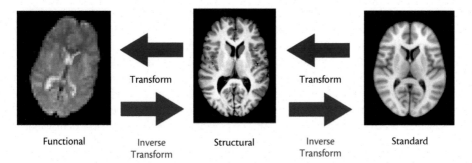

Functional   Inverse   Structural   Inverse   Standard
                    Transform   Transform

Figure 5.5: Illustration of transforming images/masks between spaces. The three spaces depicted here are functional space (left), structural space (middle), and standard space (right). In each case a representative image is shown (potentially one of many images that are aligned together in that space). Registrations between the spaces provide spatial transforms (blue arrows) that establish anatomical correspondences between the spaces. Inverse transforms (red arrows) can easily be calculated from the forward transforms and, together, these transforms allow images to be resampled from any one space to another. This resampling is demonstrated by the mask of the caudate nucleus (red), which is initially defined in the standard space (on the basis of an atlas in the standard space), then transformed into the structural space, and then into the functional space (where it could be used to define an ROI for a specific analysis).

in between these, they are all considered to have their own space initially: that is, in this case, structural space, diffusion space, and functional space. After registrations have been performed between these images it is possible to transform images (and the information they contain) between spaces. Analysis pipelines sometimes start by moving the images into a different space, or might analyze them in their *native space* and then transform the results into another space. For example, diffusion quantities—say, fractional anisotropy (FA)—are usually calculated in the native diffusion space and can then be transformed into structural space (or MNI space) afterwards, for further analysis. Before this transform, the FA image is in the diffusion space, aligned with the original diffusion images and with any other results from the diffusion analysis. It is common for analysis results to be created in the same space as the input images but then to be transformed into other spaces for further analysis (especially group analysis) or interpretation.

The concept of spaces is helpful because registration needs to be established only once between each space (per subject). So in our example we would only need registrations between (i) the diffusion space and the structural space; (ii) the functional space and the structural space; and (iii) the structural space and the MNI space (if we wanted to go to a standard space for group analysis). After we have these three registrations we can transform any image from one space into another, regardless of whether it contains anatomical detail or not.

To be able to transform images from one space into any other space, we often join several transformations together, so that the transforms effectively go via an intermediate space in order to improve the final image quality (more information on this in the next section). In the example we only mentioned getting registrations between the diffusion and structural spaces and the functional and structural spaces, but not between the diffusion and functional spaces. If we had wanted to transform something from functional space into diffusion space (e.g., to seed tractography with an area that had significant functional activation), we could have gone from functional to structural space and then from structural to diffusion space. Joining transformations together like this, or *concatenating* them, is a common and useful operation that serves to make transformations between spaces more consistent and accurate, as well as to improve the quality of the resampled image. It is also possible, as indicated in Figure 5.5, to go in either direction, for example from functional space to structural space *or* from structural space to functional space. The registration only needs to be run once, and this establishes a spatial transformation to go in one direction, but generating an *inverse transformation* is a straightforward operation and may already be provided by the registration tool or may require you to run a supplementary, but simple, operation.

The concept of "spaces" is a little abstract but is a very helpful convention, and one that you will hear often. Knowing that it is necessary to establish registration only once between a limited number of spaces is crucial if you are to be able to understand how results are generated and moved around in analysis pipelines. Quite often images will be transformed between spaces automatically within a pipeline, and knowing how to recognize the different spaces is not only useful but very important, in case you ever need to do something outside of the pipeline—for example, to quantify something specific in your results, like the average of some quantity in an ROI, or to produce a scatter plot.

5.3.2 Resampling and interpolation

Applying a spatial transformation to an image (i.e., resampling) is needed in order to move information from one space to another, for example, statistical fMRI results from an individual functional space to standard space for group analysis. The operation of applying the spatial transformation is called *resampling* and creates an image in the new space. This is different from *registration* in that a registration seeks to work out the best alignment of the images by determining parameters of the spatial transformation (e.g., the rotation angles and translations). Generating a new image using a spatial transformation is conceptually separate and requires a supplementary resampling step, although that may be done automatically by the registration software. For instance, we may know (from having done a registration) that the transformation between the functional and the standard space is a rotation of 11°, but we need to *apply* this to the images in the functional space (e.g., to the statistical outputs) in order to get an *image* in the new space that contains this information. Crucially, resampling requires the use of an *interpolation* method, which we will describe in this section.

Before describing interpolation, there is one point about spatial transformations that needs to be explained: the size of the transformed image. Although a spatial transformation specifies how a coordinate in one image is related to a coordinate in another image, it does not specify the voxel size or FOV of the other image. These properties (resolution, or voxel size, and FOV) are arbitrary choices that you, the user, must make, although it is very common just to take the same resolution and FOV as those of the image used for registration in the destination space. For example, when transforming an image from the functional space (where the voxel size of the image might be 3 mm) into the structural space, it is typical to adopt the voxel size and FOV of the structural image (e.g., a voxel size of 1 mm) rather than retain the lower resolution voxel size of the original image in the functional space, although either option is possible. Once we have specified the size of the transformed image, we need to calculate the intensities of this image, which is where interpolation comes into play.

It is necessary to calculate, rather than copy, intensities in the transformed or resampled image. This is because all the images we work with are discrete and so the intensities are only actually defined at certain points, typically taken to be at the centers of the voxels. The intensities themselves still refer to averages over the whole voxel, but when transforming an image we need to know what intensity value should represent the new voxel. For instance, consider a shift of half a voxel in one direction (see Figure 5.6, center). In this case a voxel in the transformed

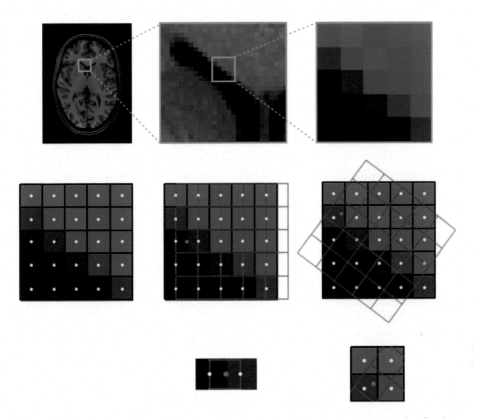

Figure 5.6: Illustration of interpolation in a 2D example. The first row shows an example of a slice from an image at three levels of zoom, with the final 5 × 5 patch used in the lower rows to demonstrate interpolation. In the second row the voxels in the 5 × 5 patch are shown in grayscale, together with black boundary lines (a grid) and a yellow dot at the center of each voxel. The center panel shows a second grid in red that represents the grid of a spatially transformed image where the transformation is a horizontal translation by half a voxel. The right panel shows the situation for a large rotation. In both cases, for illustration purposes, the center of a single voxel in the new grid is marked by a red dot (e.g., center row, left column of the 5 × 5 grid). The role of the interpolation function is to calculate the intensity value at the new grid points, such as this red dot. In the third row a single voxel (red dot) is isolated as an example, showing the voxels surrounding it and how they overlap with the new voxel. For the translation case (middle), the new voxel is split into two halves and one interpolation option (linear) would use the mean intensity of these voxel intensities (at the yellow dots) as the new intensity. In the rotation case (right) the overlap is more complicated and linear interpolation would calculate a weighted average on the basis of the distance between the voxel centers (yellow dots and the red dot), whereas nearest neighbor interpolation would pick the intensity of the closest original voxel (yellow dot in the bottom left) and spline and other interpolation functions would use a more complicated function of a larger set of neighboring voxels.

image overlaps with two voxels in the original image, with a 50 percent overlap in each. The intensity associated with this new voxel is, then, some combination of the intensities from the original voxels, and the precise combination used is specified by the *interpolation function*. For example, a simple approach in this case would just be to average the intensities from the two voxels being overlapped, and this is what a linear interpolation does. However, there are also other interpolation options, each with some advantages and some disadvantages.

Interpolation is a standard problem in mathematics and the choice of interpolation is often prespecified within an analysis pipeline. The choice depends on the type of image information being transformed; however, sometimes you will need to apply transformations outside a standard pipeline, in which case you need to be able to choose the most appropriate interpolation option yourself. Furthermore, it is helpful to be aware of the limitations of each interpolation method when viewing and interpreting results.

The simplest interpolation method is nearest neighbor interpolation, which just takes the intensity value from the closest voxel (the one with the center closest to the center of the new voxel) and copies the intensity value of this voxel. This has the advantage that the final intensities cannot end up with different values from those in the original image, which is useful for images that are discrete labels. For instance, if a label image contained nonconsecutive values for some reason (say, 10, 20, 30) then using nearest neighbor interpolation guarantees that only these values will exist in the resampled image (a value of, say, 15 would not occur). This is a big advantage when transforming certain types of label image. However, when working with other images (statistical results, structural images, etc.) the use of nearest neighbor interpolation generates poor edges with a blocky appearance and leads to errors and biases in the statistical values or locations of anatomical boundaries.

An alternative interpolation method is *linear interpolation* (also known as *bilinear* in 2D and *trilinear* in 3D). This method takes the surrounding voxel centers (8 of them in 2D, or 26 in 3D) and calculates a weighted average of the intensities from those voxels, the weighting depending on how close the centers are; the closest ones have the highest weighting. One advantage of linear interpolation is that it is highly localized and better at representing spatial boundaries or statistical values than nearest neighbor interpolation; but its disadvantage is that a small amount of blurring is induced. An additional property of linear interpolation is that the intensity values in the resampled image are restricted to the same range as in the original image. For example, resampling an FA image, where the values are all between 0 and 1, results in a resampled image where the values also lie between 0 and 1. This is not the case for all interpolation methods.

The last type of interpolation that we will discuss is the *spline* method, which is a close approximation to the slower *sinc* method and creates a weighted average from a much larger neighborhood of voxels, with weights again determined by distance, but in a nonlinear fashion. Such methods have the advantage that they preserve sharp boundaries very well; but they have the disadvantage that they can create small amounts of ringing artifact (like ripples) near strong edges, and these cause the final intensities to go outside the original intensity bounds. For example, resampling an FA image can create values smaller than 0 or greater than 1, and the same is true for binary masks.

All interpolation options have advantages and disadvantages and all of them involve some degradation of the image, as some information from the original image is lost. As a consequence, repeated interpolation (or resampling) should be avoided whenever possible. One common way to reduce the amount of interpolation is to combine (concatenate) spatial transformations together, when possible, and only perform a single resampling step from one space to a destination space, regardless of whether some intermediate spaces were involved. By using concatenated transformations, the spatial transformation can be done without generating intermediate images, only intermediate coordinates, and so the original intensities only need to be interpolated once. This type of concatenation and single resampling (or *all-in-one resampling*) is applied in many analysis pipelines.

In summary, different interpolation options are available and appropriate for resampling different types of images. The type of spatial transformation chosen (rigid-body, nonlinear, etc.) does not matter in this case, as it is the contents of the image being resampled that counts. For label images with multiple integer values, the nearest neighbor method is most often used. For structural images, spline methods (or similar ones) are most often used, whereas for other images (e.g., original functional or diffusion images) or for derived data (e.g., statistical values) either linear or spline interpolations are often used. Additional blurring, or smoothing, associated with linear interpolation should be taken into account in any subsequent analysis, but this is less of an issue when the pipeline already involves some additional spatial smoothing. Another operation that occurs in practice is the resampling of a binary mask, but this involves some extra considerations that are discussed in the next section.

Box 5.4: Symmetric registration and halfway spaces

Registration can be formulated in a fundamentally symmetric way, so that, instead of one image being transformed but not the other, both images are transformed in an equal and opposite way, in order that they "meet in the middle." All the basic registration principles are the same, but the cost function is written in such a way that switching the two images makes no difference (i.e., it is invariant to the order of the images) and a spatial transformation is applied to both images. This has particular advantages in longitudinal studies, where it is desirable to avoid a bias toward either the baseline or the follow-up scan. By using a symmetric registration approach, the analysis of longitudinal differences can be done in a *halfway space*, where both images (baseline and follow-up) are transformed to an equal and opposite amount—that is, by applying a forward transformation to one image and the inverse transformation to the other. As a consequence, the required interpolation is smaller (by half, on average) and is applied equally to both images, which helps minimize bias and increase sensitivity.

5.3.3 Transforming ROIs and masks

It is a common situation to have a binary mask that represents an ROI (voxels inside the ROI have a value of 1 in the mask, and those outside have a value of 0), which needs to be transformed into another space (e.g., see Figure 5.5). In this case there are several options available, which relate to interpolation and also to a potential thresholding step. This extra step is needed for some interpolation options and allows you to choose how to deal with ambiguous voxels at the edge of the transformed mask.

Thresholding with *binarization* (i.e., an operation where values lower than the threshold result in 0 and values greater than or equal to the threshold result in 1) is necessary whenever the interpolation can produce nonbinary values (i.e., values not equal to 0 or 1). For instance, linear interpolation produces nonbinary values at the edges of a transformed binary mask. Using thresholding (with binarization) ensures that the final result is another binary mask, which can then be used to define an ROI in the destination space.

When transforming a mask, the voxels in the transformed mask will only partially overlap with the original voxels near the boundary (see Figure 5.6). Therefore the transformed mask effectively suffers from partial voluming near the boundary, and to turn it back into a binary mask requires some choices to be made. One option is to use nearest neighbor interpolation, which produces a binary result for each voxel by only using the value from the closest voxel center. Another option is to use linear interpolation, which creates values in the resampled image that are an approximate estimate of the partial volume associated with the overlap. However, this means that the intensity values now take on nonbinary values (e.g., 0.7 rather than either 0 or 1). Thresholding and binarizing these values can then create a binary mask, and the most appropriate threshold to choose depends on the situation where the mask will be used.

Three common situations are as follows:

- The resampled ROI/mask will be used to calculate summary values/statistics *within* a particular structure. In this case it is often desirable to exclude voxels with contaminated partial volume contributions from outside structures and to restrict the mask to "pure" voxels from within the structure. This can be achieved by setting the threshold high (e.g., a threshold of 0.9 would exclude any voxel with 10 percent or more estimated partial volume contamination).

- The resampled ROI will be used to *exclude* some region (e.g., lesion, pathology, artifact) from an analysis. In this case it is better to include, as part of the resampled mask, any voxels that might have signal contributions from this region, in order to stop the signal from "leaking out" of the region into the surrounding areas. This can be achieved by setting the threshold low (e.g., a threshold of 0.1 would include any voxel where the "leaked" signal contribution, via partial voluming, was 10 percent or more).

- The resampled ROI should be the closest anatomical representation of that region, with accurate border placement and a similar volume. In this case a threshold of 0.5 is the most appropriate. However, note that this does not guarantee that the volume will be the same as the mask in the original space, since the resampling process is approximate.

See Figure 5.7 for an illustration of these different thresholds when applied to a transformed mask.

Although nearest neighbor interpolation is an easy way to resample a binary mask, we recommend that you consider your application and choose linear interpolation together with one of the above thresholds instead, as they give you more direct control over partial volume effects. In some applications this may not be important, but in many cases it does make a difference.

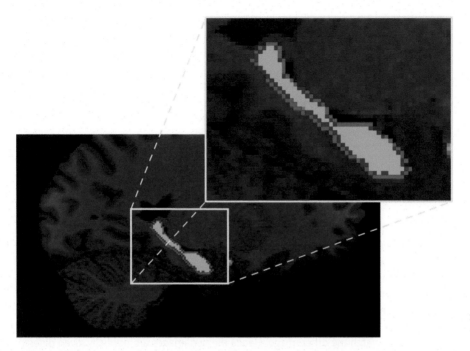

Figure 5.7: Demonstration of the effect of different thresholds when transforming a binary mask (hippocampus) from standard space to an individual structural space. A threshold of 0.9 includes only voxels in green. A threshold of 0.5 includes voxels in green and blue. A threshold of 0.1 includes voxels in green, blue, and red.

5.3.4 Downsampling

When downsampling—that is, transforming images or masks into a lower resolution—additional challenges are involved by comparison to upsampling images to a higher resolution. For example, downsampling a 1 mm (isotropic) image to a 3 mm resolution means that the destination voxels have 27 times (3 × 3 × 3) the volume of the original voxels and will overlap with at least 27 voxels in the original image. In this case the simple interpolation methods mentioned already do not lead to good results when used on their own, as they will consider only the intensities in a small region near the new voxel center and will not cover the full extent of the new, larger voxel, which will end up effectively ignoring a large amount of the original data. Instead it is better to include the values from all the overlapping voxels in a suitable average. A better interpolation can be achieved by using methods that include an explicit averaging within them, or by spatially smoothing the high resolution source image before interpolation. Such a smoothing step achieves a similar result, by averaging over neighborhoods to give representative values that can be interpolated as usual, since each individual value (after smoothing) represents an appropriate (larger) local average.

Both approaches (explicit averaging and presmoothing) are commonly used for downsampling, and different tools will implement one or the other—or possibly neither one. If an explicit downsampling procedure has not been implemented, then it will be expected that the user will apply an appropriate presmoothing or similar operation and you should find out whether this is necessary for the software you use (either check the documentation or make a simple test case and see what happens: for example, a 1 mm thick line that is rotated will have substantial gaps when you resample to lower resolutions unless averaging or presmoothing is implemented). Although most software tools will automatically perform such operations when you are downsampling, it is worth realizing the limitations of this process and the fact that it can induce even more smoothness into the data.

5.4 Case studies

In this and the previous chapter we have covered the main elements of the registration process—brain extraction, spatial transformations, cost functions, interpolations—and explained how these can cater for a very wide range of situations. In this section we will consider some common case studies that indicate how these elements are put together in specific circumstances.

Registration aligns two images and establishes a link between the coordinates, but resampling is usually applied to only one image. That is, one image is transformed or resampled to match the other image. Hence the two images are normally given different names, to clarify which is which. Unfortunately there are quite a few different names commonly used, such as *fixed, reference, target,* or *destination* image for the one that is not resampled (and hence remains the same) and *moving, input,* or *source* image for the one that is resampled (and hence transformed/moved). We will call them input and reference images here (using conventional FSL names), but it is useful to be able to recognize the other names too.

Not all software makes this distinction between the two images, as some use *symmetric registration* methods (which can have advantages—see Box 5.4), so that both images are transformed to "meet in the middle" in a *halfway space.* There are some big advantages in using the halfway space in certain circumstances (e.g., in longitudinal studies, so that results are not biased toward either the baseline or the follow-up scans), but most of the time registration or resampling is performed in order to move information into a known destination space (e.g., standard space). However, methods that are based on symmetric underpinnings can still apply transformations from one space directly to the other, bypassing the halfway space, if requested by the user. Here we will describe how the nonsymmetric methods work, but symmetric methods can also be applied.

For the following case studies we will assume that all images have been reoriented and cropped, as described in section 3.1. This is done in order to increase the robustness of the registration and reduce the chances of large errors; but it is not essential and, depending on the quality and type of images, it may make no difference whether these steps are performed or not. However, in general we recommend them, as it is rare for them to fail or cause problems; it is much more common that they prevent failures in subsequent registration steps from happening.

Case 1: Two structural images of the same subject

In this case study we will assume that there is one T_1-weighted image and one T_2-weighted image from a particular subject in the same session. However, what will be said here applies very well to other combinations of images with sufficient anatomical detail, and also to cases involving different sessions but the same subject.

The two key pieces of information to use here are that (i) both images are from the same subject and (ii) the images are different modalities. From this we can determine the most appropriate type of spatial transformation (namely the rigid-body type as it is within-subject; same anatomy), and cost function (correlation ratio, mutual information, or boundary-based registration, BBR; different MRI modalities). As a rule of thumb, when given a choice of cost functions, using the more restricted one may offer extra robustness. So, in this case, using the correlation ratio might help, as mutual information is the more general (BBR is less commonly used in this context but is also likely to work well and may sometimes be the best option, although it requires extra processing to obtain a segmentation or boundaries from one image).

Another consideration is whether or not to perform brain extraction, which in this case is likely to be helpful, as both images should have sufficient anatomical detail to produce good brain extractions but are likely to have very different intensity contrasts in the nonbrain tissues. That is, some nonbrain tissues may show up distinctly in one image but not in another, and this could possibly cause some inaccuracies in the registration if nothing was done. Hence brain extraction is recommended for this case, though if it is not possible to obtain a good enough brain extraction then performing the registration without it is a reasonable alternative, as long as neither image is brain-extracted. One thing that should always be avoided is registration when one image is brain-extracted and the other is not (since in this case there would be very large mismatches of intensities in nonbrain areas—zero in one image and a value very different from zero in the other).

In addition, some artifacts can cause problems in structural image registration, and the most likely one is bias field. For rigid-body registration, bias field is unlikely to cause noticeable inaccuracies, unless it is very strong. Nevertheless, removing this bias field with a specific tool or as part of a tissue-type segmentation (see section 3.2.3) is most likely to be helpful and to improve the accuracy and robustness of the registration.

Example Box: **Evaluating registrations**

Evaluating the quality of a registration is an important skill, and we strongly recommend that you always check your registration results. This is important because sometimes registration can fail or contain inaccuracies that could significantly affect your later results. The best way to check is to view the results by eye. To do this requires a viewing tool where you can overlay the transformed version of the input image on top of the reference image, as these should have been aligned by the registration. There are several techniques for visualizing the alignment, and the best approach is determined partly by the type of images being examined and partly by personal preference. One technique is to "flick" between the two images (e.g., by turning the transparency/opacity on and off, or by sliding smoothly between the two extremes); the flicking can draw the eye to areas that "move" between the two—although this really only works well for images of the same modality and contrast. If the images are of different modalities, then flicking between them causes huge intensity changes all over the image and is perceptually difficult to work with; in these cases it can be better to place a cursor at a certain location and compare this location between the images. Doing this for a range of locations across the brain can help give a sense of the registration accuracy—and it can be done on side-by-side images or by turning the topmost image overlay "on and off." It is also possible to extract edges from one image and show them on top of the other (usually with colored edges); this highlights whether the grayscale boundaries in one image coincide with the boundaries extracted from the other image, for example boundaries from the reference image in red overlaid on the grayscale display of the transformed input image. Some static examples are shown in Figure 5.8. Other techniques include making one image partially transparent, so that the intensities of both can be seen, which can be combined with false coloring in order to highlight intensity changes with different colors. However you do it, visually checking registration quality is an important step in the analysis and you should do it for all registrations. With experience you will learn how much inaccuracy is typical for your images and analysis pipeline, and thus you will become able to single out and improve poor registrations—for example by identifying artifacts, by improving brain extraction, or by using alternative cost functions. If you are unsure about the quality of your registrations, then consult a colleague or compare them with other example registrations, such as those available on the primer website and referenced in the example boxes.

Visually inspecting registration results is the best way to determine the accuracy and should always be carried out, as there is no automated, quantitative assessment of registration accuracy that is anywhere near as general and reliable. In fact, if such a measure did exist, it could be used as a cost function, to drive the registrations. Although cost functions provide a form of quantitative assessment, they do not quantify the accuracy in terms of a geometric measure of misalignment. However, the biggest problem with cost functions is that, although they are useful for comparing candidate transformations between the pair of images being registered, they are not good at comparisons between registrations with a different pair of images. That is, registrations performed using different subjects can lead to substantial differences in cost function value for the same quality of alignment. This is because the artifacts, noise, and anatomy are not the same across images and subjects, which affects the cost function; hence the value of a cost function reflects both the quality of the alignment and the quality of the images themselves and is not particularly meaningful when comparing registrations with different images or subjects. Consequently it is not that useful to treat cost functions as a quantitative assessment of registration accuracy; for example the minimum cost function value from a within-subject registration of two images from one subject, as in case study 1, and the minimum cost function value from the same kind of registration but with images from another subject do not necessarily reflect the relative accuracy of each of the within-subject registrations, and the subject where the cost function is lower may actually have a less accurate alignment. Thus no absolute thresholds or ranges can reliably be established for an accurate or "good quality" registration that holds in general with respect to cost function values. Nonetheless, cost functions are

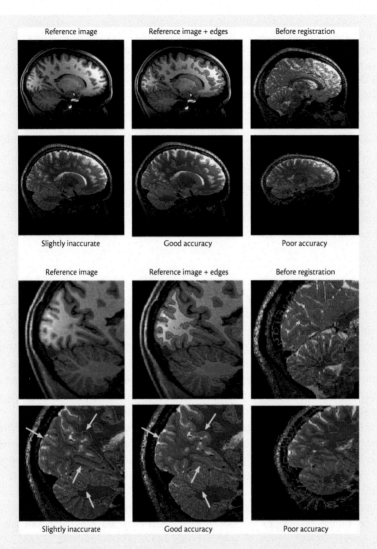

Reference image   Reference image + edges   Before registration

Slightly inaccurate   Good accuracy   Poor accuracy

Reference image   Reference image + edges   Before registration

Slightly inaccurate   Good accuracy   Poor accuracy

Figure 5.8: Illustration of within-subject registration and of ways of viewing the results. First row shows the T_1-weighted reference image (left) and this image together with the red edges (middle) that were extracted from it (derived from the boundary of a white matter segmentation). The edges align perfectly with the anatomy, as they are calculated from this image; and they are very useful for overlaying on the transformed versions of the T_2-weighted input image in order to visualize the quality of the registration result. The next image (top row, right) shows these red edges from the reference image overlaid on the input image prior to registration, where the alignment is clearly poor. The second row shows three registration outputs, each overlaid with the red edges from the reference image, which demonstrate various levels of accuracy obtained: slightly poor (left), good (middle), and very poor (right). The last two rows show zoomed-in portions of the images in the top two rows, allowing the difference in the best two registrations (bottom left and bottom middle) to be seen more clearly. The yellow arrows highlight some locations where the improvement between the left and the middle cases can be seen. These registrations are illustrative examples but give an indication of the level of accuracy that can be obtained from good-quality within-subject registration.

sometimes used as part of quality assessment procedures; but they tend to be most useful in identifying gross failures and not so useful for assessing the finer degrees of accuracy. This means that it is still necessary for you to look at your data, as that really is the best way to evaluate the performance.

Case 2: Structural image of one subject and the MNI152 template

In this case study we will assume that there is a T_1-weighted image of a subject to be registered to MNI space (e.g., for group analysis). The T_1-weighted MNI152 template is to be used as the reference image, which is the most commonly used version, although other MNI templates also exist.

The two key pieces of information to use here are that (i) the images represent different anatomy and (ii) the images are the same MRI modality. From this we can determine the most appropriate type of spatial transformation (namely nonlinear spatial transformation; different anatomy) and cost function (any of them, except unnormalized sum of squared differences; same modality). Here we exclude the unnormalized sum of squared differences because the range of intensities, or scaling, will almost certainly be different between the two images. Once again, as a rule of thumb, the more restricted cost functions are likely to work better—such as normalized correlation or (normalized) sum of squared differences. To use the latter requires extra normalization of the intensities, in order to ensure that they have the same range, which is sometimes applied within the registration method or can be done as a separate preprocessing step. Many nonlinear registration methods only offer a limited range of cost functions, such as sum of squared differences (with prenormalization) or normalized correlation.

For the nonlinear registration to work robustly, it is also necessary to perform an initial affine registration, in order to get the location, orientation, and scale of the image approximately the same as the MNI template (see Figure 5.9). The affine transformation parameters are typically passed into the nonlinear registration directly, so that we avoid having to perform any image resampling.

Brain extraction and bias-field correction are also recommended, as in case 1, where brain extraction should be applied to both images (brain-extracted MNI templates are readily available) and bias-field correction needs to be applied only to the structural image (as the MNI template is already bias-corrected). Given that the nonbrain structures in the MNI template will be different from the nonbrain structures in the subject's structural image, brain extraction (whether explicitly done beforehand or implicitly done within the registration tool) is important for accurate registration in this case.

Once the registration has been completed, you should evaluate the quality visually, as discussed in the Example Box "Evaluating Registrations." All the same principles apply here, but with the caveat that the standard template image (MNI152) will be sharper in some areas and blurrier in others, on the basis of how variable the anatomy is across the population in that region and how well it can be aligned with nonlinear registration methods (see Figure 5.10). Therefore there will be regions where it will be difficult to determine the accuracy of the alignment, as not all folds will be present in the template image. Many of these areas are regions with high anatomical variability, which cannot be aligned perfectly with current methods. This

Before Registration

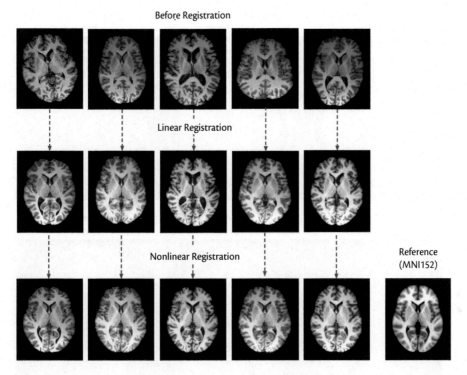

Linear Registration

Nonlinear Registration

Reference
(MNI152)

Figure 5.9: Illustration of registration in a group analysis: five subjects with different brain sizes and folding patterns, each registered to a common reference template (MNI152). The top row shows slices from the original images, while the middle row shows the corresponding images after linear (affine) registration and the bottom row shows the corresponding images after nonlinear registration. Note how the linear registration makes the images similar in brain size and overall shape, while the finer anatomical details are well matched only after nonlinear registration.

should be kept in mind when evaluating the registration quality, and also when interpreting the final results of the analysis.

Case 3: EPI image (fMRI or dMRI) and structural of one subject and the MNI152 template

In this case study we will assume that there is an fMRI 4D image (though dMRI would work the same way) and a T_1-weighted image from the same subject, and that a registration to MNI space is desired (e.g., for functional group analysis). This involves three spaces: functional, structural, and MNI. As explained in section 5.3.1, these spaces can all be brought into alignment with two registrations and the various combinations of their spatial transformations. We will take a common approach here, which is to register in two stages: (i) the functional and structural spaces; and (ii) the structural and MNI spaces (see Figure 5.11 for an illustration of this two stage registration). As the details of the second stage of this registration have already been dealt with in the second case study, we only need to discuss the first stage here.

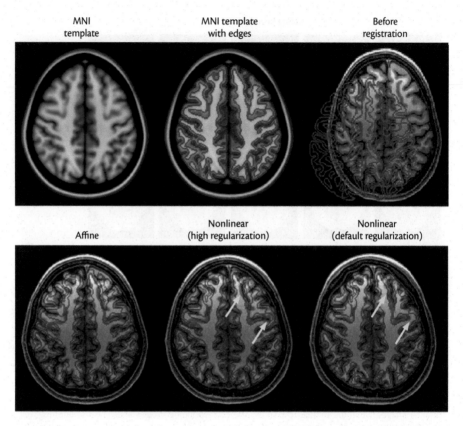

MNI template | MNI template with edges | Before registration

Affine | Nonlinear (high regularization) | Nonlinear (default regularization)

Figure 5.10: Illustration of registration to the MNI152 template. The first row shows the reference image—the MNI152 template (left) and the same template overlaid with red edges from a gray matter segmentation (middle). The T1-weighted image from the individual subject is shown (right) prior to any registration, along with the edges from the reference image. In the bottom row are the registration results from initial affine (left), nonlinear with high regularization (middle), and nonlinear with default regularization (right). These results correspond to the nonlinear transformations shown in Figure 5.3, the default (lower) regularization generally giving better alignment (as highlighted by the yellow arrows).

For the functional to structural space registration, we will take one 3D image from the functional 4D image (typically the middle image, but it is not important which one, as long as it is not corrupted by any bad artifacts). The registration of this functional image to the structural image of the same individual has (i) the same anatomy, (ii) different modalities, and (iii) distortions in the fMRI. We will deal with distortion correction separately in Chapter 6; for now we will assume that the distortions have already been corrected (and tools for this exist, especially in dMRI). The main purpose of this case study is to illustrate the two-stage approach that will also be used (in a modified way) in Chapter 6.

In the first stage (functional to structural space) the anatomy is the same, and so a rigid-body spatial transformation is appropriate. Due to the different modalities, a multimodal cost function is appropriate—such as correlation ratio, mutual information, or BBR. Few nonbrain structures are visible on the fMRI images, due to the fat suppression applied in all EPI acquisitions, and

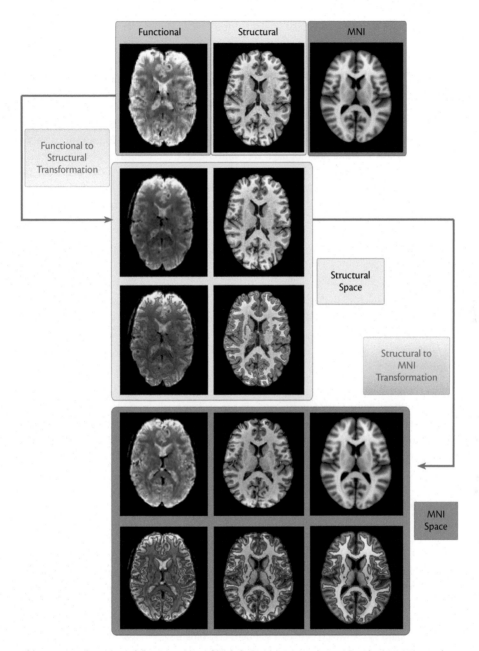

Figure 5.11: Illustration of the registration of both fMRI and structural images to the MNI152 template. The first row shows the original images (still in their own spaces, each one color-coded: green for functional, yellow for structural, and blue for MNI). The second row shows the results of registering the fMRI and transforming it into structural space (left), along with the original structural image (right). The third row shows the same images as in the second row, but overlaid with red boundaries extracted from the structural image. The fourth row shows the results of transforming both the fMRI and the structural images (left and middle, respectively) to the MNI152 template (right), using the registration of the structural image to the MNI template. The fifth row shows the same images as in the fourth row, but overlaid with red boundaries extracted from the MNI template. The transformation of the fMRI to the MNI (standard) space is performed with one resampling, from the fMRI space to the MNI space, by combining the transformations of fMRI to structural and of structural to registration, as illustrated by the red arrows.

therefore brain extraction should be applied to the structural image (or something equivalent should be done within the registration tool).

Once a registration has been performed for each stage separately and their quality checked visually, the spatial transformations can be combined together to allow any image in the functional space (including statistical results) to be resampled directly into MNI space. Note that any inaccuracy that occurs in this combined transformation will have its source in one or both of the transformations that contribute to it. That is, if the fMRI does not look like it is well aligned with the MNI152 template, this is because the fMRI did not align well with the structural or the structural did not align well with the MNI152 template—or both. Hence, if any troubleshooting needs to be done, then it needs be done for one, or both, of the original registrations. Once good-quality registrations have been obtained for the individual stages, it is the combined transformation that is used from then on in the pipeline. Each of these cases is illustrated with real data in the Example Box "Registration case studies."

Example Box: **Registration case studies**

On the primer website there are illustrative datasets suitable for any software and instructions on how to apply FSL tools for each of these case studies. These materials will also illustrate how to visually assess the quality and what steps to take when troubleshooting problematic results.

One case that we have not considered is how to register two (or more) EPI scans of the same subject. If these come from separate acquisitions, it is normally best to register them to the structural scan as a common, and higher quality, anatomical reference, as described in Case 3. However, if the scans are two 3D volumes from a 4D acquisition (e.g., fMRI), then that is given a special name, motion correction, which we will discuss in the next chapter.

5.5 Standard space and templates

In group analyses it is necessary to register all the subjects to a common space in order to have consistent anatomical alignment and be able to identify an anatomical location with a voxel coordinate. This is achieved by registering images to a template image, which can either be created from the set of subjects in the study or be a population-derived template. A standard template is one that has been derived from a certain population, is distributed publicly, and can be used as the reference for many studies, such as the MNI152. These templates are associated with a standard space, which defines a standard coordinate system that is useful for reporting the location of results in a quantitative way that does not rely on potentially inconsistent, subjective descriptions of anatomical location.

The first commonly used standard space in neuroimaging was the one developed by Talairach and Tournoux, which was based on a careful postmortem examination and annotation of a single elderly subject. This examination defined a set of coordinates throughout the brain that were centered on the anterior commissure and oriented so that the x axis was left–right, the y axis was posterior–anterior and the z axis was inferior–superior. These definitions have been adopted in all subsequent standard neuroimaging spaces.

Limitations of the standard space of Talairach and Tournoux include the fact that there is not an associated MRI template image for registration and that it does not represent a population but only a single individual. To address these issues, researchers at the Montreal Neurological Institute, along with colleagues in the International Consortium for Brain Mapping (ICBM), created an MRI-based template by aligning a set of subjects together in such a way that the coordinates were very similar to those of Talairach and Tournoux, although not exactly the same. Several generations of the MNI templates have now been created, and the most widely used one at present is the MNI152 (also known as the ICBM152). This is an average of structural MRI images from 152 young healthy adult subjects that have been aligned with nonlinear registration to create a template that has very similar coordinates to the original Talairach and Tournoux coordinates but better captures the anatomy of this population of young healthy adults. It shows sharp boundaries in areas where the registration has been able to accurately align the subjects' anatomy, but is blurry in areas where the individual variations in anatomy were too great for the registration to be able to find a consistent alignment (see Figure 5.12).

There are several different MNI152 templates with different resolutions (e.g., 2 mm, 1 mm, and 0.5 mm) and that are based on different acquisition modalities (e.g., T_2-weighted and PD). Every MNI152 template is in the same space, meaning that the world (or mm) coordinates associated with a particular anatomical location are consistent across all template images. Therefore it does not matter which template is used for registration purposes in order to align a subject with this standard space, as long as the registration result is sufficiently accurate. Hence you will find some pipelines using templates with different resolutions or with different modalities.

Not all studies use the MNI152 space or templates; some software tools align to the Talairach and Tournoux space instead. There are some subtle differences in these coordinates and in how they relate to anatomical locations, which should be kept in mind when reporting and interpreting results. However, the main reason for not using the MNI152 is that the subjects being studied do not fit the population used to create the template. Nonetheless, the MNI152 has been used in a huge number of studies, including ones involving children, elderly subjects, and pathological patients. Whether the MNI152 template should be used for a particular study depends partly on the desired degree of anatomical accuracy, partly on the ability to relate to other studies (to make direct comparisons to their standard coordinates), and partly on the difficulty of obtaining a more appropriate template. A number of alternative templates (and hence spaces) do already exist for different demographics (different ages, ethnicities, etc.), although none is presently as widely used as the MNI152.

One alternative to using a standard template is to build one from the set of subjects in the study. Such study-specific templates can be created automatically in some analysis pipelines (e.g., VBM) or can be created separately, usually by running registrations several times, in a loop, to iterate towards a better average image. These templates can more accurately represent the population from which the subjects were drawn, provided that there are sufficient subjects, since generating a template from a small number of subjects does not work too well. A potential difficulty with using a study-specific template is that the

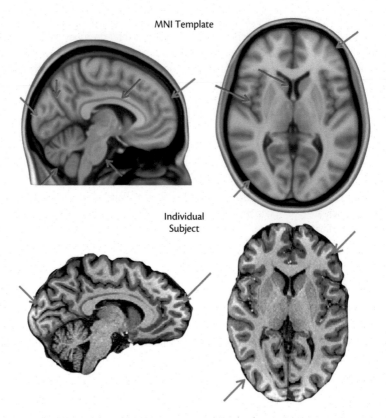

MNI Template

Individual
Subject

Figure 5.12: Illustration of slices from the MNI152 template (top) and of approximately matched slices from an individual subject (bottom). The red arrows indicate areas where the MNI template has sharp boundaries, corresponding to structures that were precisely aligned across the set of subjects used to form the template. Blue arrows indicate areas that are blurry in the MNI template due to unresolved variations in individual anatomy; these areas can be compared with the individual subject's image where the boundaries are sharp.

coordinates are no longer exactly the same as the MNI152 standard coordinates. This should be kept in mind when reporting and interpreting results. Thus there are possible advantages and disadvantages to using study-specific templates and this is one of the many decisions and trade-offs to be considered when planning and analyzing your own experiments.

5.6 Atlases

Apart from template images, you will frequently encounter *atlases* in standard space. These atlases are in the same space as the template images and are stored in the form of images where the intensities are used to encode other forms of information. For example, discrete labels that correspond to different anatomical structures such that the left thalamus is labelled with the number 4, the left caudate with the number 5, and so on. When visually displayed, these discrete labels look like maps with solid colors or patches rather than looking like MRI acquisitions—just as a political map of the world shows countries with solid colors rather than looking like a satellite photo. This makes atlases very helpful for learning about anatomy and for quantitatively identifying structures (see the top row of Figure 5.13). Atlases are often used to automatically label the location of results of interest and to create ROIs within the analysis or in the investigation of results.

Information that is stored in an atlas depicts anatomical or functional subdivisions of the brain, and these divisions are collectively known as a *parcellation*. A parcellation may cover the whole brain or a limited portion. In addition, the information can come from a number of different sources, such as expert manual labelings of MR images, analyses of MRI data (segmentations, tractography, ICA), or histological data. In each case the data are derived in some fashion from a set of subjects, and hence each atlas is specific to the population that this set represents. Most often this is the young, healthy, adult population, although atlases for many other populations, with different demographics, exist as well. However, the data usually come from a set of subjects that is separate from the set used to form the template of the standard space. For example, there are numerous atlases in the MNI152 space that derive their underlying data from a different set of subjects, and may represent slightly different populations (see Table 5.2), though they all must be registered to an MNI152 template in order to get into the MNI152 space. When using an atlas it is also necessary to use a template that corresponds to the atlas space (e.g., the T_1-weighted MNI152 template) for the registration, rather than to the atlas images themselves. It is therefore worth keeping in mind the demographic characteristics relevant for each of these atlases and making sure that they are appropriate for the subjects you are working with.

There are two main types of atlas image: *discrete* and *probabilistic*. A discrete atlas image provides a single integer (discrete) label value per voxel, where the label value corresponds to a particular structure or parcel. This is like a hard parcellation where each voxel is either fully part of one structure or not, and a visualization of such an atlas can show multiple regions, each with a solid color, all stored in one 3D image (see the top row in Figure 5.13).

A probabilistic atlas provides a value between 0 and 1 at each voxel that represents the probability of that voxel belonging to a particular structure. This is the most common type of atlas, as it can represent more information about the variation in anatomy in the population; see the Example Box "Probabilistic atlas construction." That is, areas that are very consistent between subjects and very accurately aligned will have sharp boundaries (probabilities that change from 0 to 1 over a short distance), as opposed to areas where there is substantial variation between subjects and less precise alignment, which will have diffuse boundaries (probabilities that change from 0 to 1 over a much greater distance); see the bottom row of Figure 5.13. Probabilistic atlases are usually stored as 4D images, with each 3D volume (image) corresponding to the probability map for a single structure, the same way that PVE images were stored for tissue-type segmentation (see section 3.2.3).

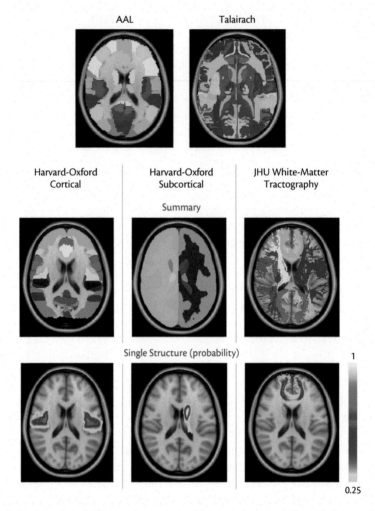

Figure 5.13: Examples of different atlases: AAL and Talairach (top row: left to right); Harvard–Oxford cortical and subcortical atlases, and JHU white matter tractography atlas (bottom rows: left to right). The atlases in the top row are discrete ones, while the other three are probabilistic. For the probabilistic atlases, the probability distribution for just one of the structures within each atlas is displayed in the bottom row: central opercular cortex (left); caudate (middle); forceps minor (right). A separate 3D image of this type exists for each structure within a probabilistic atlas. A summary label image of all the structures within a probabilistic atlas (middle row; same order as in bottom row) is also typically provided, where the color coding is determined by the structure that has the maximum probability at each voxel. In both cases, voxels where the probability is lower than 0.25 are not shown here, for display purposes.

Example Box: **Probabilistic atlas construction**

The Harvard–Oxford atlas was created by aligning MR images from 37 subjects to the standard MNI152 template, then transforming manual labelings from each of these subjects to the standard space, and finally averaging the transformed labels. This was done separately for each structure. For instance, the left hippocampus is one of the structures in the atlas, and for each of the subjects a manual label was created that corresponded to the left hippocampus (e.g., the number 9 is the label for the left hippocampus). A binary image was then created by extracting only this label (i.e., by generating an image where all voxels inside the left hippocampus have a value of 1 and all others have a value of 0). This binary image was then transformed into standard space using the spatial transform derived from the registration of that subject's T_1-weighted image with the MNI152 T_1-weighted template. This procedure was repeated for each subject and the transformed images were then averaged to yield a final probabilistic image. In this image, voxels that were clearly inside the hippocampus for all subjects ended up with a value of 1, whereas voxels near the border were considered part of the hippocampus in some subjects, but not in all, and hence ended up with a value between 0 and 1.

It is possible to create a discrete label image from a probabilistic atlas (see the middle row in Figure 5.13). This is done by assigning a label to each voxel on the basis of the structure that has the highest probability at that location. That is, if the atlas contains 20 structures, there will be 20 separate 3D images, and so each voxel will be associated with 20 different probabilities (one per structure). The structure associated with the largest probability then has its label value stored at that voxel (e.g., if the left thalamus is the fourth structure on the list and has a label value of 4, a voxel would be labeled with a value of 4 if that location had a higher probability of being in the left thalamus than all other structures). There is also one additional operation that is often performed when assigning the labels, which is to exclude any voxels where the maximum probability is smaller than a certain predefined threshold. For example, a threshold of 0.25 might be applied so that the borders of structures do not extend too far from the average boundary. This is done because the probabilities can sometimes extend well beyond the average boundary position, with low values representing a small minority of subjects with very extended, unusual boundaries. These subjects cause some more distant voxels to have nonzero probabilities, and so, when converting to a discrete label, they might create an unrepresentative position of that structure's boundary.

In summary, many different atlases are available that cover a wide variety of information; but each one is either a discrete or a probabilistic atlas. A probabilistic atlas usually comes with a discrete, summary version of itself—a version based on labeling voxels according to the structure or region with the maximum probability. Each atlas typically uses different information in its construction (histology, manual labels based on T_1-weighted images, etc.) and is appropriate for a population that is matched to the subjects used to create the atlas. Many atlases, though not all, exist in the MNI152 space and therefore require registration to the MNI152 template in order for information from that atlas to be used in a particular subject or study. Atlases are

Table 5.2 A small set of example atlases that illustrate the range of regions and methods of atlas creation. All examples here are probabilistic atlases, except the Talairach and AAL atlases. References and links to these atlases are available on the primer website.

Atlas Name	Standard Space	Original Source of Information	Structures Included
Talairach	MNI152	Histology: a digitized version of original Talairach and Tournoux atlas, based on one postmortem brain.	1105 cortical and subcortical structures
Jülich	MNI152	Histology: detailed microscopic and quantitative histological examination of 10 human postmortem brains	52 gray matter and 10 white matter structures, divided into 121 subregions
Harvard–Oxford	MNI152	Manual labels (based on T_1-weighted images): averaged over 37 healthy adult subjects	48 cortical and 17 subcortical structures
AAL	MNI152	Automatic labeling of a set of scans from a single healthy adult subject (provided by the MNI)	116 cortical and subcortical regions
HCP Multi-Modal Cortical Parcellation (MPM)	fs_LR (standard HCP surface space)	Automated parcellation of multimodal data from 210 young healthy adult subjects from the Human Connectome Project	180 cortical regions per hemisphere
JHU White-Matter Tractography	MNI152	Deterministic tractography: results averaged from 28 young healthy adult subjects	20 major white matter tracts
Oxford Thalamic Connectivity	MNI152	Connectivity-based segmentation (from diffusion MRI tractography): results averaged from probabilistic tractography parcellations in 8 young healthy adult subjects	7 thalamic subregions
Cerebellar	MNI152	Manual labels (based on T_1-weighted images): averaged from 20 young healthy adult subjects	28 regions of the cerebellum

particularly useful for defining ROIs in order to study effects (e.g., average FA value or fMRI activation) within these regions, or as part of the analysis (e.g., seeding tractography from an anatomical structure/region). They are also useful for interpreting results and learning about brain anatomy.

5.7 Atlas-based segmentation

The anatomical information contained in an atlas or in multiple atlases can be used to perform segmentation. This is done by registering a subject's structural image (usually but not necessarily a T_1-weighted image) to a template image in the space of the atlas, and then transforming the atlas information into the native, structural space of that individual subject. If discrete labels from the atlas are used, then transforming the labels is the same as transforming binary ROIs or masks for a particular structure (see section 5.3.3) and the result is a labeled image (or a binary mask, if only one structure is of interest). If one structure's probability image from a probabilistic atlas is transformed, then the result is a probability map of that structure, now in the space of the individual subject. Depending on the application, this probability information may be useful in itself or may be thresholded (and binarized) so as to create a mask.

The accuracy of atlas-based segmentations is based on several factors: the accuracy of the registration, the sharpness of the template, the variability of the anatomy, and the match of the subject to the demographics of the atlas and template. The most obvious factor is the accuracy of the registration, and this is strongly influenced by the sharpness of the template. For example, in areas where the template is blurry, the registration will have reduced accuracy, which is usually a consequence of large variability in the anatomy of that area. Using a probabilistic atlas can help quantify some of the variability in anatomy but does not take everything into account.

An alternative approach, which has been shown to substantially improve accuracy, is to use segmentations or parcellations from a set of individual subjects rather than an average atlas and a template. A labeled image together with a structural image from a single subject is called a single "atlas" in this case, and combining a set of these constitutes *multi-atlas segmentation*. This method therefore requires access to the individual datasets (one structural image and one label image per subject), as opposed to access to just a probabilistic average. To perform the segmentation, the label image from each subject is transformed into the native structural space of the query subject (the query subject is the one being segmented by the multi-atlas method), and this provides a set of labels for the query subject, each of which is usually slightly different from the others. The final result is then obtained by combining these individual labels—for example into some form of weighted average.

One advantage of multi-atlas segmentation is that no template image is required, since an individual structural image is used for each subject, and this then avoids some registration inaccuracies induced by the blurring that is seen in template images. However, registration accuracy in areas of large anatomical variation (such as differences in the number of folds) is still limited. To improve on accuracy even further, multi-atlas segmentation methods also tend to select a subset of the atlases (subjects), using only the ones that best match the query subject. After this selection, the remaining labels are combined, often with weighted averaging. A range of methods exist for atlas selection and the calculation of weights. These methods are based on cost function values (an approximate estimate of overall alignment quality), demographics (e.g., age), local quality measures, or more sophisticated machine-learning techniques.

Multi-atlas segmentation can perform well when the registrations are accurate and the subject to be segmented fits with the demographic characteritics of the set of subjects (atlases). However, the availability of suitable multiple atlas datasets (which consist of many individual subjects) is more limited than for other types of atlases. Whether this form of segmentation is superior to other alternatives will depend on the structures you are interested in, on the image quality, and on the availability of appropriate tools and atlases. To find the best method requires trying different alternatives on your own data and evaluating the quality of the results with respect to what matters for your application.

SUMMARY

- Registration is a fundamental tool in all areas of neuroimaging, for structural, functional, and diffusion analyses.

- A number of options and parameters need to be specified—in particular, choosing appropriate types of spatial transformations and cost functions. The range of options available will depend on the software package being used.

- Applying a spatial transformation, or resampling an image, requires the interpolation of intensity data that degrade the data quality to some degree. Resampling steps are therefore minimized and transformations are often combined to enable a single, all-in-one resampling to be done.

- The results of registration should be checked visually, to guard against major failures and also to get an impression of the level of accuracy attained with your data. This will help you to optimize the performance of your pipelines by tuning the registration. It will also help with the interpretation of your results (e.g., it will help with knowing how trustworthy the detailed localization is).

- Registration between multiple spaces (functional, structural, and standard spaces) is often done using a multistage registration (e.g., functional to structural and then structural to standard) with one resampling step at the end.

- The most common standard space is the MNI152 and several templates exist for this space, but there are also benefits to using study-specific templates, especially for cohorts that are not well matched to a young healthy adult population.

- Many atlases exist, most of them in the MNI152 space, and they can encode information about anatomy or function that can come from a wide variety of sources (e.g., histology, MRI analysis, manual tracings). These are widely used for automatically labeling locations and for deriving ROIs.

■ Registration and resampling of atlas-based information can be used for the segmentation of individual images. This can be done with standard-space atlases or, if available, with a set of individual subject segmentations that use multi-atlas segmentation methods.

FURTHER READING

■ Keszei, A. P., Berkels, B., & Deserno, T. M. (2017). Survey of non-rigid registration tools in medicine. *Journal of Digital Imaging*, 30(1), 102–116.
  ▫ *General overview of a range of available registration tools, with some technical details.*

■ Viergever, M. A., Maintz, J. A., Klein, S., Murphy, K., Staring, M., & Pluim, J. P. (2016). A survey of medical image registration—under review. *Medical Image Analysis*, 33, 140–144.
  ▫ *A general overview of the field of registration—this paper take a well cited review paper from 1998, updates the content and charts the development of the registration field over time.*

■ Friston, K., Ashburner, J., Frith, C. D., Poline, J. B., Heather, J. D., & Frackowiak, R. S. (1995). Spatial registration and normalization of images. *Human Brain Mapping*, 3(3), 165–189.
  ▫ *Paper describing the registration methods used in the SPM package (with technical details).*

■ Jenkinson, M., & Smith, S. (2001). A global optimisation method for robust affine registration of brain images. *Medical Image Analysis*, 5(2), 143–156.
  ▫ *Paper describing the linear registration method used in the FSL package (with technical details).*

■ Glasser, M. F., Sotiropoulos, S. N., Wilson, J. A., Coalson, T. S., Fischl, B., Andersson, J. L., et al. (2013). The minimal preprocessing pipelines for the Human Connectome Project. *Neuroimage*, 80, 105–124.
  ▫ *Paper describing the general HCP analysis pipeline, with information about registration, using FSL and FreeSurfer tools.*

■ Evans, A. C., Janke, A. L., Collins, D. L., & Baillet, S. (2012). Brain templates and atlases. *NeuroImage*, 62(2), 911–922.
  ▫ *Overview paper describing a range of atlases, including many of those contained in Table 5.2.*

■ Glasser, M. F., Coalson, T. S., Robinson, E. C., Hacker, C. D., Harwell, J., Yacoub, E., et al. (2016). A multi-modal parcellation of human cerebral cortex. *Nature*, 536(7615): 171–178.
  ▫ *Paper describing a recent atlas from the HCP, using a multimodal parcellation technique.*

■ Iglesias, J. E., & Sabuncu, M. R. (2015). Multi-atlas segmentation of biomedical images: A survey. *Medical Image Analysis*, 24(1), 205–219.
  ▫ *A paper that provides a survey of multi-atlas segmentation methods.*

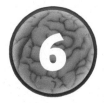

Motion and Distortion Correction

In the previous chapter we discussed registration in its general form and with specific applications, predominantly involving structural images. This chapter will discuss two other uses of registration that are particularly relevant for functional and diffusion imaging: motion correction and distortion correction. These corrections are needed because for both fMRI and dMRI a series of images based on the echo planar imaging (EPI) sequence is acquired, so that motion between volumes and image distortion are commonplace and have the potential to cause substantial confounds in later analyses. Both of these effects are related to spatial transformations, and hence can be corrected for by the use of specially adapted registration-based methods.

6.1 Motion correction

When acquiring a series of 3D volumes, it is necessary to compensate for any subject motion that occurs between the acquisitions. This kind of motion always occurs in functional or diffusion acquisitions, where tens to hundreds of 3D volumes are acquired in rapid succession, but it can also can occur when scanning multiple repeats of a structural sequence (e.g., several T_1-weighted volumes, each acquired relatively quickly, in order to increase robustness with respect to artifacts by allowing badly affected volumes to be rejected). Furthermore, even very small motions (< 0.3 mm) in a functional series can induce signal changes of the order of 10 percent, which is much more than the typical changes in the neuronal signals of interest: those change only by around 1 percent . Therefore motion correction is a very important step in fMRI preprocessing (see section 3.4.2) and would be recommended even if prospective motion correction methods are also used in the acquisition.

Within a scanning session the brain rotates and translates as the head moves, and therefore rigid-body transformations are used to model this motion. It is common to implement motion correction as a series of pairwise 3D registrations, using the same fixed reference image for all registrations, with a cost function tuned for within-modality registration (e.g., sum of squared differences or normalized correlation). The reference image can be the first 3D image in the series, the middle one, or an average; the method is the same and the effect on the results is normally minor, as long as the chosen reference image does not suffer from bad artifacts. Most motion correction tools implement this type of registration-based method, though other varieties also exist (see section 6.1.2).

6.1.1 Motion parameters and summary measures

The outputs from motion correction include values of the rotation angles and translations for each volume, obtained from the rigid-body transformations. These parameters are often plotted as a function of time, to show the (estimated) motion that occurred and to quantify its extent (see Figure 6.1). It is common to use these parameters (and other functions of them, such as squared and/or delayed versions) as regressors, in order to denoise data (see section 6.1.2 and the online appendix titled *Short Introduction to the General Linear Model for Neuroimaging*), particularly for functional data. Although there are no universally accepted conventions for how to represent motions in terms of parameters (some tools use different units, different centers of rotation, etc.), this does not make much difference to their use as regressors for denoising.

It is common to summarize these parameters into a quantity that expresses some form of average distance moved, for example by averaging the voxelwise displacement between 3D images—a quantity known as *framewise displacement* (FD). This summary measure can represent the displacements either with respect to the fixed reference image or with respect to the next image in the sequence. The summary using the fixed reference is sometimes known as an absolute measure and shows both rapid changes in position and slower changes (or drifts). In contrast, the summary using the next image is a relative measure and only highlights rapid changes, with slow changes usually being negligible (see Figure 6.1). These summary measures provide information that can be used to assess whether motion is correlated with functional stimuli or is different across subject groups.

There are also other, independent measures that are used to assess motion in a dataset. These do not depend on the motion correction parameters but can play a role similar to that of the motion summaries. The most well known example is DVARS, which is essentially the root mean square difference between intensities in successive images and highlights any signal changes. These intensity changes are typically dominated by motion-induced changes, as those are large by comparison with neuronally induced changes. The advantage of using such metrics is that they do not rely on the accuracy of motion correction; and in challenging data, especially with a number of artifacts, accurate motion correction can be difficult to achieve at all times. The disadvantage is that these metric values are not specific to motion and may be driven by other artifacts as well as by motion. Using such measures (or metrics) in combination with ones generated by motion correction (such as framewise displacement) is a good way to get an understanding of what motion there is in the data.

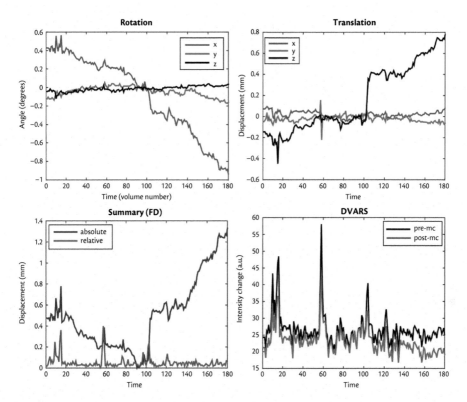

Figure 6.1: Examples of various motion correction plots. Rotation and translation parameters (angles in degrees and displacements in millimeters), plotted as a function of time (in terms of volume number, where this example dataset had 180 volumes), are shown in the top row. Summaries of the motion are provided in the bottom row: average displacement (or framewise displacement) is shown on the left for both absolute and relative displacements (i.e., with respect to a fixed reference point or with respect to the next time point in the series respectively); DVARS (root mean squared intensity change between successive 3D images) is shown on the right, both before and after motion correction is run.

6.1.2 Motion artifact correction

Unfortunately there are several common artifacts in fMRI (see sections 3.4.1 to 3.4.4) and in dMRI (see sections 3.3.1 to 3.3.4). The main ones are geometric distortions caused by B_0-inhomogeneities; slice-timing effects; eddy-current distortions (diffusion only); and signal loss (functional only). These all interact, both among themselves and with the motion, so that independent correction methods for individual artifacts provide an approximation to the full correction but (in principle) cannot do as well as more sophisticated correction methods, which combine all corrections simultaneously. That being said, individual serial corrections are still very common and give an accurate approximation in many cases, especially when the amount of motion is small. However, because of the potential advantages of combined corrections, such tools are becoming increasingly available. For instance, in diffusion MRI there are tools for simultaneously correcting for eddy-current distortions, B_0-inhomogeneity distortions, and motion. Slice-to-volume registration methods, which relax the constraint that slices must stay parallel (see Figure 3.18), are also available. Methods that perform such combined corrections often require good-quality data in order to drive the estimation of the distortions and motions.

Apart from these distortions, motion in the scanner induces a range of additional changes and artifacts in the signal intensity (such as spin-history effects; see Box 3.5 in section 3.4.2), and these cannot be removed by spatial transformations alone. Hence corrections for such motion artifacts are often implemented in addition to the motion correction (or combined correction) stage. These artifact corrections are particularly important for fMRI, as the analysis is more sensitive to motion-related artifacts. The three main approaches to additional motion artifact correction (performed after motion correction) are *regressing out motion parameters, outlier rejection*, and *ICA-based denoising*. Different pipelines and situations call for different approaches or combinations of approaches to be used, and this may be something that you need to decide upon yourself. We will briefly describe each of these approaches here and give an indication of their advantages and disadvantages, as well as an indication of when they can be most useful.

Regressing out motion parameters from the data involves taking the six motion parameters (three rotation angles and three translation parameters) and using them as regressors in order to find matching signals and "throw them away" (i.e., treat them as confounds; more details can be found in the online appendix titled *Short Introduction to the General Linear Model for Neuroimaging*). These regressors are also sometimes augmented by squared or delayed versions (to make a set of 12, 18 or 24 regressors) to account for signal changes that are not linearly related to the amount of motion or do not happen instantaneously (these are approximations of what is a highly complex relationship between motion and signal intensity). This approach to "cleaning" the data is very common in resting state fMRI, as it aggressively eliminates a lot of the signals that could be motion. It is an attractive approach in resting state analysis, because such confounds are particularly problematic where the nature of the neuronal signal and timings is not known and hence neuronal signals could easily be confused with motion-induced changes. However, this approach has some problems for task fMRI in situations where the motion is correlated with the stimulus timings. In such cases—that is, cases of *stimulus-correlated motion*—this approach can be too aggressive and throw away a lot of useful neuronally related signals too, which are sparser in task fMRI than in resting state. Hence in those cases this approach is best avoided; it is preferable to use alternatives instead.

Detecting outliers is often done on the basis of the summary measures, for example framewise displacement (FD) or DVARS. In cases where the motion is very large and artifacts are prominent, it can be better to use DVARS or other metrics that are based on intensities, since the estimates of motion are likely to be poor and hence framewise displacement can be very inaccurate and fail to identify the outliers reliably. Alternatively, a combination of both can be used. Either way, some form of thresholding is typically required, to differentiate between outliers and non-outliers, and there is no universal way of determining such thresholds, as they depend on the type and quality of the imaging data. In fact, the threshold may be something that is left for the user to set, and this can be done on the basis of inspecting the data or of comparing them with other datasets or with literature values. Once the outliers have been identified, they can be either deleted from the 4D image (which reduces the number of timepoints) or corrected for in regression models. For task fMRI, there are some disadvantages to deleting images (volumes/timepoints), as this can impact on preprocessing steps such as temporal filtering and on the estimation of crucial noise parameters. For resting state fMRI, deleting images (an operation also called *scrubbing*) is more common, particularly in high-motion populations such as children and patients. As outliers associated with large motions can contain very large intensity changes, removing them, either through deletion or through regression, can have huge benefits. Their removal is also less likely to throw away a lot of true neuronal signal by comparison to motion parameter regression; one exception is in task fMRI, if each stimulus coincides with a large motion, although in that case the data are likely to be too contaminated to be useful anyway.

The third approach to motion artifact correction is ICA-based denoising, which uses independent component analysis to decompose the data into different components (or sources) and then identifies the ones that are noise and can be removed. This was previously discussed in section 3.4.6, in the context of physiological noise correction, and the principle is exactly the same. In fact ICA-based denoising typically corrects for multiple sources of noise, such as physiological noise and motion-related artifact. Identification of neuronal and non-neuronal components can be done either manually or automatically (with suitable training data, which might need to be generated manually). ICA-based denoising can be more effective at separating motion effects from real neuronal effects, as it takes into account both the spatial distribution of the artifact and its timecourse. As a consequence, it is commonly used and is often the best approach, especially for the difficult case of stimulus-correlated motion in task fMRI.

These approaches can be applied separately or in combination, and there can be advantages in combining them, particularly in situations where data quality is limited or the degree of motion is challenging. They are still limited in how much of the motion artifact they can correct for, and if motion is very problematic it might be necessary to use the ultimate fallback: to exclude that subject from your analysis. However, this should be a last resort, as often these correction methods can do a very good job. There is no useful rule of thumb about how much motion is "too much," as the effects vary hugely, depending on the nature of the motion (the speed, the type of rotation, and so on), on the interaction with the process of acquisition, and on data quality. In general we recommend that you stay alert to motion-induced artifacts (knowing that motion artifacts tend to be worse near boundaries such as the edge of the brain and the edge of the ventricles), and that you try different methods for correcting for them, and report and interpret your results accordingly.

6.2 Distortion correction

EPI acquisitions, used for fMRI and dMRI, are sensitive to imperfections in the B_0 field. This results in substantial geometric distortions of the images and, for the gradient-echo versions used in fMRI, in localized signal loss (or *dropout*) as well (see Figure 6.2). In addition, the EPI images have relatively low spatial resolution and potentially poor tissue contrast. Consequently, registering them accurately to a structural image, even with the same anatomy, is challenging and requires more than just the approach outlined in case 3 of section 5.4.

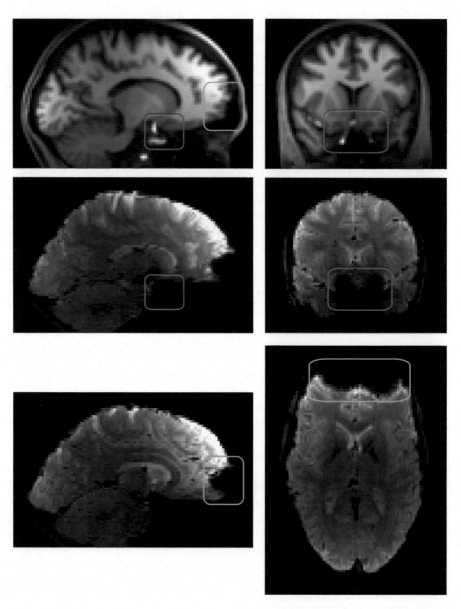

Figure 6.2: Illustration of distortion and signal loss in EPI. The first row shows a T_1-weighted structural image (included here in order to provide a comparison with the undistorted anatomy) that was resampled and reoriented to match the functional EPI acquisition (from the same subject), which is shown in the second and third rows. Signal loss, or dropout, is prevalent in the inferior frontal and temporal lobes, as highlighted by the red boxes (i.e., in the EPI shown in the second row, where a large amount of signal is lost within the boxes by comparison to the T_1-weighted structural in the top row). The geometric distortion is highlighted by the blue boxes and is most prominent in the orbitofrontal cortex (it appears as though a bite has been taken out of the frontal cortex in the EPI: third row). Note that the bright parts in the T_1-weighted structural image, in and near the boxes, correspond to blood vessels.

Of all of these challenges, the one that often causes the biggest issues is the geometric distortion that results from the B_0 inhomogeneities. These inhomogeneities are mainly caused by the air-filled sinuses and air cells in the skull. The phenomenon is largely problematic, because the changes are localized in specific areas of the brain and, in fMRI, accompanied by signal loss. These inhomogeneities change the nature of the spatial transformation and cost function required for obtaining accurate alignments. There are two main approaches for dealing with this distortion: to correct it before registration, as a separate step in the preprocessing pipeline; or to incorporate the distortion correction into the registration step. We will describe both approaches in this section.

To begin with, we will describe the method of incorporating distortion correction into registration. In the most general case, this requires you to have information about the B_0 inhomogeneities, so that you may calculate the geometric distortion, which is provided via separate images that measure or map this field—a B_0 *fieldmap*. Such images require separate acquisitions and can be acquired using a specific gradient-echo acquisition sequence (see section 3.4.1) or calculated from acquisitions of one or more phase-encode reversed spin-echo EPI (i.e., b = 0) pairs (see section 3.3.2). Either way, the resultant fieldmap contains values that represent the deviations from the ideal, uniform B_0 field—usually in units of frequency, as the change in field affects the frequency of the signal from the hydrogen nuclei. These units can be either Hz or radians per second (the latter is simply 2π times the former).

6.2.1 Using fieldmaps

Fieldmap values (in frequency) provide information about the amount of distortion, which can then be converted into a fixed, nonlinear spatial transformation. The inverse of this transformation can be applied to the EPI image (e.g., to the functional or diffusion image) to correct the distortion or to *unwarp* it. This transformation can be calculated from the following information:

- the direction of the distortion:

   this is a known property of the image to be corrected, as the distortion occurs along the *phase-encode axis* of the EPI image due to the physics of the acquisition, and this axis is specified by the scanner operator at acquisition;

- the size of the B_0 inhomogeneity, at each voxel:

   this value is taken from the fieldmap, in units of Hz or rad/s, and converted to a shift, which is proportional to the B_0 field: see next point;

- some timing information about the EPI acquisition (e.g., the fMRI or dMRI image):

   in particular, the echo spacing is needed (or the effective echo spacing, if there is in-plane acceleration), as this is used to determine the scaling of the fieldmap values in order to obtain the shift in voxel units.

More details about the calculation can be found in Boxes 6.1 and 6.2.

The important point is that a fieldmap provides us with the necessary information to fully calculate the geometric distortion and that it is not necessary to try and estimate the distortion from the EPI images. Avoiding estimation from the EPI images is an advantage, since the estimation of distortion from the images alone is often very problematic in fMRI due to signal loss, low resolution, and limited tissue contrast.

Box 6.1: Gradient-echo fieldmap acquisitions

One common form of fieldmap acquisition involves acquiring two undistorted images with relatively low resolution. Each image is acquired with a sequence that is more like a structural MRI sequence (i.e., not EPI), so that it is undistorted (or has negligible distortions). In addition, the images are gradient-echo ones, like in fMRI, so that the signal intensity is sensitive to the effects of B_0 inhomogeneities, but in this case the effect on the intensity is not accompanied by noticeable geometric distortion or signal loss. The acquisition is low resolution, unlike a typical structural image, so that each image can be acquired in less than a minute. The two images that are acquired differ in one parameter—the *echo time* (TE)—as this represents the amount of time that the magnetization of the hydrogen nuclei rotates (or precesses) in the B_0 field before being measured. Taking the difference in the *phase* (i.e., the angle that the magnetization has rotated) between the two images, at each voxel, gives a rate of change of phase. This rate of change of phase (difference in phase divided by the difference in echo times) is equal to the value of the B_0 field, expressed in units of frequency (e.g., radians per second). Thus it is the phase part of the image that contains the most important information for such fieldmaps; and this needs to be saved. Normally the phase part of an image is thrown away by the scanner when reconstructing images, as it is the magnitude that is of interest in most cases, but in this type of fieldmap acquisition both the magnitude and the phase *must* be saved, since we will use each one (see Figure 6.3).

As hydrogen nuclei precess at a frequency that is proportional to the B_0 field, the change in phase in a given time interval is linearly related to the B_0 field. However, the initial phase can also be influenced by other (static) factors, such as the phase of the RF field, which is why two gradient-echo images are acquired and the difference in their phase values is used, rather than just the phase from one image. This difference in phase will then be proportional to the B_0 field but independent of the initial phase. More precisely, at a location $\mathbf{x}$:

$$\Delta\theta(\mathbf{x}) = 2\pi\,\gamma\,.\,\Delta B_0(\mathbf{x})\,.\,\Delta TE$$

where $\mathbf{x}$ is a 3D coordinate; $\theta(\mathbf{x})$ is the phase of the signal (magnetization) at this location; γ is the gyromagnetic ratio (42.6 MHz per tesla [T] for hydrogen nuclei); $\Delta B_0(\mathbf{x})$ is the inhomogeneity in the B_0 field at this location; and ΔTE is the difference in echo times of the two acquisitions. As no complete cycles of phase can be detected from two measurements (although multi-echo methods do exist that can detect them), it is customary to arrange for the difference in TE to be small in order to keep the expected phase changes under 2π radians. A typical value for the difference in TE would be 2.6 ms (this particular value is common at 3T in order to prevent any residual signals from fat from corrupting the phase measurements, since both water and fat signals are in phase at multiples of this period, on the basis of the known fat-water frequency separation). The most important point here is that the fieldmap, $\Delta B_0(\mathbf{x})$, can be calculated from the measured phase difference, $\Delta\theta(\mathbf{x})$, by using the above equation.

When acquiring the fieldmap, there are a couple of important points to note. First, it is sufficient to use a similar resolution to the EPI (as the B_0 inhomogeneities are relatively smooth) but the resolution does not need to be matched precisely to the EPI acquisition. Using a low resolution helps keep the acquisition time short, usually around a minute or less. Second, it is important that there is no re-shimming of the scanner in between the fieldmap and the EPI acquisitions, as re-shimming changes the B_0 field, and for the fieldmap to be useful it must measure the same field that is present when the EPI images are being acquired. Furthermore, large changes in the orientation of the head can have a substantial impact on the B_0 field. These factors affect all forms of measuring the field or distortion, including the phase-encode reversed method (discussed in the next section). Consequently it is advisable to acquire fieldmaps either immediately before or after the EPI acquisitions, to minimize the potential movements of the head and the chances of re-shimming. Your scanner operator, physicist, or radiographer can also help to avoid re-shimming, so make sure to discuss this matter with them so that they appreciate that it is important.

Box 6.2: Calculating distortion from gradient-echo fieldmaps

The geometric distortion that a change in field induces is related to the change in phase during the EPI acquisition (which is separate from the change in phase during the fieldmap acquisition). In all MR images, spatial gradient fields are used to deliberately induce changes in phase that vary with the spatial coordinate; and this is the basis of how the MRI signal is localized in space. However, additional changes in phase induced by a B_0 inhomogeneity are very similar to those that would result from the hydrogen nuclei being in a different location. More precisely, when acquiring one slice of an EPI scan, one gradient (let us call it "the x-gradient") is switching between positive and negative values, while the other gradient for that slice (call it "the y-gradient") always has the same sign once the signal measurements begin (it is off most of the time but is turned on for a short interval—a "blip"—at the end of each line in k-space). This means that the phase induced by the position along the y-axis will change in a consistent direction during the acquisition (it may increase the whole time or decrease the whole time, depending on the location on the y-axis). The field inhomogeneity, $\Delta B_0(\mathbf{x})$, will also have the same effect, as it is will consistently increase the phase with time if ΔB_0 is positive and consistently decrease the phase with time if ΔB_0 is negative.

If the phase changes by one whole cycle between each line of the EPI acquisition, then there is no discernible difference in the signal and the image is unchanged, which is equivalent to a shift of one full FOV. That is, if there are N voxels in the y direction, then a change of phase of 2π per line of k-space would be the same as a shift of N voxels, as the shift is actually a cyclic one, so that, if things are pushed off the top of a slice, they wrap around to the bottom, and vice versa. The shift is linearly proportional to the amount of phase change per line, and this leads to:

$$\text{shift}(x) = N\,\Delta\theta(x)/2\pi = N\,\gamma\,\Delta B_0(x)\,T_{EES}/2\pi$$

where shift(x) is the geometric distortion along the *phase-encode direction* (what we have been calling the y-direction) in units of voxels; N is the number of voxels in the phase-encode direction; and T_{EES} is the time associated with the *effective echo spacing*. The echo spacing is the time taken between the acquisition of one line in k-space and the next line, for the EPI. If there is in-plane acceleration (e.g., GRAPPA or SENSE), then lines are skipped during acquisition and we need an effective echo spacing, which is the actual echo spacing (the time between the lines that are actually measured) divided by the acceleration factor (which is designed to take into account the difference between the number of lines acquired in k-space and the number of voxels in the image along the phase-encode direction). This equation is the one that we use to calculate the geometric distortion from the fieldmap, $\Delta B_0(x)$.

Once the geometric distortion is calculated, it can in principle be applied directly, as a spatial transformation, but in practice the head may have moved between the acquisition of the fieldmap and the EPI scans. Therefore it is necessary to account for a rigid-body transformation between the EPI and the fieldmap. This can be done by building the distortion correction into a rigid-body registration tool—that is, a registration where the spatial transformation is a combination of an unknown rigid-body transformation with a known nonlinear transformation. However, the fieldmap scan is typically low resolution and can have very poor tissue contrast, which makes the direct registration between the fieldmap and the EPI quite difficult.

An alternative (used in FSL) is to do the registrations of both EPI and fieldmap images to the structural image through a three-stage approach:

- Perform a rigid-body registration of the fieldmap (magnitude) to the structural image. For this we use the magnitude part of the fieldmap image, which is acquired along with the phase part in a gradient-echo fieldmap (see Figure 6.3) or is an image calculated from the halfway transformation of phase-encode reversed pairs (see top center image in Figure 6.5 and section 6.2.3).

- Next we apply the rigid-body transformation to the fieldmap image (i.e., the one in units of frequency, not the magnitude image) in order to get the B_0 information into structural space.

- Finally we register the EPI to the structural image using the fieldmap information (now in the structural space).

Since both the fieldmap magnitude and the structural images have negligible distortions (and no signal loss), a rigid-body transformation is sufficient for the alignment of the fieldmap to the structural image and for transforming the fieldmap (B_0) information into structural space.

As we noted in section 2.4.3, signal loss in the gradient-echo EPI acquisitions used for fMRI causes parts of the image (e.g., inferior temporal and frontal areas) to be unusable, because they contain negligible signal and this cannot be recovered in the analysis. Furthermore, we noted in section 3.4.8 that signal loss can also cause global registration inaccuracies, since it results in parts of the image that cannot be matched well, even after a good alignment of the rest of the

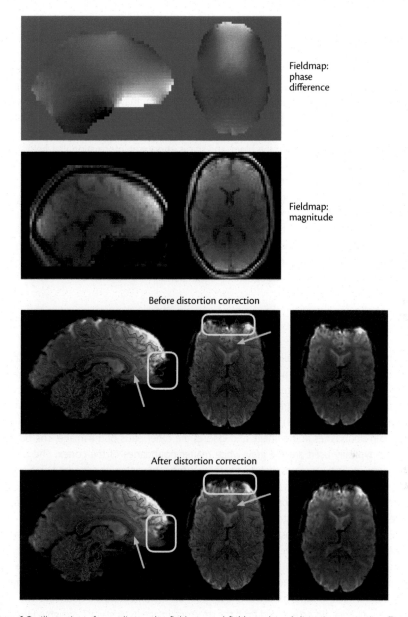

Fieldmap: phase difference

Fieldmap: magnitude

Before distortion correction

After distortion correction

Figure 6.3: Illustration of a gradient-echo fieldmap and fieldmap-based distortion correction. Top two rows show slices from a gradient-echo fieldmap acquisition: phase difference in the first row (linearly proportional to the fieldmap in Hz or radians per second) and magnitude in the second row (used for registering the fieldmap to other images). Both the phase and the magnitude images are reconstructed from the same fieldmap acquisition (the phase part of most acquisitions is thrown away, but for fieldmaps it is crucial to keep it). Bottom two rows show a functional EPI before and after distortion correction (third and fourth rows respectively). The right-hand column shows a single slice of the EPI, while the left panel shows two slices of the same EPI along with red edges transformed from a registered structural image (white matter boundaries). The blue arrows highlight areas where the distortion correction results are most evident, while the yellow boxes highlight areas that contain signal loss that cannot be reversed and where, although geometric changes are evident, the boundaries still do not align well due to this signal loss.

brain structures. This will be an issue for distortion correction, since the method we are using here relies on registration to the structural image; hence this is an instance of a situation where cost function masking is very useful (see section 5.2.1). The areas of signal loss can be calculated from the fieldmap values themselves, as signal loss is associated with areas where there is a rapid change of the B_0 field in one or more directions. Being able to calculate the signal loss helps distinguish between areas where there is low signal that should have been high signal and areas where the signal should have been low (e.g., in the skull). Simply masking out all the areas of low signal would be a bad thing to do, as it would remove all the information about the boundaries at the edge of the brain, and this is important information that helps drive the registration. Therefore a signal loss mask, calculated from the fieldmap, is another input to the registration we create as part of distortion correction.

Using the fixed nonlinear spatial transformation and the signal loss mask, the registration can then search for the unknown rigid-body transformation in order to both correct distortions and align the EPI with the structural image. A number of cost functions could be used in this situation, such as correlation ratio, mutual information, or boundary-based registration (BBR). However, the BBR cost function has some advantages in this case, as it was developed for precisely this application: EPI to structural registration.

6.2.2 Boundary-Based Registration

The registration method called BBR was briefly introduced in section 5.2 but is presented in more detail here, as it is most often applied in EPI to structural registration, either directly incorporating distortion correction (with gradient-echo fieldmaps) or after distortion correction (as alternative methods are used for distortion correction with phase-encode reversed fieldmaps; see section 6.2.3). It is based on a cost function that concentrates on the alignment at certain boundaries in the image and ignores the other parts of the image. The boundaries that are typically used are the gray–white matter boundaries of the cortex. The use of this boundary implicitly assumes that the anatomy is the same across the images being registered, as it is sensitive to the details of the cortical folding. It also ignores other boundaries, such as the outer gray matter boundary of the cortex, since there can be artifacts and non-brain structures there that show up inconsistently between the structural and the EPI.

BBR is based on an intensity model where, for well aligned images, the intensities in the EPI should be consistently higher on one side of the anatomical boundary (e.g., higher in gray matter than in white matter in BOLD fMRI, given that the images are T_2^*-weighted; see Box 6.3 for technical details if you are interested). That is, the intensity inside the white matter is always lower than it is outside the white matter, and changes most rapidly across the boundary. The location of the boundaries are determined from the structural image (typically, a T_1-weighted image) and are mapped onto the EPI using the candidate spatial transformation (i.e., the spatial transform that the cost function is currently evaluating during the search/optimization phase; see Figure 6.4). Two consequences of this are (i) that it is necessary for the EPI to show some degree of intensity contrast between white and gray matter, and (ii) that it is possible to derive anatomical boundaries reliably from the structural image. The intensity contrast in the EPI does not have to be very strong, as long as it is consistent, since only six parameters (of the rigid-body transformation) need to be found by considering the whole image (see Box 6.4 for a discussion of registrations for

EPI with low contrast). Extracting tissue boundaries from the structural image can be done with a simple tissue-type segmentation or can use the results of cortical modeling. As we are trying to find a rigid-body registration that applies globally across the whole image, such registration will be relatively insensitive to small errors in the tissue segmentation and boundary location.

Box 6.3: Intensity model for BBR

The mathematical form of the BBR cost function is: $\sum_v h_v(1 + \tanh(M_v Q_v))$

where v is a boundary point projected from one image (structural) to the other image (EPI)—the red points in Figure 6.4; $Q_v = (I_1-I_2)/(I_1+I_2)$ is the normalized intensity difference across this boundary, I_1 and I_2 being intensities on either side of the boundary in the EPI image (pairs of yellow points in Figure 6.4); M_v is a pointwise scaling factor; and h_v is a pointwise weighting factor. Often both h_v and M_v are set to constant values. The tanh function acts to make the cost function robust to outliers by limiting the influence of large intensity differences. When aligned, this normalized intensity difference (from the EPI) across the boundary (which is projected from the structural image) should be maximized.

T1w	T1w + boundaries	EPI + boundaries	EPI

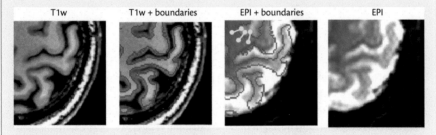

Figure 6.4: Illustration of how the BBR cost function works by overlaying boundaries extracted from the T_1-weighted structural image (in red) on the EPI and by calculating the intensity difference across the boundary (yellow dots). A function of the intensity difference (which caps the contributions of very large differences) is then summed over every boundary point. This sum is the heart of the cost function (the maximum difference occurs when the boundary is well aligned).

Box 6.4: Low contrast EPI and registration

Some EPI acquisitions have an extremely low contrast-to-noise ratio (CNR) for tissues of interest (e.g., when using high multiband accelerations). One way to improve registrations in this case is to acquire a separate image that matches the standard EPI for distortions and resolution but has better contrast. This can often be done for free, by retaining the calibration scans or any preparation scans from the EPI sequence rather than letting them be deleted (as is normally the default—in fact they are sometimes called "dummy scans" and are thrown away). Calibration scans (such as single-band reference scans) or preparation scans (at the start of the 4D EPI acquisition) have different signal intensities from those in the main EPI acquisition, as the main acquisition takes place after the magnetization has settled into a steady state. Either calibration or preparation scans are very useful for registration. They can be used in place of the standard EPI when obtaining a registration between the functional and structural spaces and for distortion correction. It then also becomes necessary to register the standard EPI to the calibration/preparation image in order to account for any movement, but this is easily done with a simple rigid-body registration, without worrying about distortions and signal loss, as both are well matched in the two images.

It is possible to apply the BBR cost function either with or without fieldmap information. Since BBR is finely tuned to the anatomy of the individual folds in the cortex, it works better when distortion correction is done and more of the boundary can be aligned accurately. Hence it should be applied either without a fieldmap to undistorted images (i.e., images where there was no distortion to start with, or where the distortion has already been corrected for, as in diffusion MRI: see section 6.2.3) or with a fieldmap when the images are distorted (see the Example Box "Distortion correction with fieldmaps"), to correct the distortions at the same time as the registration is done.

Box 6.5: Combining fieldmap-based distortion correction and registration

The registration that we have been describing has two functions: (i) to correct for the distortions caused by B_0 inhomogeneities; and (ii) to align the corrected EPI with the structural image. Therefore many outputs are possible, such as the following:

- a nonlinear transformation (warp) from EPI to structural space that corrects for the distortion in the EPI and aligns it to the structural image;
- a rigid-body transformation between the functional and structural space (relating the distortion-corrected EPI to the structural image);
- a nonlinear transformation that corrects for the distortion to the EPI within the functional space.

These last two transformations can be combined to give the first one, that is, correcting a distortion within the functional space (nonlinear) and then transforming to structural space (linear).

In addition, several types of output image may be generated, for example:

- a single 3D EPI, transformed (and distortion-corrected) to structural space;
- a single 3D distortion-corrected EPI in functional space;
- the 4D distortion-corrected EPI dataset in structural space;
- the 4D distortion-corrected EPI dataset in functional space.

All of these options are possible as outputs from such a tool or pipeline, but all of them are also easily generated if the fundamental spatial transformations are saved. Whether the EPI should be transformed into structural space (or standard space, by concatenating with the structural to standard space transformation) depends on the pipeline and on the choices made in the analysis. Both options are used in practice and lead to similar results. The most important point here is that a range of outputs are possible and any of them can be easily generated from the original images and the derived spatial transformations.

Although we have described the BBR cost function in some detail here, it is not the only option. Other cost functions have also been developed for, or applied to, EPI to structural registration (e.g., Local Pearson Correlation) and these can also produce accurate results. In addition, nonlinear registration is capable of correcting for distortions, although it should be constrained to operate only along the phase-encode direction. However, accurate nonlinear registration is difficult to achieve when the EPI resolution and contrast is poor, and hence the more constrained and informed alternatives, using fieldmaps, typically have advantages so long as the fieldmaps themselves are accurate. The best option for your particular experiment will depend on your image quality and on the software tools you have available, although we strongly recommend the acquisition of a fieldmap or an equivalent (as described next) that will allow you to use a wide range distortion-correction methods.

> ### Example Box: Distortion correction with fieldmaps
>
> On the primer website there is an illustrative dataset containing a gradient-echo fieldmap, structural, and fMRI images. Instructions are given to demonstrate how to calculate a fieldmap in appropriate units from the original acquisitions, and then to apply the fieldmap to correct distortions in the fMRI images and to register these images to the structural image.

6.2.3 Phase-encode reversed (blip-up–blip-down) images

An alternative to using gradient-echo fieldmaps is to use a pair of spin-echo EPI images (the same as b = 0 diffusion images) acquired with reversed phase-encode directions.[1] These are also referred to as *blip-up–blip-down scans*, because the gradients applied in the phase-encode direction are "blipped" during the acquisition (but this is a technical detail). From a pair or multiple pairs of such images it is possible, by a different method, to determine the distortion, and then either to use it to correct the images directly or to calculate a fieldmap image and use the fieldmap with the methods described previously.

The distortion can be calculated from these images because the direction of distortion is reversed in the two images that form the pair (see Figure 6.5). Hence the undistorted image is the "halfway" image between the two. The basic idea in calculating the distortion from these images is to perform a registration between the two that transforms both images by an equal and opposite amount, along the phase-encode direction (as that is the direction of distortions),

---

[1] Actually it is only strictly necessary to get two different phase-encode directions; they could be 90° apart rather than 180°, though we will describe here only the 180° version.

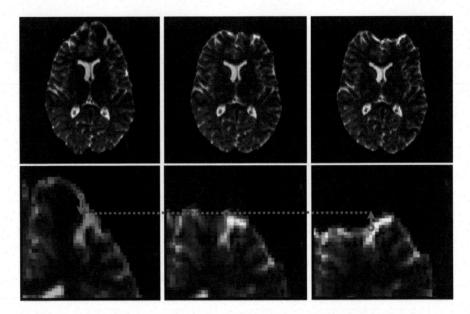

Figure 6.5: Illustration of blip-up–blip-down images used for distortion correction. These are spin-echo-based acquisitions (the same as b = 0 diffusion images) and hence they do not suffer from signal loss. Top row: blip-up and blip-down acquisitions (left and right images) show opposite directions of distortions, which is particularly visible in the top (anterior) portion of the brain, as they are stretched in the left-hand image and compressed in the right-hand image (note that intensities decrease when stretched but pile up and become brighter when compressed). The middle image is the distortion-corrected image, created by performing a halfway registration between the outer two images. The bottom row shows a zoomed-in portion of each of the images in the top row, along with an example of how halfway registration works for one particular voxel: the distortion occurs along the phase-encode direction (anterior–posterior in this particular case) and voxels are shifted by an equal and opposite amount (see arrows) along this direction to create halfway images that represent the distortion-corrected image. The shift values can then be stored as a warp field (nonlinear transformation) or converted to a fieldmap (like the one shown at the top of Figure 6.3), which can then be used to correct the distortion in other images where the B_0 inhomogeneities were the same (i.e., same subject, same session, and no re-shimming).

so that the images are made to align with each other at the halfway point. The distance that each voxel needs to be moved is then equal to the distortion, and this can be stored as a nonlinear transformation or converted to a fieldmap image. This transformation or fieldmap can then be applied to other images, including gradient-echo fMRI acquisitions, provided that they are distorted by the same B_0 inhomogeneities.

As any motion between these two images can cause changes in the direction of the distortion or displace corresponding phase-encode lines relative to the anatomy, a rigid-body transformation between the pair needs to be incorporated into this registration too. Hence the outputs can take multiple forms in terms of a combination of a rigid-body transformation and a nonlinear transformation (representing the distortion, or its inverse). In addition, the outputs can include various transformed or distortion-corrected images (see Box 6.5).

Use of blip-up–blip-down pairs is very common for diffusion MRI, as half of the pairs are already being acquired, namely the standard b = 0 images. Hence acquiring a few extra phase-encode reversed b = 0 images represents a very small amount of additional scanning time. Furthermore, there are advantages to applying the distortion correction using tools that are developed specifically for diffusion-weighted images and that can also incorporate corrections for other distortions—especially eddy-current-induced distortions. In addition, the distortion-corrected images and any fieldmap derived from them are automatically aligned with the reference b = 0 image, which eliminates the need for one of the rigid-body transforms.

The distortion-corrected images obtained from this approach are still in the original diffusion space (aligned to the b = 0 reference scan), and to register them to structural space requires an extra step. This is simply a rigid-body registration, given that the distortions are already corrected (just as in case 3 of section 5.4). Using the BBR cost function (see section 6.2.2), or something similar is still a good and accurate way to achieve this EPI to structural registration, even with images that are already distortion-corrected and so no fieldmap is needed in this case.

It is also possible to use the fieldmaps derived from these acquisitions as direct replacements for fieldmaps acquired with gradient-echo acquisitions; and, once the fieldmaps are obtained in the correct units, there is no difference in how they are used (see the Example Box "Distortion correction with blip-up–blip-down data"). Whether you should acquire gradient-echo fieldmaps or blip-up–blip-down pairs depends on factors such as acquisition time, image quality, and convenience, since both methods produce similarly accurate results. The most suitable method will depend on your scanner, your acquisition protocol, and the available tools. This kind of decision is best made by testing the alternatives during your piloting phase in order to determine what works best for your particular experiment.

Example Box: **Distortion correction with blip-up–blip-down data**

On the primer website there is an illustrative dataset containing blip-up–blip-down images as well as spin-echo and gradient-echo EPI acquisitions. Instructions are given to demonstrate how to perform a halfway registration, calculate a distortion-corrected image from the blip-up–blip-down images (the result of the halfway registration), create a fieldmap, and apply the fieldmap to correct the distortion in the gradient-echo EPI (fMRI) acquisitions.

6.2.4 Evaluating the results

Correcting EPI distortions is important for obtaining accurate alignment to structural and standard spaces, which also leads to reduced variability and greater statistical power in group-level analyses. However, evaluating the quality of EPI to structural registrations by eye is more difficult than in other cases, such as a registration from a structural to a standard template. The difficulty is partly due to the lower resolution and tissue contrast, but also to the presence of artifacts, such as signal loss in fMRI.

One very helpful way to evaluate a registration visually is by viewing the anatomical boundaries (obtained from the structural image) overlaid on the EPI. This mimics what is done internally in the BBR cost function, and is a useful way to visualize the registration and distortion correction regardless of whether BBR was used or not (see Figures 6.3, 6.6, 6.7, and also Example Box "Evaluating Registrations" in section 5.4). The boundaries aid the eye in determining whether the change in grayscale intensity coincides with the boundary location or not. Places where the distortion is not corrected well (see illustrations in Figures 6.6 and 6.7) will tend to have light or dark fringes near the boundary. However, it is important in fMRI not to mistake the edges of regions of signal loss for true anatomical boundaries. Being aware of where signal loss typically occurs (in the inferior frontal and temporal regions) is the best way to avoid that mistake, and you should expect that these regions will not appear to match with the anatomical boundaries due to this signal loss (see Figures 6.6 and 6.7). Some of the best places to evaluate the quality of the registration and distortion correction are the anterior portion of the ventricles and corpus callosum, the superior gyri and sulci, the caudate nucleus, the occipital lobe (but not the most inferior part), the cerebellum, and the brainstem (but be aware that the anterior portion of the brainstem often suffers from signal loss).

Structural Image

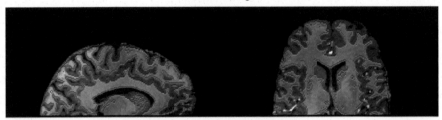

Registration without Distortion Correction

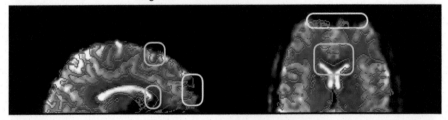

Registration with Distortion Correction

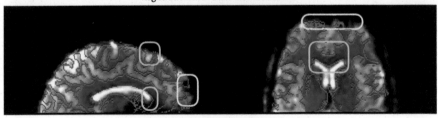

Figure 6.6: Examples of visualizing registrations with the white matter boundary (red) overlaid on the EPI. Top row shows a structural image in grayscale (not the EPI), along with white matter boundaries that are derived directly from it. Second and third rows show the results of registration of the EPI (in grayscale) to the structural image, without distortion correction (second row) and with distortion correction (third row). Areas indicated by the blue boxes illustrate regions suffering from geometric distortion, which are much better aligned when distortion correction is applied. Areas indicated by the yellow boxes illustrate regions suffering from signal loss, which are present with or without distortion correction, and the edges of these regions cannot be relied upon for evaluating registration accuracy.

Registration without Distortion Correction

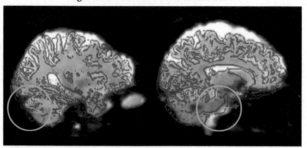

Registration with Distortion Correction

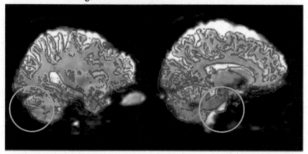

Registration without
Distortion Correction

Registration with
Distortion Correction

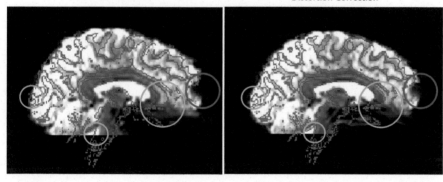

Figure 6.7: Example of visualizing registrations with the white matter boundary (in red) overlaid on the EPI (in grayscale). Top two rows show EPI acquisitions (lower resolution than previous figure) where the registration is done without distortion correction (top row) and with distortion correction (second row). The green circles highlight the areas where the distortion correction shows the greatest improvement in this case. In the third row an example using a higher resolution EPI acquisition is illustrated, and the left panel shows the results of a registration without distortion correction, while the right panel shows the results of a registration with distortion correction. The areas where the improvement with distortion correction is most noticeable are highlighted by the green circles, whereas the area where the mismatch due to signal loss remains is highlighted by the blue circle.

SUMMARY

- Functional and diffusion imaging are based on collecting a set of EPI acquisitions (a 4D dataset) that need to be corrected for motion between images and for geometric distortion.

- Motion correction is often performed using a rigid-body registration between each 3D volume within the 4D dataset, although more sophisticated methods also exist that can additionally correct for the motion that occurs during the volume (slicewise motion correction) and/or for motion artifacts (changing distortions, MR physics artifacts, etc).

- The amount and type of motion present in a dataset is often visualized or quantified using the rigid-body motion parameters, summaries of these parameters (e.g., framewise displacement) or separate, intensity-based measures (e.g., DVARS).

- Motion causes a range of artifacts in the data, and many of these affect the intensities and the subsequent analyses. Three common methods of motion artifact correction are motion parameter regression, outlier regression/removal, and ICA-based denoising.

- Geometric distortion, due to B_0 inhomogeneities, is common and substantial in EPI acquisitions and requires correction if you want to obtain an accurate spatial localization of your results, which will also substantially improve the statistical power for group analyses.

- Signal loss, or dropout, is also present in functional MRI, and eddy-current distortions are present in diffusion MRI.

- Fieldmaps can be used to estimate geometric distortion and to correct for it, either as part of a registration step or in a separate process. Two main options exist for acquiring fieldmap information: gradient-echo fieldmap acquisitions and phase-encode reversed spin-echo EPI (or blip-up–blip-down) acquisitions. Both can be used to create a fieldmap suitable for general distortion correction, though phase-encode reversed acquisitions can be used for more direct corrections in diffusion MRI. Either way, extra images must be planned for and acquired in each session.

- BBR is a cost function that is based on maximizing the intensity change across certain anatomical boundaries—often the white matter boundary. This function is well suited to the registration of EPI to structural images, as it is less affected by artifacts and nonbrain tissue near the outer gray matter surface.

FURTHER READING

- Poldrack, R. A., Mumford, J. A., & Nichols, T. E. (2011). *Handbook of Functional MRI Data Analysis*. Cambridge University Press.
    - *This is an accessible text that focuses on task-based fMRI and contains information on both motion correction and distortion correction.*

- Power, J. D., Schlaggar, B. L., & Petersen, S. E. (2015). Recent progress and outstanding issues in motion correction in resting state fMRI. *Neuroimage*, 105, 536–551.
    - *This paper discusses a range of motion correction and motion artifact correction methods and their implications for resting state fMRI.*

■ Friston, K., Ashburner, J., Frith, C. D., Poline, J. B., Heather, J. D., & Frackowiak, R. S. (1995). Spatial registration and normalization of images. *Human Brain Mapping*, 3(3), 165–189.
  ▪ *The original paper on the motion correction method used in the SPM package (www.fil.ion. ucl.ac.uk/spm), containing technical details.*

■ Jenkinson, M., Bannister, P., Brady, M., & Smith, S. (2002). Improved optimization for the robust and accurate linear registration and motion correction of brain images. *Neuroimage*, 17(2), 825–841.
  ▪ *The original paper on the motion correction method used in the FSL package (fsl.fmrib. ox.ac.uk), containing technical details.*

■ Glasser, M. F., Sotiropoulos, S. N., Wilson, J. A., Coalson, T. S., Fischl, B., Andersson, J. L., et al. (2013). The minimal preprocessing pipelines for the Human Connectome Project. *Neuroimage*, 80, 105–124.
  ▪ *Paper describing the HCP (Human Connectome Project) pipeline, with considerable details on distortion and motion correction, for both fMRI and dMRI (with some technical details).*

■ Jezzard, P., & Balaban, R. S. (1995). Correction for geometric distortion in echo planar images from B_0 field variations. *Magnetic Resonance in Medicine*, 34(1), 65–73.
  ▪ *Original paper describing the principle behind fieldmap-based distortion correction methods.*

■ Andersson, J. L., & Sotiropoulos, S. N. (2016). An integrated approach to correction for off-resonance effects and subject movement in diffusion MR imaging. *Neuroimage*, 125, 1063–1078.
  ▪ *Recent paper describing a combined approach for distortion and motion correction in dMRI, with technical details.*

■ Greve, D. N., & Fischl, B. (2009). Accurate and robust brain image alignment using boundary-based registration. *Neuroimage*, 48(1), 63–72.
  ▪ *Original paper describing the boundary-based registration method, with technical details.*

■ Cusack, R., Brett, M., & Osswald, K. (2003). An evaluation of the use of magnetic fieldmaps to undistort echo-planar images. *Neuroimage*, 18(1), 127–142.
  ▪ *Paper describing one of the first approaches to using fieldmap-based distortion correction.*

■ Smith, S. M., Jenkinson, M., Woolrich, M. W., Beckmann, C. F., Behrens, T. E., Johansen-Berg, H, et al. (2004). Advances in functional and structural MR image analysis and implementation as FSL. *Neuroimage*, 23, S208–S219.
  ▪ *General paper describing the FSL software package (fsl.fmrib.ox.ac.uk), with a specific section on fieldmap-based distortion correction.*

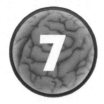

Surface-Based Analysis

I n the previous chapters we have mainly discussed volumetric image analysis methods, which work at the voxel level. That is, they treat the image data as a 3D or 4D regular array of voxels and usually produce 3D spatial maps of results. *Surface-based analysis* is an alternative approach that takes points (otherwise known as *vertices*) on the surface of an anatomical structure and performs analysis using data from these anatomical locations, creating outputs in the form of surface maps. It is possible to perform surface-based analysis on the surface or boundary of any anatomical structure, but it is the surface of the cerebral cortex that is of the greatest interest and benefits the most from surface-based methods, due to the complicated geometry of the folding patterns. In this chapter we will discuss surface-based analysis for the cerebral cortex, starting with methods for extracting and analyzing structural data and finishing with functional MRI applications, where surface-based techniques have many useful advantages.

7.1 Cortical surface extraction

As briefly discussed in section 3.2.5, cortical surface extraction involves fitting separate boundaries to the inner and outer surface of the cortical gray matter. This typically involves an analysis pipeline that starts with tissue-type segmentation and registration to a standard space. These pipelines normally use these steps for initializing the surfaces and do not expect those results to be perfect, given that it is extremely difficult to detect small amounts of cerebrospinal fluid (CSF) within many sulci (especially in children and young adults) and that volumetric registration is limited in its ability to deal with variations in folding patterns. However, large errors in either the initial segmentation or the registration steps can cause problems with the surface fitting, and so it is important that the results be checked to ensure that they are reasonably accurate. Documentation for the specific cortical surface analysis package you are using (e.g., FreeSurfer) is the best source of information on what initial stages require checking and how to fix any major errors that might occur.

The surfaces are represented by *mesh models*, which are a collection of points (vertices) on the surface that are joined together by edges to form triangles (see Figure 7.1), much like a net. Vertices can be placed anywhere on the surface, unlike voxels, which are arranged in a fixed grid. This means that the density of vertices can, and does, vary across the surface. Surface-fitting algorithms typically aim to keep the spacing between vertices relatively even, to minimize the variations in density. Spatial resolution of a mesh model is therefore not a fixed quantity, and hence it is common to refer to the number of vertices used in a model rather than to the spacing. To represent the geometry of the human cortex, it is common to have somewhere between 20,000 and 200,000 vertices, corresponding to average spacings of approximately 2 mm to less than 1 mm. The analysis software will normally choose an

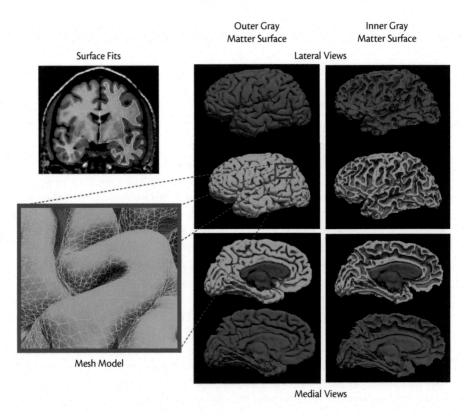

Figure 7.1: Illustration of surface meshes of the left hemisphere. Top left image shows a coronal section with the inner and outer gray matter surfaces shown in yellow and red respectively. The middle column shows views of the outer gray matter (pial) surface, and the right column shows views of the inner gray matter (white matter) surface. The top panels show surfaces of the lateral side and the bottom panels show surfaces of the medial side. Color coding for the surfaces in the second and third rows depicts the sulcal depth (from green at the outermost surface to red in deeper locations). The gray area on the medial surface (third row) represents the area associated with central structures (corpus callosum, brainstem, etc.) that cannot be split between hemispheres and is therefore excluded from the surface. The inset on the left shows a zoomed-in portion of a surface; it depicts the vertices and triangles that constitute the mesh model of the surface.

appropriate number of vertices itself, but may output results in several different "resolutions" (i.e., with different numbers of vertices).

Although the cortex is highly folded, it has a fixed *topology*, equivalent to a sphere. In the same way, a paper bag always has the same topology, even when it is crumpled and folded, so long as it is not torn. The topology of the entire gray matter cortex is essentially the same as two spheres—one for each hemisphere—although this is only an approximation, since the corpus callosum and brainstem both cut across them. For the purposes of cortical surface modeling, each hemisphere is treated as a folded or crumpled sphere with a portion on the medial surface that is excluded, where the corpus callosum, the brainstem, and other subcortical structures would be (see Figure 7.1). When the surface is fit to the image it maintains this topology, avoiding holes or loops (handles) in the surface, and this is one of the constraints that are applied by the surface-fitting methods; it helps correct for any small errors in the segmentation. Errors in the surface-fitting methods, where this topology is not constrained correctly, are known as *topological defects* and can cause many problems in a pipeline if not detected and fixed.

Two cortical surfaces are fit to the original, or native, image: (i) the inner gray matter surface, also known as the *white matter surface*; and (ii) the outer gray matter surface, also known as the *pial surface*. These surfaces are often initially molded to fit segmentation boundaries obtained from a T_1-weighted image, although inclusion of additional intensity information (such as a T_2-weighted image) can help in determining precise boundary locations, especially for the outer gray matter surface.

The two surfaces are usually fit in relation to each other (i.e., not independently), which helps reduce the effects of noise and artifacts. It is common for the inner gray matter surface to be fit first and then for the outer gray matter surface to be obtained by deforming the inner gray matter outwards, so as to fit the segmentation or intensities or both (although other methods of fitting also exist). Vertex-to-vertex correspondence is also established (or maintained) between these surfaces more easily by not fitting them independently. This means that each vertex on the inner gray matter surface has a corresponding vertex on the outer gray matter surface, and vice versa (see Figure 7.2). The line joining a corresponding pair can be seen as an approximation of where the cortical column (an arrangement of neurons spanning the cortical layers, between the inner and the outer gray matter surfaces) would be. However, as only MRI is used to determine these locations, and not histology, the correspondence with the true cortical columns will have limited accuracy; it is based purely on geometry. From the inner and outer surfaces a *mid-thickness surface* can also be calculated by averaging the location of corresponding vertices from the inner and outer gray matter surface.

Several quantities can be calculated from these surfaces that describe the geometry of the anatomy, such as *cortical thickness*, *sulcal depth*, and *curvature*. Cortical thickness is the most commonly used and is a measure of the distance between the inner and the outer surfaces, although this is not necessarily the same as the distance between corresponding vertices. There are several methods of calculating cortical thickness, based on minimum geometric distances or on solving differential equations, and the details of these methods are beyond the scope of this primer. The most important point is that cortical thickness is derived purely from the surfaces and is commonly used in structural analyses—an alternative to volumetric voxel-based morphometry (VBM). This is because cortical thickness is a relatively direct measure of the local quantity of cortical gray

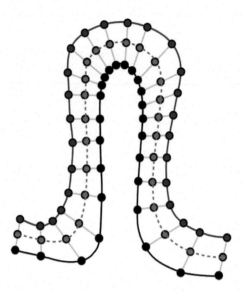

Figure 7.2: A 2D illustration of part of the cortical gray matter, showing corresponding vertices on the inner (black) and outer (blue) gray matter surfaces, joined by gray lines (approximations to the cortical columns). The mid-thickness points (red) are halfway between corresponding points and define the mid-thickness surface (red dashed line).

matter and is independent of how much folding there is, unlike VBM, where the amount of folding and even the proximity of adjacent folds (gyri) influence the measure of local gray matter volume.

Sulcal depth and curvature are quantities that measure the geometry of the cortical folding. Curvature is a local measure of how flat or curved that part of the surface is, whereas sulcal depth can be considered as an approximation of how far a vertex is from the skull, or outermost membrane surrounding the brain. In general, the curvature contains more local, fine detail and is more variable between subjects, whereas the sulcal depth tends to highlight more stable features, such as the major divisions between lobes.

Both sulcal depth and curvature can be useful for registration purposes, as they provide information about the geometry or folding of the local anatomy, which can drive the alignment. For instance, the largest and deepest sulci are the most common and consistent features of the cortical folding pattern and should be aligned between subjects. Finer and finer details can then be picked out from the sulcal depth and curvature, which provide a way to progressively match up common aspects of the folding patterns.

These quantities also provide crucial information for parcellation (segmentation) purposes, as cortical parcellations are defined by the positions of key sulci and gyri. Almost all cortical parcellation methods rely on some form of surface modeling, as volumetric methods are less accurate and reliable at identifying appropriate surface landmarks and boundaries (e.g., postcentral sulcus) that are needed for parcellation.

Both surface-based registration (see section 7.3) and surface-based parcellation, for the cerebral cortex, are powerful tools and have been shown to have substantial advantages over volumetric alternatives.

7.2 Inflated, spherical, and flattened surfaces

All the surfaces we have discussed so far have been in the native space of the original image and show the folded structure. These surfaces can be deformed to improve visualization; we do this by stretching and expanding them, like inflating a crumpled paper bag. The most common of these is the *inflated surface*, which is expanded enough so that the bottom and sides of the sulci, as well as the tops of the gyri, are all visible while still maintaining the rough shape of the brain, to help provide visual cues about the overall anatomy. To provide further cues for anatomical location it is common to show either the sulcal depth or the curvature values as shades of gray on this surface, with other information (e.g., statistical results) in color on top of this (see Figure 7.3). These surfaces are often used to display information such as statistical results (e.g., from a cortical thickness analysis, or from fMRI), as they allow everything on the cortical surface to be seen with only a couple of views per hemisphere. The volumetric alternative, showing 2D cross-sectional slices of a 3D image, makes it more difficult to visualize how things are connected in 3D and requires many more images to show all the relevant locations (e.g., all the statistically significant locations), so that often only a subset of the results is shown in most papers when using cross-sectional slices.

Flattened surfaces are also used for visualization but require more distortion of the surface. In particular, strategic cuts need to be made in the surface in order to flatten it. A similar thing is done when making flat maps of the world—cuts typically going down the Pacific Ocean, separating this ocean into two parts, on either side of the flat map. Furthermore, whenever we make flat maps like this, some distortions (of distance and area) are incurred; for maps of the world, this occurs most around the poles, stretching out the apparent size of the arctic and antarctic regions. When we flatten brain surfaces, or even inflate them, the algorithms used strive to minimize these distortions, though distortions will always be there to some degree. Despite the fact that it is harder to orient yourself with respect to the anatomy when looking at flattened surfaces, especially for the first time, they are very useful for viewing retinotopic maps and other topographically organized sections of cortex.

Another surface that is created is the *spherical surface*, which is basically an extension of the inflated surface, where the whole surface is inflated even more, in order to become a sphere. This surface is not very useful for visualization, as it is extremely difficult to orient yourself with respect to the anatomy. However, this surface is useful for registration, since it enables a surface constraint to be applied during the registration by using a simple geometry. More details about surfaced-based registration, which is a generally powerful tool, are presented in the next section.

7.3 Registration of surface data

The large amount of variation between folding patterns in different individuals makes between-subject registration difficult, especially for volumetric methods. Moving voxels in 3D to match the cortical geometry can require a large amount of folding or unfolding, which the

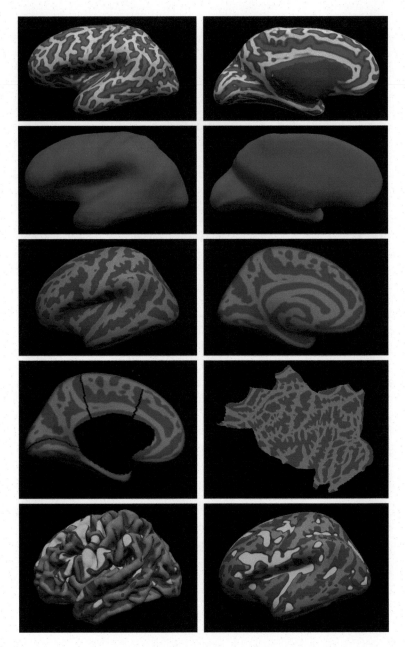

Figure 7.3: Illustration of inflated and flattened surfaces of the left hemisphere. Top row shows inflated versions of the cortical surface; sulcal depth is depicted in grayscale (light to dark for shallow to deep), with the lateral view on the left and the medial view on the right. Second row shows the same inflated surfaces, without coloring. Third row shows the inflated surface of another subject, with curvature depicted in grayscale (lateral view on the left, medial view on the right). The fourth row shows cuts made in the medial surface (left) in preparation for the flattening of the surface, along with the final, flattened version of this surface (right). The fifth row shows results from a statistical analysis on the native surface (left) and on the inflated surface (right), demonstrating the usefulness of the inflated surface for visualization.

regularization in 3D nonlinear registration methods tries to prevent (as regularization is there to encourage smoothness in the deformations). As a consequence, volumetric registration methods tend to generate small mismatches between cortical gray matter and nearby white matter and CSF. A more natural way to ensure that cortical gray matter is only registered to other cortical gray matter is to enforce a correspondence between the cortical surfaces.

Surface-based registration can use the surface geometry as constraints, to enforce the correspondence between the cortical surfaces of two subjects. This still allows the corresponding point to move around on the surface, but not to move off the surface. A convenient way to represent the spatial transformation between two surfaces is by using the spherical versions of each surface. By doing so, the mathematical representation is simpler for the algorithm to work with, but the final correspondence between points can be transferred easily to any related surface of that individual—native, inflated, or flattened.

Any available information on the surface can be used to drive the surface-based registration. The most commonly used information is the sulcal depth, which results in the alignment being based on the geometry of the folding pattern. Similarly, driving the registration with curvature also aligns the folding patterns, though sulcal depth is often used to initialize the registration, since sulcal depth more robustly picks out features that are stable across subjects (e.g., main sulci between lobes, such as the lateral sulcus or the central sulcus).

Using the cortical surface constraint has been shown to improve the accuracy of registration, not only with respect to the geometry of the surfaces but also with respect to functionally and histologically defined areas of the cortex. However, the accuracy varies according to the location in the cortex. For instance, Fischl and colleagues showed that cytoarchitectonic boundaries were more accurately aligned for areas in the occipital cortex than for areas in the frontal cortex, when using surface-based registrations driven by geometrical features. This is partly because there is a stronger relationship between functional areas and structure (folding patterns) in the occipital cortex and partly because such registrations are still not able to "solve" difficult biological correspondence problems of structure in a consistent way. For example, if there is a different number of gyri in the two subjects, there is no consistent result that is based only on structure. However, the surface constraint always prevents clearly erroneous solutions, such as aligning gray matter with other tissues.

It is also possible to drive registration by using information besides geometric structure, and recently developed methods are able to take advantage of quantities such as estimates of cortical myelination, functional activity, and connectivity. It is still uncertain what the best features for driving registration are, but there appear to be advantages to using information about functional organization (via resting state fMRI, or via fMRI that uses rich tasks, such as watching movies), especially when analyzing functional data on the surface. However, care needs to be taken if the functional analysis is using the same (nonindependent) data that were used to drive the registration, as that may be circular and create statistical biases.

7.4 Surface-based fMRI analysis

One type of analysis that can benefit greatly from being done on the cortical surface is fMRI analysis. This analysis proceeds in a very similar way to volumetric fMRI analysis, except that, instead of analyzing the data at each voxel separately (*voxelwise analysis*), we analyze the data at each vertex separately *(vertexwise analysis)*. To do this we need to *project* the fMRI data from the spatial 3D grid (voxels) onto the surface (vertices). Depending on the resolution of the volume and on the surface mesh, this step may just involve interpolation of the volumetric data at each vertex on the mid-thickness surface, on the basis of the vertex coordinates (see Figure 7.4). This would be done separately for each time point, by effectively taking the 4D image and creating a timeseries from it for each vertex. However, if the resolution of the functional data is high enough, there can be several voxels that span the distance between the inner and the outer gray matter surface, and in this case the data from several voxels can be appropriately averaged together to give a data value that represents a mean value over the different layers of the cortex (from inner to outer). When the resolution is sufficient, it is also possible to decide whether certain voxels are contaminated by signals from outside the gray matter and then exclude these voxels from the average. That way a purer gray matter signal can be obtained, which is a distinct advantage of a surface-based analysis approach.

It is still necessary to perform volumetric registration of the fMRI and structural images in order to be able to do the projection of the functional data onto the surface. In fact it is more important for this step to be accurate when doing surface-based analysis because, if a true gray matter voxel in the fMRI data is not aligned with the surface from the structural data, then the data at this voxel will not be projected onto the surface and will be lost to the analysis. Hence it is very important to correct for geometric distortions by applying the methods described in section 6.2, such as using boundary-based registration (BBR) with appropriate fieldmaps.

In addition to obtaining a purer gray matter signal (if the fMRI has sufficient resolution), there are three other main advantages to surface-based analysis by comparison to its volumetric counterpart. These are (i) a reduced multiple comparison problem (see the online appendix

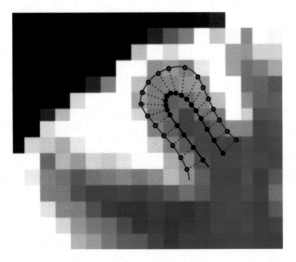
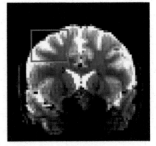

Figure 7.4: Illustration of projecting fMRI data onto the cortical surface. The right panel shows a functional image (2 mm isotropic resolution) and the borders of the zoomed panel shown on the left. In the zoomed portion one gyrus of the surface meshes is shown as an example, illustrating that for this resolution it is possible to interpolate the gray matter signals onto the surface, but this will be influenced by partial voluming. For higher resolution functional data and/or thicker portions of cortex, it is possible to identify and average several voxels per (approximate) "cortical column," shown by the dotted red lines.

titled *Short Introduction to the General Linear Model for Neuroimaging*); (ii) surface-based smoothing; and (iii) improved registration. The first of these advantages is quite straightforward, as restricting the analysis to the cortical surface means that the number of statistical tests (comparisons) being performed is equal to the number of vertices on the cortical surface, and not the number of voxels in the brain. For example, 32,000 vertices are often used to represent the cortical surface with a mean within-surface spacing of approximately 2 mm, which is normally sufficient to cater for typical fMRI resolutions. By comparison, for volumetric analysis the number of voxels within the brain at a resolution of 3 mm is roughly 75,000 and, at 2 mm, roughly 250,000. Therefore there is an increase in statistical power for surface-based analyses simply because they do not have to correct for as many multiple comparisons.

The second advantage relates to smoothing on the surface, and this is the one preprocessing step that is significantly different for surface-based analysis versus volumetric analysis. This smoothing is different because it is performed purely on the surface; hence only signals from neighboring gray matter vertices are included in the smoothing, and no confounds from white matter or CSF signals are introduced. In addition, smoothing on the surface is more biologically meaningful, since regions of the cortex are grouped according to neighboring cells within a two-dimensional sheet-like structure; how close cells are in 3D is not particularly relevant. For example, cells on opposite sides of a sulcus can be very close in 3D and would typically be averaged together by a 3D smoothing operation (see Figure 7.5). However, these cells would be far apart when viewed on flattened or inflated cortical surfaces, and this is the relevant distance biologically—because, when they are on opposite sides of the sulcus, they are less likely to be performing the same functions as when they are on the same side; hence they would not be averaged together by a 2D smoothing operation that works on the surface. Thus surface-based

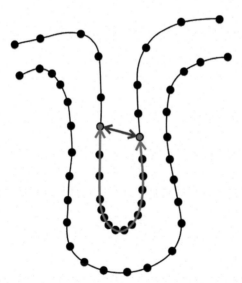

Figure 7.5: Illustration of the difference in 3D distance (blue) and 2D within-surface distance (red) between points on opposite sides of a sulcus. Surface-based smoothing methods will use this within-surface distance and hence will treat these two points as relatively distant, whereas 3D (volumetric) smoothing would treat them as nearby and closer than the points at the bottom of the sulcus.

smoothing is advantageous because there is less contamination from surrounding non-gray matter signals and because the smoothing only considers nearby locations on the cortical surface that are more likely to perform a biologically similar function.

The third advantage is the surface-based registration that we discussed in the previous section. This has been shown to provide more accurate alignments of functional areas, even when driven from geometric information alone. However, it is also possible to drive registrations with functional information from a separate acquisition (e.g., some additional resting state fMRI) in combination with geometric and other quantities (e.g., myelination), and this has been shown to increase the accuracy even further. This type of registration is what is used in the pipelines for the Human Connectome Project (HCP; see the Further Reading section).

In general, the surface-based analysis of fMRI data has considerable advantages; however, it does require the acquisition of a high-quality T_1-weighted image in order to extract the cortical surfaces. As well as this, the fMRI data should have a reasonably high spatial resolution (2.5 mm or better), or many of the benefits of surface analysis will be lost. It should also be remembered that not all functional activity occurs in the cerebral cortex and that subcortical structures and the cerebellum are excluded from surface-based analyses of the cortex. It is therefore important to also do a volumetric analysis for these parts of the brain, unless you have a strong hypothesis that only concerns the cortex. In theory, the cerebellum could also be analyzed with surface-based methods, but cerebellar structures are smaller and more fine-grained than those of the cerebral cortex, and only highly specialized, cutting-edge structural and fMRI acquisitions have sufficient resolution to make cerebellum surface modeling feasible. However, formats and analysis methods for dealing jointly with surface and volumetric data (which represent the cortex and subcortical structures/cerebellum respectively) are being developed and becoming more common, especially due to the work done in the Human Connectome Project.

With advances in acquisition techniques, especially accelerated imaging and simultaneous multi-slice methods, higher quality scans with better spatial resolution and SNR are now possible for most studies. This, combined with improvements in the quality and availability of analysis methods, is promoting a growing trend in the use of surface-based analyses for fMRI data.

SUMMARY

- Cortical surface modeling involves fitting surface models to the inner and outer cortical gray matter surfaces on the basis of information from the volumetric structural MR images. Good-quality structural images are required to get accurate surface models.

- Cortical thickness can be calculated from surfaces, and this can be analyzed (as an alternative to VBM) in order to examine differences between groups or relationships with covariates of interest.

- Surfaces can be inflated or flattened for viewing purposes.

- Spherical versions of the surfaces are also generated internally, as they are useful for surface-based registration.

- Surface-based registration has been shown to be more accurate than volumetric registration even when driven only by geometric information, but it can be even better if driven by additional modalities (e.g., resting state fMRI).

- Projecting functional data onto the cortical surface can minimize contamination from non-gray matter signals and allow more biologically based smoothing, provided that an accurate fMRI to structural volumetric registration, with distortion correction, is done.

- Surface-based analyses of fMRI have several advantages and can be combined with volumetric analyses of subcortical structures with recent pipelines and formats.

FURTHER READING

- Fischl, B. (2012). FreeSurfer. *Neuroimage*, 62(2), 774–781.
  - *General paper giving an overview and history of the FreeSurfer software package (surfer.nmr. mgh.harvard.edu).*
- Saad, Z. S., & Reynolds, R. C. (2012). Suma. *Neuroimage*, 62(2), 768–773.
  - *General paper giving an overview and history of the SUMA software—the surface-based part of the AFNI package (afni.nimh.nih.gov/Suma).*
- Fischl, B., Rajendran, N., Busa, E., Augustinack, J., Hinds, O., Yeo, B. T., et al. (2008). Cortical folding patterns and predicting cytoarchitecture. *Cerebral Cortex*, 18(8), 1973–1980.
  - *This paper demonstrates the benefits of surface-based registration methods for aligning functional boundaries.*
- Van Essen, D. C., Smith, S. M., Barch, D. M., Behrens, T. E., Yacoub, E., Ugurbil, K., & the WU-Minn HCP Consortium. (2013). The WU-Minn Human Connectome Project: An overview. *Neuroimage*, 80, 62–79.
  - *General paper giving an overview of the entire HCP project.*
- Robinson, E. C., Jbabdi, S., Glasser, M. F., Andersson, J., Burgess, G. C., Harms, M. P., et al. (2014). MSM: A new flexible framework for multimodal surface matching. *Neuroimage*, 100, 414–426.
  - *This paper demonstrates the benefits of driving surface-based registration from combined structural and functional information (containing technical details).*
- Glasser, M. F., Smith, S. M., Marcus, D. S., Andersson, J. L., Auerbach, E. J., Behrens, T. E., et al. (2016). The human connectome project's neuroimaging approach. *Nature Neuroscience*, 19(9), 1175–1187.
  - *Overview of the HCP approach to acquisition and analysis, with a general description of the combined surface- and volume-based processing methods.*

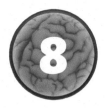

Epilogue

This chapter concludes our introduction to the field of MRI neuroimaging analysis, but this should only be the beginning of your journey in this area. Before we finish this primer there are a number of important points that we would like to reiterate and summarize.

8.1 Planning

As you will have read many times throughout this primer, it is important to consider analysis, acquisition, and experimental design together when planning your experiments. These topics are presented separately in most classes and books, but they are all intertwined and it is important to think about how decisions made in one area affect other areas. For instance, failing to acquire a calibration image or a fieldmap can severely hamper your later analysis. Piloting your experiment, including acquisition and analysis, is a great way to see how things work together and to optimize all the parts of your experiment, making them work as a whole.

There is often a lot to be gained by incorporating new techniques and modalities into your experiments. Do not assume that an experiment that was previously performed in your lab or that you read about in a paper is the best way to do it. Even if it was the most optimal experiment at that point in time, there are often improvements and innovations in this field. You certainly do not want to find out that you could have done it better at the point where a reviewer asks why you are using an out of date technique! Looking at previous designs is still a good starting point, but do not just blindly copy them. Instead, stay up to date with developments and talk to your colleagues, scanner operators, and so on, to find out what other options there are, and consider them carefully when planning your work.

Along these lines, we would encourage you to consider the benefits of including a rich set of modalities in your experiments. That could involve enlarging the set of MRI modalities used (e.g., adding a resting state fMRI scan, or acquiring dMRI data in order to explore connectivity), adding complementary modalities (e.g., MEG/EEG), or employing interventional methods (e.g., TMS). Increasingly, studies are widening the set of information that they acquire, so that they are able to more deeply explore effects and make precise interpretations.

8.2 Analysis

It is hopefully clear to you, after having read this primer, that there is no single way of doing most neuroimaging analyses. This is mainly because the analysis methods are very flexible in order to accommodate the wide variety of MRI acquisitions and experimental designs. Consequently, there are often several potential ways to analyze data, each of which has some advantages and disadvantages, and these need to be weighed up on a case-by-case basis. However, there are also ways of doing things that are bad or wrong, and one of the skills you need to learn is to be able to differentiate between acceptable alternatives (i.e., similarly good options but with with slightly different trade-offs) and alternatives that have major drawbacks or lead to invalid analyses.

For example, a study-specific template and the standard MNI152 template are often similarly good alternatives when you have a reasonable number of subjects that are not too dissimilar from young healthy adults. However, if you are studying subjects with moderate to advanced neurodegeneration, in an elderly population, then the advantages of study-specific templates can become greater. Or, if you are studying very young children, the standard MNI152 template would probably be a bad idea.

Another example would be what amount of smoothing to use in an analysis (e.g., for VBM, or for task fMRI). This typically involves a trade-off between using more smoothing to increase statistical power and using less smoothing to improve spatial localization. Very large amounts of smoothing usually lead to uninterpretable or underpowered results, since the maps may show incredibly broad areas of the brain as "significant" even though many parts did not contribute to the result, or there may be no significant results at all if the relevant effects become too diluted. Therefore very large amounts of smoothing should be avoided. Doing no smoothing at all may be a good option in some cases, as long as the registration is very accurate and the images have high SNR. Most of the time, however, some amount of smoothing is beneficial. Given that there is no "right amount" to choose, you have to weigh up the effects of smoothing in combination with your study hypothesis (e.g., how large is the brain region in which you expect to find a result), in order to make the most appropriate decision for your study.

Hopefully these examples help to reiterate and clarify that, although there is scope to choose between different ways of doing analysis, care must be taken to avoid poor approaches. Gaining a thorough understanding of the analysis decisions and of their impact (through these primers, as well as from papers, colleagues, talks, discussion forums, blogs, and other resources) will help you to differentiate between the possible approaches.

A further instance of where care is needed is in checking your data, both the raw image data from the scanner and the output of the various analysis stages in your pipelines. Care is necessary here because analysis methods sometimes fail to produce acceptable results (e.g., there can be gross misalignments after registration), especially across the wide range of possible acquisitions and experiments. Therefore it is crucial that you get into a regular habit of checking for unusual or problematic images. Usually problems are very obvious and so a quick check is normally all that is needed. If problems are found, then check for mistakes in what you were doing, and if you cannot find the source of the problem (or if it is an artifact or an incidental finding in the data), then seek help from someone with experience. And remember that the best way to check things is to *look at your data*!

8.3 Interpretation

When you have finished your analysis, make sure that you think about the limitations of the acquisition and analysis as you interpret your results. For example, the resolution of functional images and the degree of accuracy of the registrations will determine how precisely you can locate any functional activation. Or, as another example, you might be testing the hypothesis that a disease is causing axonal loss in an area of white matter, and you may measure a decrease in fractional anisotropy (FA) in that area. Such a finding is consistent with this hypothesis, but it does not definitively show that there is axonal loss, as other changes (e.g., myelination, axon diameter, or extent of crossing fibers) could also have been responsible for this measurement. As you read the literature, be on the lookout for good papers in which the authors discuss the limitations of their study, including the choices they made in their analysis, and be wary of those that include speculative conclusions about the underlying mechanisms.

8.4 Next steps

Reading this primer should have given you a broad overview of how neuroimaging is used in research and of the types of analysis that can be done, particularly for structural, diffusion, and functional MRI. This is the first step in learning how to do neuroimaging analysis in practice. The next step is to learn more about the specific modality, or modalities, that you want to use in your studies. This can be done by reading more textbooks (including other primers in this series), general review papers, and papers on specific topics, as well as educational talks and a variety of online resources.

One choice that you will need to make when it comes to doing analysis in practice is what analysis software or tools to use. In general we would recommend that you make your choice on the basis of the kinds of analysis that you want to do (which will rule out some tools) and, importantly, on the basis of the local expertise that is available. It is extremely helpful to have people nearby who already know how to use a particular tool and can help you with it. You should also learn about how to use the tools from the documentation, discussion forums, and any online or in-person courses; but often the most valuable source of information and assistance will be your colleagues. Becoming familiar with the tools and with the options available from them is crucial for being able to do good research.

If you have not looked at them already, we strongly encourage you to do the online practical examples referred to in the example boxes (these are available through the primer website: www.neuroimagingprimers.org). These will really help explain, clarify, and extend the material presented in the text as well as giving you some practical skills in analyzing neuroimaging data. Although instructions are only provided for FSL tools, the datasets can also be analyzed by many other software tools.

Finally, we would like to highlight the increasing amount of data that are being made publicly available as neuroimaging joins the push toward open science and big data. We have mentioned some of these datasets before—for example the Human Connectome Project (HCP; humanconnectome.org), which provides a wealth of MRI and other data from 1,200 young healthy adults and is now adding to this via Lifespan extensions. There is also the well-established Alzheimer's Disease Neuroimaging Initiative (ADNI; adni.loni.usc.edu) dataset, which is targeted at Alzheimer's disease and contains MRI and PET images a well as genetics, cognitive tests, CSF, and blood biomarkers on over 1000 subjects. Another big data sharing effort is fronted by the 1,000 Functional Connectomes Project powered by the International Neurolmaging Data-Sharing Initiative (INDI; fcon_1000.projects.nitrc.org), which includes the Autism Brain Imaging Data Exchange (ABIDE). In addition, the UK Biobank imaging study (www.ukbiobank.ac.uk) is due to make available brain (and body) imaging data for 100,000 subjects as well as a wide range of genetic, psychological, clinical, and lifestyle data. These are just some examples of the many excellent datasets that are available, which are too many to be mentioned individually. There is great potential for these valuable resources to play an increasingly important role in the future of neuroimaging and to enhance our understanding of the brain in health and disease. This is an exciting area to pay attention to in the coming years.

Appendix A
Short Introduction to Brain Anatomy
for Neuroimaging

This appendix is a very simple and very short overview of gross neuroanatomy. If you have done any courses that touched on brain anatomy or physiology in the past, just skip this or skim through it very quickly—but have a look at the information more specific to neuroimaging (such as the terminology related to image views) in section A.2 if you have not previously worked with images. The intended readership for this appendix is someone without a background in biological sciences beyond school level (e.g., many mathematicians, engineers, and physicists), and its aim is to introduce some basic concepts and terminology that will help you understand the material in this and other primers.

A.1 Brain cells and tissues

There are several different types of cells present in the brain, but the most well known and most interesting (for most of us) are the "little gray cells"—that is, the *neurons*. Neurons are highly interconnected and their electrical activity is what underlies all actions and mental processes. In addition to the neurons there are also glial cells, blood vessels, membranes, and fluid that support the neurons both structurally and nutritionally.

Each neuron has an *axon*, which transmits the output of the cell as an electrical current. The axon is the longest component of the cell, being anything from a fraction of a millimeter to hundreds of millimeters long. The axon is connected to the neuronal body (the soma), and the neuronal body accumulates inputs through an array of *dendrites*, which connect it to a large number of other neurons via *synapses* (points where the axon terminal and the dendrites connect). See Figure A.1 for an illustration.

Within the brain, most axons are surrounded by insulating layers of *myelin*, also known as the *myelin sheath*; the myelin is created by cells called oligodendrocytes. This myelin covering is made from a fatty substance and greatly improves the transmission of electrical signals down the axons. The breakdown of myelin is a major factor in several neurodegenerative diseases.

The diameter of a typical axon is of the order of one micrometer (1 μm), although this varies with the type of neuron, while the neuronal cell bodies are an order of magnitude bigger. However, as the resolution of a structural MRI scan is typically 0.5 mm to 1 mm, we cannot resolve individual cells and we have a view that is similar to what can be seen by looking at

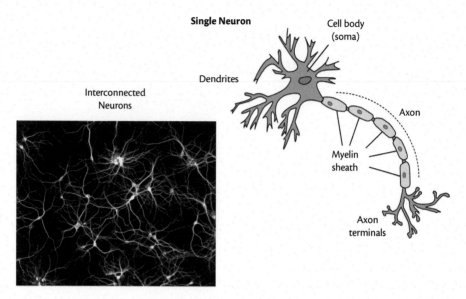

Figure A.1: Schematic of a neuron (top right), showing the constituent parts, especially the cell body (soma), the dendrites, the axon, and the myelin sheath. Neurons are very densely connected together via synapses between axon terminals and dendrites, as shown in the image (bottom left).

Left panel: Reproduced under the terms of the Creative Commons Attribution-Share Alike 4.0 International. Source: Else If Then/CC BY-SA 4.0. Right panel: Reproduced under the terms of the Creative Commons Attribution-Share Alike 3.0 Unported license. Source: "Anatomy and Physiology" by the US National Cancer Institute's Surveillance, Epidemiology and End Results (SEER) Program, https://training.seer.cancer.gov/

an individual brain with the naked eye. At this resolution there are two obvious types of gross brain "tissue": *gray matter* and *white matter*. The gray matter is mainly comprised of neuronal cell bodies, though it contains a mixture of other cells and structures (e.g., some axons, glia, blood vessels, membranes), while white matter is mainly comprised of axons, often collected together in *axonal fiber bundles*, but, again, a mixture of some other cells and structures is present. White matter gets its name from the fact that it is the tissue with the lightest color when seen in a postmortem brain; this is due to the fatty content of the myelin. In addition, we commonly refer to *cerebrospinal fluid* (CSF), for convenience, as the third "tissue" type in the brain, though really this is just fluid and not an actual tissue. See Figure A.2 for an illustration.

These "tissues," although they seem visually distinct, are a simplification of the microstructure. For instance, different relative proportions of axons and neuronal bodies exist in various regions, as well as different subtypes of neurons (e.g., pyramidal neurons); so there is variation within both white matter and gray matter across the brain. This variation is particularly pronounced in the deeper structures (e.g., the thalamus), as these tend to have a higher proportion of axons to neuronal bodies than other areas of "gray matter" in the brain. Nonetheless, these "tissues" are a very widely used and convenient concept in both gross anatomy and MRI.

That is all we will say here about these tissues and cells; we will not discuss glial cells, blood vessels, and other structures (e.g., meninges, choroid plexus, falx cerebri) although it is useful to keep in mind that there are a variety of cells and structures in brain tissue beyond neuronal

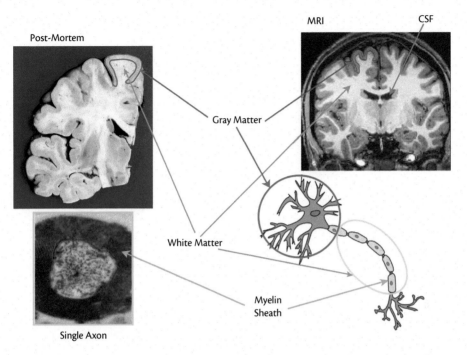

Figure A.2: Illustration of gray matter and white matter tissues in a postmortem brain section (top left) and in an MRI (top right), together with how they relate to the neuronal cells (bottom right). The white matter is predominantly full of axons, each surrounded by a myelin sheath (bottom left).

Left panel: Reproduced under the terms of the Creative Commons Attribution 4.0 International (CC BY 4.0). Source: Liu XB, and Schumann CM (2014). "Optimization of electron microscopy for human brains with long-term fixation and fixed-frozen sections," *Acta Neuropathologica Communications*, Volume 2, Issue 42, doi: 10.1186/2051-5960-2-42, Copyright © 2014 Liu and Schumann. Right panel: Reproduced under the terms of the Creative Commons Attribution-Share Alike 3.0 Unported license. Source: "Anatomy and Physiology" by the US National Cancer Institute's Surveillance, Epidemiology and End Results (SEER) Program, https://training.seer.cancer.gov/

bodies and axons. A great deal is known about these various cells and structures, but we will not discuss any of it here, as this introduction is only intended to give you the essential information that you will need in order to do neuroimaging analysis.

A.2 Navigating around brain images

Besides knowing something about the small scale of the biological constituents of brain tissue, it is also important to know something about how to navigate around the brain at the large scale. To start with, we will consider how directions in the brain are named, as in neuroimaging you will encounter these terms regularly. There are, unfortunately, two standard naming conventions that are applied to the brain and both are in active use, so you need to be familiar with both.

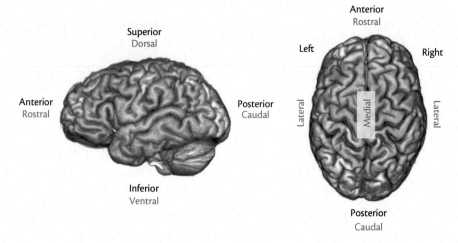

Figure A.3: Illustration of the main anatomical axes of the brain, showing both sets of terms; each set is commonly used and hence worth memorizing.

The terms that name the major anatomical axes within the brain, in one convention, are *superior–inferior, anterior–posterior*, and *left–right* (or S–I, A–P, and L–R for short). In the other convention the equivalent terms are respectively *dorsal–ventral, rostral–caudal*, and *left–right*. See Figure A.3 for an illustration of these directions in the human brain. For those of you who are not Latin scholars, the second set can be harder to remember; you may find it helpful to think of dorsal fins of a fish, dolphin, or shark being at the top and of the word "rostral" as rhyming with "nostril." In addition to these axes, there are also the terms *lateral–medial* for describing whether locations are near a side edge (lateral) or near the center (medial).

In imaging we also commonly use standard terms for the different planes that are used to virtually slice through the brain (in neuropathology labs the slicing is more literal). The terms for these planes are *coronal* (showing superior–inferior and left–right), *sagittal* (showing superior-inferior and anterior–posterior), and *axial, horizontal, transverse*, or *transaxial* (showing anterior–posterior and left–right). These are illustrated in Figure A.4. In this figure the planes are shown at a fairly standard orientation, but it is also possible to have imaging planes at other angles and, when a plane is very different from the ones illustrated (e.g., when an axial plane is tilted by 30–45° toward the coronal plane), it is described as *oblique*, though such cases are relatively rare.

It is also worth noting that, when displaying 2D slices, there are two different conventions for the orientation that are commonly used: *radiological* and *neurological*. These terms refer purely to the way the left and right sides of the brain are displayed (on a screen or on paper); the neurological convention having them consistent with the viewer's perspective (i.e., left on the left), whereas on the radiological convention they are flipped (i.e., left on the right). The reason why these exist is historical and based on whether they reflect the view that you would have of the brain (head) if facing a person as opposed to standing behind them (see Figure A.5). Neuroimaging did not invent either of these conventions—they come from medical practice—but we are stuck with them. In the literature you will see both conventions used, and hence it

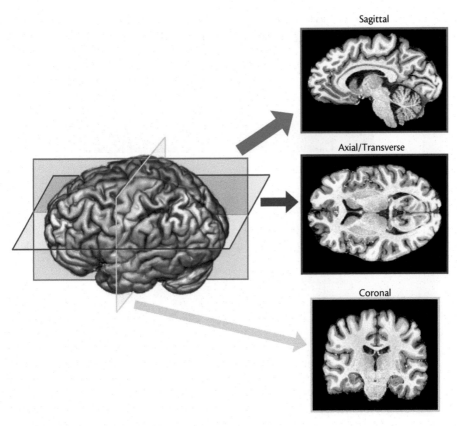

Figure A.4: Illustration of the anatomical axes of the brain and of the three cross-sectional planes that are very commonly used in imaging.

is very important to label your images with "L" and "R" symbols if the reader needs to know what convention you are using.

Other useful terms for navigating around the brain at the large scale are associated with the major lobes. The names for these lobes are *frontal, occipital, parietal*, and *temporal* (see Figure A.6). Although they are easy to distinguish in nice colored images, finding the boundaries between them on an individual brain varies between easy (e.g., between the temporal and the frontal lobes) and highly difficult (e.g., between the parietal and the temporal lobes) and determining them requires some experience. These lobes are very common and their names are very useful for navigating around the brain, as a lot of the more specific names are really just compound terms made from them and the anatomical axes. For example, the dorsolateral prefrontal cortex (or DLPFC) is an area that is in the top (dorsal) and outside (lateral) part of the start (pre-) region of the frontal lobe (that is, in the most anterior part of the frontal lobe). It is worth spending a little time to become familiar with all the terminology in this section, as this will help you a lot with understanding what other people are talking about and what is written in the literature. It certainly does not cover everything, but it is the most important basis to start with.

Radiological

Neurological

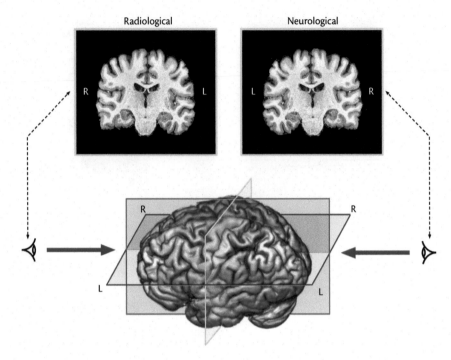

Figure A.5: Illustration of radiological and neurological conventions for viewing images, which are originally based on whether the brain is viewed from the front (radiological) or from behind (neurological). The labeling "L" and "R" in the images is necessary for making it clear which convention is being used when showing images.

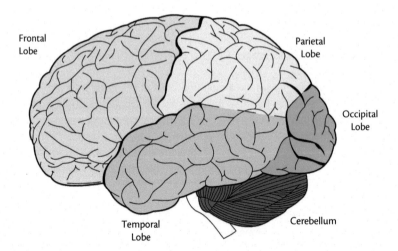

Figure A.6: Illustration of the four main lobes of the human brain and of the cerebellum.

Reproduced from Gray H (1918) *Anatomy of the Human Body*, 20th Edition, Warren H. Lewis (ed.), Philadelphia and New York: Lea and Febiger.

A.3 Brain structures

There are a lot of finer, more detailed, structures and terminology associated with brain anatomy. However, learning about all of these is not necessary in order to start in neuroimaging. You will soon become familiar with the structures that are of the greatest relevance to your own area of interest and to that of your closer colleagues. That being said, we will now discuss a set of *very* common terms and structures that it is helpful to know a little about.

The most essential and general structures[1] to know about next are the lateral ventricles, the spinal cord, the brainstem, the cerebral cortex, the corpus callosum, and the cerebellum. A very brief description of these structures is given here, as well as in Figure A.7, which depicts where they are in the brain.

- The *lateral ventricles* are the main fluid-filled spaces in the middle of the brain, where the fluid is cerebrospinal fluid (CSF). These usually provide the most obvious visual indication of brain atrophy (brain tissue loss due to typical ageing or pathology), as the ventricles increase in size to take up the extra volume due to fluid pressure.

- The *spinal cord* is primarily a collection of axonal fibers linking the brain to the rest of the body and running from the base of the brain down the spinal column. It also contains areas of gray matter and not only acts as a relay of signals from the brain and peripheral nerves but also does some basic processing of the signals itself.

- The *brainstem* is a medial structure at the base of the brain, continuous with the spinal cord, and contains substantial amounts of white matter and gray matter, organized into various smaller structures or nuclei.

- The *cerebral cortex* is the outer layer of gray matter that covers most of the human brain and, roughly speaking, represents higher level cognitive functions in the human (less evolved brains have less of it). This layer is typically between 2 mm and 5 mm thick, primarily consisting of neuronal cell bodies (though it contains some strongly myelinated areas as well, such as the stria of Gennari) and the whole cortex is very highly folded. Each fold consists of a *gyrus* (the top/crown/crest/ridge of the fold) and a *sulcus* (the bottom/pit/valley/depression/furrow/fundus); see Figure A.7. Certain gyri and sulci (these are the plural forms) are useful landmarks or have special roles. However, due to the large variability in folding patterns between individuals, not all gyri or sulci have specific names, which is why the large-scale terminology of directions and lobes is still very useful.

- The *corpus callosum* is an obvious white matter structure, easily seen on a medial sagittal slice, sitting on top of the lateral ventricles. It is a large array of axons that constitute the primary connections between the two hemispheres (halves of the brain).

- The *cerebellum* or "little brain" is a structure that sits underneath the occipital lobe and is like a mini version of the cerebral cortex, having an outer layer of gray matter that is very highly folded and white matter tracts running within, which connect it to the rest of the brain.

---

[1] Consensus will never be reached on such lists, so apologies to anyone who has a favorite structure that did not make it into this section.

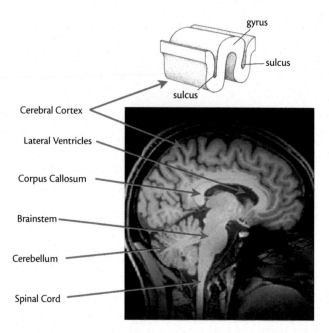

Figure A.7: Illustration of some of the main features of brain anatomy. At the top is a diagram showing a small section of the 3D folded gray matter cortex.

Contains material that has been released into the public domain. Source: Albert Kok.

In addition to these structures there are some very notable subcortical structures (or deep gray matter structures) that will be mentioned in the primers. These are the thalamus, the hippocampus, the amygdala, the putamen, the globus pallidus (or the pallidum), the caudate nucleus (or the caudate), and the nucleus accumbens; see Figure A.8. They are also referred to in groupings (e.g., the striatum or the basal ganglia) or in terms of subdivisions (e.g., internal and external parts of the globus pallidus). Their anatomy and function are complicated, but they have prominent roles in brain function and structure, especially in disease, and so it is useful to have at least a passing familiarity with their names.

After this, things get more and more detailed. For instance, a set of anatomical areas, or *parcellation*, of the cortex that is commonly referred to is the set of *Brodmann areas* (BA), though these are based on cytoarchitecture (microscopic cellular structure) and are not easily or accurately defined on MRI. Nonetheless, Brodmann areas are well-known structures in brain anatomy and you are likely to come across at least some of them. The good news is that it is not necessary to go into details about further anatomical terms and definitions at this stage, and some are likely to remain relatively unfamiliar, depending on the areas that you work with most. If you are new to neuroscience, we recommend that you consult one of the texts listed in the Further Reading section at a later date in order to get a better overview and understanding of brain anatomy and to use the digital atlases in order to learn about them (see Example Box "Learning anatomy with digital atlases").

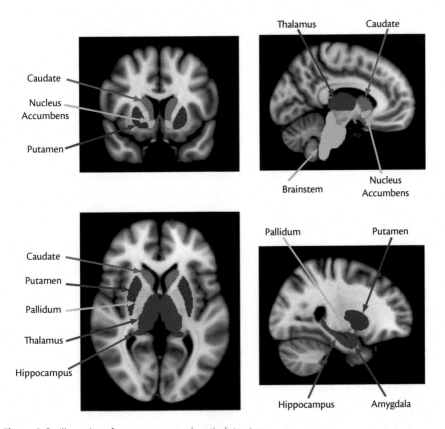

Figure A.8: Illustration of some common subcortical structures.

Example Box: **Learning anatomy with digital atlases**

A very good way, either for beginners or for experienced researchers, to learn about brain anatomy and to delve into more details is to use existing digital atlases. These are available in all major neuroimaging software toolsets; but they are usually generated by independent research groups. The structures and details depicted in each atlas are different and each atlas normally concentrates on a particular aspect of brain anatomy or on a technique used to derive the information. The kinds of techniques that are used include manual tracing of MRI scans by experts; histology results aligned to MRI; and data-driven imaging results derived from diffusion or functional parcellation methods. Each technique brings with it certain advantages and disadvantages in terms of what determines the boundaries between areas and what kind of areas are included. For example, the Harvard–Oxford atlas is based on probabilistic averaging of expert manual tracings of MRI scans of a group of subjects; hence it is driven by features in the MRI scans, combined with some higher level expert knowledge about structure shape, as not all boundaries are clear on an MRI scan. In contrast, the Jülich histological atlas is based on probabilistic averaging of multisubject postmortem cyto- and myelo-architectonic segmentations, while the Oxford thalamic connectivity atlas is based on probabilistic averaging of parcellations calculated using diffusion tractography.

On the primer website you will find instructions for viewing several different atlases and ways to explore them. We strongly recommend this for people new to the field; and we suggest that the more experienced researchers also take a quick look, as the number of available atlases and tools for interacting with them improve over time.

SUMMARY

- The three main "tissue" types in the brain are: gray matter, white matter, and CSF.
- Gray matter and white matter are actually a complicated mixture of cells and other structures, and variations exist within each tissue.
- There are two naming conventions for large-scale directions in the brain: superior–inferior or dorsal–ventral; anterior–posterior or rostral–caudal; left–right; lateral–medial.
- The main imaging planes are sagittal, coronal, and axial.
- The main brain lobes are frontal, temporal, parietal, and occipital.
- Be aware that there are many structures and areas in the brain and that it is difficult to identify some cortical areas, given individual variability in the folding patterns.
- Digital atlases are a great tool for improving your knowledge of anatomy and of how it relates to MRI scans.

FURTHER READING

The following is just a small sample from the many excellent texts available in the field of neuroanatomy, including several that had personal recommendations from our colleagues.

- Swanson, L. W. (2012). *Brain Architecture: Understanding the Basic Plan*. Oxford University Press.
- Nolte, J. (2008). *The Human Brain: An Introduction to Its Functional Anatomy* (6th ed.). Elsevier.
- Siegel, A., & Sapru, H. N. (2011). *Essential Neuroscience*. Wolters Kluwer Health/Lippincott Williams & Wilkins.

- Martin, J. H. (2012). *Neuroanatomy Text and Atlas* (4th ed.). McGraw-Hill.

- Bear, M. F., Connors, B. W., & Paradiso, M. A. (Eds.). (2007). *Neuroscience* (Vol. 2). Lippincott Williams & Wilkins.

- Gould, D. J., & Brueckner, J. K. (2007). *Sidman's Neuroanatomy: A Programmed Learning Tool*. Lippincott Williams & Wilkins.

Index

Tables, figures, and boxes are indicated by an italic *t*, *f*, and *b* following the page number.